MCAT® Prep

Lesson Book

FIFTH EDITION

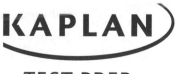

KAPLAN

TEST PREP

Materials in the CARS chapters were adapted from the following sources:

Daniel C. Dennett, *Elbow Room: The Varieties of Free Will Worth Wanting*, © 1984 The MIT Press
Irving Howe, Politics and the Novel, © 1957
Milan Kundera, *The Book of Laughter and Forgetting*, © 1980 Alfred A. Knopf, Inc.
Alice M. Rivlin, "Economics and the Political Process," © 1987 *American Economic Review*
Miriam Silverberg, "The Modern Girl as Militant," *Recreating Japanese Women, 1600–1945*
Gail Lee Bernstein, ed. © 1991 The Regents of the University of California

Published by Kaplan Publishing, a division of Kaplan, Inc.
750 Third Avenue
New York, NY 10017

ISBN: 978-1-5062-3784-8
10 9 8 7 6 5 4 3 2 1

Kaplan's MCAT Team

Alexander Stone Macnow, MD

Content Manager, MCAT

Tyler Fara

Content and Curriculum Manager, MCAT

Samantha Fallon

Content Manager, MCAT

Alexandra Côté

MCAT Faculty, Writer/Editor

Elizabeth Flagge

Content and Curriculum Manager, MCAT

Christopher Durland

Content and Curriculum Manager, MCAT

Matthew Dominic Eggert

Content and Curriculum Manager, MCAT

MCAT faculty writers/contributers:

Mikhail Alexeeff; Laura Ambler; Jesse Barrett; Erik Bowman; Eric Chiu; Brian Cohen; Alisha Crowley; Marilyn Engle; Tyler Fraser; Kimberly Gold; Adam Grey; Joe Hazel; Samer Ismail; Ae-Ri Kim, PhD; James Leach; Casey Lester; Christopher Lopez; Keith Lubelcy; Petros Minasi, Jr.; Jason Pfleiger; Deeangelee Pooran-Kublall, MD/MPH; Derek Rusnak; Kristen Russell; Neha Rao; Thomas C.C. Sargent, II; Komal Shah; Noah Silva; Logan Stark; Stephen Sylwestrak; Nandini Verma; Christopher Vestuto; Michael Welch; Pam Willingham; Valerie Yeung

Countless thanks to Kim Bowers; Potoula Chresomales; Owen Farcy; Dan Frey; Robin Garmise; Rita Garthaffner; Joanna Graham; Allison Harm; Beth Hoffberg; Aaron Lemon-Strauss; Jennifer Moore; John Polstein; Adam Ray; Rochelle Rothstein, MD; Larry Rudman; Sylvia Tidwell Scheuring; Carly Schnur; Bob Verini; Lee Weiss; and many others who made this project possible.

Contents

SECTION II: MCAT SKILLS

CHAPTER 7

CARS MCAT Expertise

CHAPTER 8

Know the Test

SECTION III: EXTRA PRACTICE

SECTION I

High-Yield Science

CHEM/PHYS 1

High-Yield Science:

Stereoisomers

VSEPR Theory

Fluid Dynamics

STEREOISOMERS

In this lesson, you'll learn to:

- Differentiate between constitutional, conformational and configurational isomers
- Determine whether a double bond is a source of isomerism
- Contrast the types of optical isomers (enantiomers and diastereomers)

Ibuprofen (isobutylphenylpropionic acid), known widely by its trade-name Advil, is a non-steroidal anti-inflammatory drug (NSAID) taken to alleviate pain. Only one of its two isomers is biologically active. In fact, the active isomer was once isolated and marketed but was quickly withdrawn due to its adverse side effects: consumers failed to account for its increased potency and took too much of it. Ibuprofen is currently produced industrially as a mixture of both isomers.

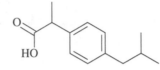

Isobutylphenylpropionic acid

Interestingly, *in vivo* testing revealed the existence of an isomerase, AMACR, that is able to convert 50-65% of the inactive isomer to the active one via a bond-breaking mechanism. Where does AMACR act on the ibuprofen molecule, and aside from their biological activity, how do these two isomers differ?

What are the defining characteristics of the three major classes of isomers?

The 3C isomers (conformational, configurational, constitutional)		
3D (stereo) isomers ("*conf*-isomers")		Constitutional
Conformational	Configurational	
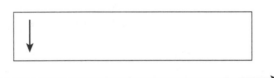		
Bond-breaking?	Bond-breaking?	Bond-breaking?
Connectivity? (Substituents)	Connectivity? (Substituents)	Connectivity? (Substituents)

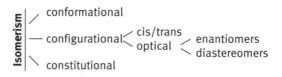

How can we eliminate the options of conformational and constitutional isomers in this case?

Conformational:

Constitutional:

There are two types of configurational isomers: optical and *cis/trans* (geometric). Are the double bonds in ibuprofen a potential source of *cis/trans* isomerism?

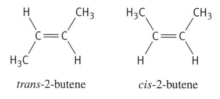

trans-2-butene   *cis*-2-butene

Why must the two isomers of ibuprofen be enantiomers, and what part of the ibuprofen molecule must be the target of AMACR?

Besides the fact that the active isomer is biologically active, how else do the isomers differ?

Stereoisomers are covered in:
Organic Chemistry, Chapter 2: Isomers

VSEPR THEORY

In this lesson, you'll learn to:

- Contrast trigonal planar and trigonal pyramidal geometries
- Explain how deviations from ideal bond angles affect molecular stability
- Use VSEPR theory and molecular geometry to explain molecular reactivity

Penicillin is a β-lactam antibiotic, meaning that its functionality as an antibiotic depends on a central β-lactam ring. In the case of penicillin, that β-lactam ring is fused to a second, five-membered ring:

β-lactam

Penicillin

Penicillin kills bacteria by irreversibly binding to the active site of transpeptidases, a class of essential bacterial enzymes, disabling these enzymes through competitive inhibition. In this reaction, penicillin's nitrogen-carbonyl bond is broken:

Transpeptidase

Transpeptidase

In a normal amide, this nitrogen-carbonyl bond is quite strong. However, penicillin's β-lactam structure and its fused five-membered ring both weaken penicillin's nitrogen-carbonyl bond, enabling penicillin's activity as an antibiotic. According to VSEPR theory, why do these factors weaken the nitrogen-carbonyl bond?

Why do the bonds around the nitrogen in a normal amide assume a trigonal planar geometry?

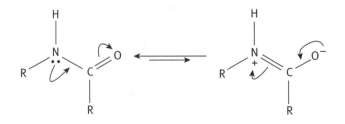

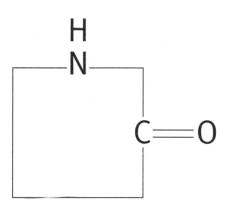

Why are the bond angles in a normal amide distorted from the ideal bond angle?

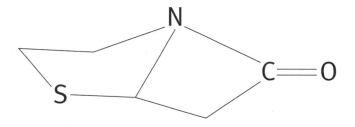

How does the β-lactam structure destabilize the nitrogen-carbonyl bond?

How does penicillin's fused five-membered ring affect the resonance of the amide functional group?

VSEPR Theory is a topic covered in:
General Chemistry, Chapter 3: Bonding and Chemical Interactions

7

FLUID DYNAMICS

In this lesson, you'll learn to:

- Eliminate unnecessary variables in conservation of energy problems
- Describe the connection between Bernoulli's law and conservation of energy
- Use the continuity equation to describe the movement of fluid in a pipe

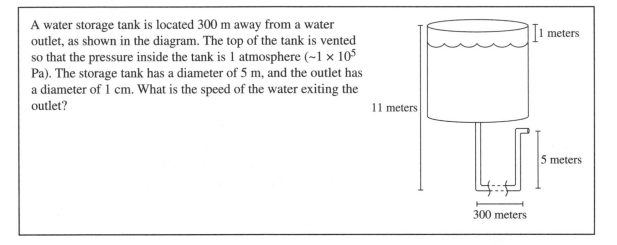

A water storage tank is located 300 m away from a water outlet, as shown in the diagram. The top of the tank is vented so that the pressure inside the tank is 1 atmosphere (~1 × 10⁵ Pa). The storage tank has a diameter of 5 m, and the outlet has a diameter of 1 cm. What is the speed of the water exiting the outlet?

1 meters

11 meters

5 meters

300 meters

In what ways is this situation similar to a rock rolling down a hill?

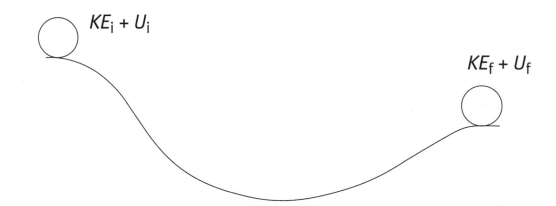

$KE_i + U_i$

$KE_f + U_f$

How does Bernoulli's law express conservation of energy for fluids?

$$P_i + \frac{1}{2}\rho v_i^2 + \rho g h_i = P_f + \frac{1}{2}\rho v_f^2 + \rho g h_f$$

How can the pipes below the tank be simplified to eliminate the final potential energy variable?

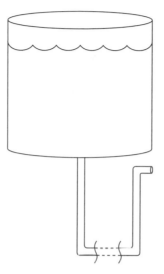

How does the continuity equation help eliminate the initial velocity variable?

$$A_i \, v_i = A_f \, v_f$$

What is the fluid's velocity as it exits the pipe?

$$P_i + \tfrac{1}{2} \rho v_i^2 + \rho g h_i = P_f + \tfrac{1}{2} \rho v_f^2 + \rho g h_f$$

Fluid Dynamics is a topic covered in:
Physics, Chapter 4: Fluids

High-Yield Science:

Enzyme Kinetics

ENZYME KINETICS

In this lesson, you'll learn to:

- Explain the significance of key aspects of the double-reciprocal Lineweaver–Burk format, including axes, intercepts, units, and slopes
- Identify V_{max} and K_M on both Michaelis–Menten and Lineweaver–Burk plots
- Plot the effects of competitive inhibition on both graph types

Enzyme activity is often graphed using a Michaelis–Menten plot. However, enzyme activity may also be graphed using an alternative format, the Lineweaver–Burk plot. HMG-CoA reductase is the rate-limiting enzyme of cholesterol synthesis. Statins, such as atorvastatin (Lipitor), simvastatin (Zocor), and rosuvastatin (Crestor) are routinely used to treat patients with high cholesterol because they are competitive inhibitors of HMG-CoA reductase. How would the use of a statin affect the Lineweaver–Burk plot of HMG-CoA reductase?

Michaelis–Menten Plot

A Michaelis–Menten plot clearly shows the asymptotic behavior of a plot of an enzyme's kinetics. What is the plot's basic shape? How does it display K_M and V_{max}?

Enzyme Kinetics are covered in:
Biochemistry, Chapter 2: Enzymes

Lineweaver–Burk Plot

$\frac{1}{V}$ (s/μmol)

$\frac{1}{[S]}$ (mM^{-1})

A Lineweaver–Burk plot shows the same information as a Michaelis–Menten plot. How does it display K_M and V_{max}? What are the benefits of a Lineweaver–Burk plot, compared to a Michaelis–Menten plot?

Why does a competitive inhibitor increase an enzyme's K_M while leaving its V_{max} unchanged?

A competitive inhibitor will have the effect of increasing the slope of a Lineweaver–Burk plot. Why?

High-Yield Science:

Organization of the Human Nervous System

Associative Learning

Theories of Emotion

Stages of Moral Reasoning

ORGANIZATION OF THE HUMAN NERVOUS SYSTEM

In this lesson, you'll learn to:

- Recognize the divisions of the nervous system
- Predict portions of the nervous system involved in response to given stimuli

Henry is a newborn infant who has been taken to his physician for a check-up. Up until now, Henry has behaved normally. His doctor tests several things to ensure that Henry is healthy.

- The doctor asks Henry's parent whether Henry is either sleeping or becoming more docile after nursing.
- The doctor tests Henry's vision and range of motion by waving a brightly colored object in front of Henry and watching his response, which should typically involve visual tracking of the object and an attempt to move extremities towards or away from the object.
- The doctor tests Henry's Galant reflex. In this test the physician taps on the infant's spine, and the infant's hips should involuntarily and immediately twitch toward the location of the tap.

Henry behaves as expected in the first two tasks, but fails to exhibit the Galant reflex. What should the physician focus on in further neurological assessment?

Why would Henry's eating and sleeping habits inform the doctor about his peripheral nervous system function?

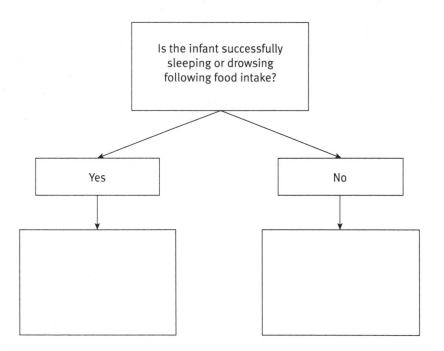

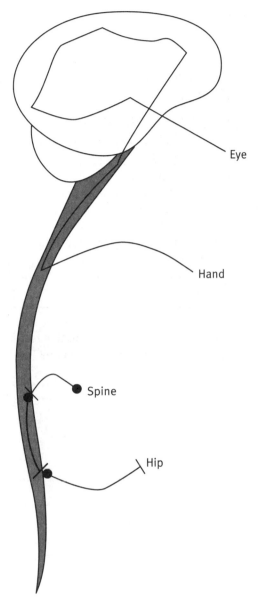

Eye

Hand

Spine

Hip

How does the bright object test assess both major divisions of the nervous system?

Why doesn't the Galant reflex test provide much information about brain function, and what does it provide information about?

If the doctor is trying to test for a potentially systemic issue, should the sensory neuron, the motor neuron, or the spinal interneuron be targeted first in testing?

The Organization of the Human Nervous System is a topic covered in:
Behavioral Sciences, Chapter 1: Biology and Behavior

ASSOCIATIVE LEARNING

In this lesson, you'll learn to:

- Recall the different types of conditioners used in operant conditioning
- Identify the conditioners in a complex operant conditioning experiment
- Identify the schedules of reinforcement used in operant conditioning experiments

A pigeon is placed in a cage with two buttons: one blue and one green. Pressing the blue button triggers the immediate release of a food pellet. However, pressing the blue button also immediately triggers an electric shock. Furthermore, each time a food pellet is released, the mechanism used to release food pellets is disabled for a period of time varying randomly between 5 and 55 seconds. The blue button's electric shock mechanism remains active during this period. And once the latency period has passed, the next press of the blue button will immediately trigger the release of another food pellet. Finally, pressing the green button will disable the electric shock mechanism until the next food pellet is released, at which point the electric shock mechanism will reactivate. What pattern of button presses will a trained pigeon use to successfully receive a food pellet without being shocked?

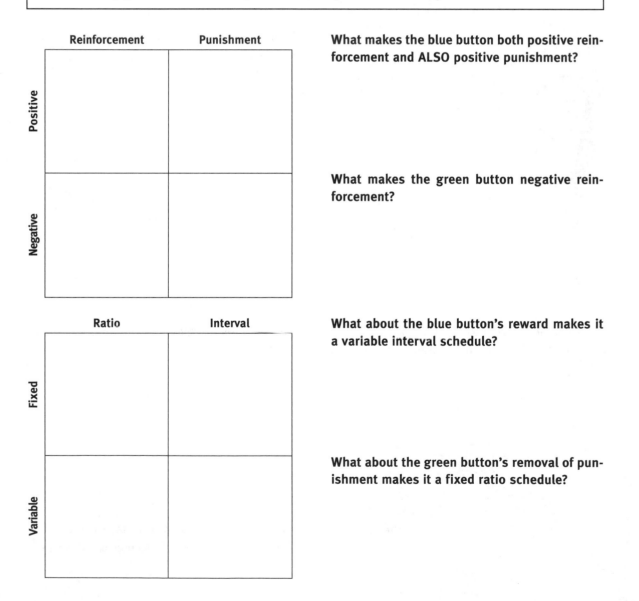

What makes the blue button both positive reinforcement and ALSO positive punishment?

What makes the green button negative reinforcement?

What about the blue button's reward makes it a variable interval schedule?

What about the green button's removal of punishment makes it a fixed ratio schedule?

After the pigeon has been trained to use the buttons and after the pigeon has been conditioned by the buttons, the pigeon will settle into an "ideal use" pattern that eliminates the possibility of electric shock, and follows the frequency of button presses that reflects a variable interval reward schedule. What is this this "ideal use" pattern?

Trained Button-Pressing Frequency

TIME

⟶

THEORIES OF EMOTION

In this lesson, you'll learn to:

- Determine the relationship between physiology and emotion in different theories of emotion
- Relate known information about brain physiology and function of the nervous system to theories of emotion

One major early attempt to explain the relationship between physiological events and emotion was made in the 19th century by William James and Carl Lange: the James–Lange theory of emotion. This theory held that a precipitating event would lead to physiological arousal, which would be followed by neural interpretation and generation of an emotional response. This (now largely defunct) theory has been strongly refuted by later research, especially that of Walter Cannon and Philip Bard. These scientists ran a series of studies in which sympathetic nervous system structures were completely removed from animal models, and stressful situations were then used to attempt to induce emotional response. Despite the elimination of physiological input, the animal models in these studies demonstrated emotional responses to precipitating events. In later experiments, subjects' viscera (when present, but detached from direct brain connection) still experienced physiological arousal in the stressful situations created by the experimenters. Based on this research and its findings, how would Cannon–Bard theory explain the generation of emotion?

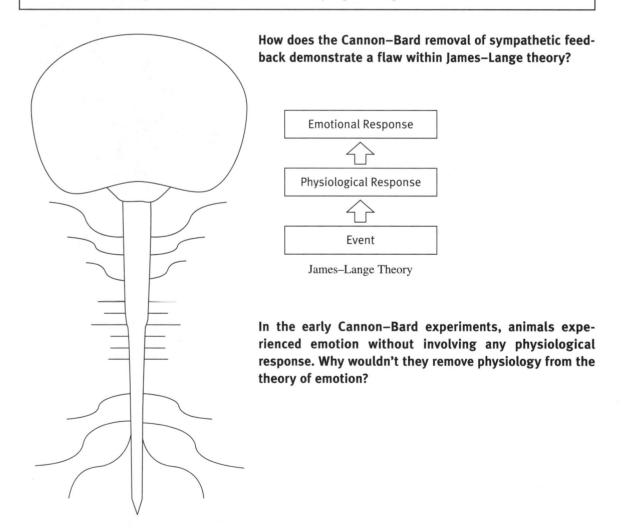

How does the Cannon–Bard removal of sympathetic feedback demonstrate a flaw within James–Lange theory?

Emotional Response

⇧

Physiological Response

⇧

Event

James–Lange Theory

In the early Cannon–Bard experiments, animals experienced emotion without involving any physiological response. Why wouldn't they remove physiology from the theory of emotion?

Given the flaw found in James–Lange theory, what should the Cannon–Bard theory look like?

Event

STAGES OF MORAL REASONING

In this lesson, you'll learn to:

- Recall the stages of Kohlberg's theory of moral reasoning
- Identify which stage of Kohlberg's theory of moral reasoning best fits a given argument

> Marvin is in his residency program for internal medicine. He encounters a patient whom he identifies as someone who can be helped by Varvipax, a new and expensive drug for her condition. However, the patient's insurance does not cover the drug, and she says she couldn't afford Varvipax at its list price. Rather than prescribe an older, less-effective drug, Marvin gives the patient dozens of the "free samples" of Varvipax he has received from the drug company—enough for a full course of treatment—despite the fact that this is against his office's policy and is against his contract with the drug company. How might Marvin justify this behavior in each of the major stages of Kohlberg's theory of moral development?

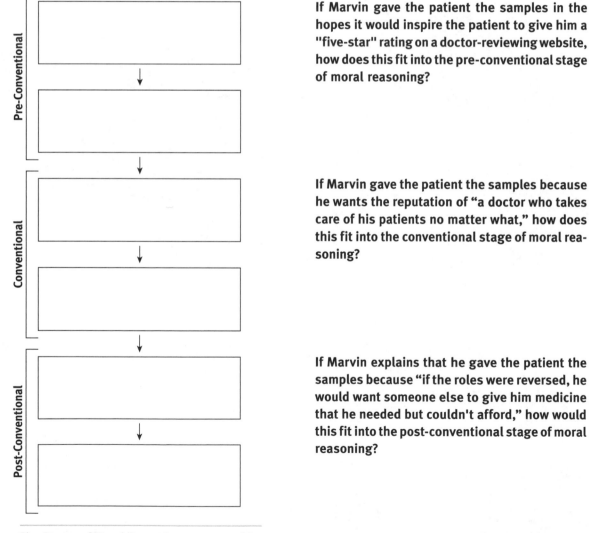

Pre-Conventional

If Marvin gave the patient the samples in the hopes it would inspire the patient to give him a "five-star" rating on a doctor-reviewing website, how does this fit into the pre-conventional stage of moral reasoning?

Conventional

If Marvin gave the patient the samples because he wants the reputation of "a doctor who takes care of his patients no matter what," how does this fit into the conventional stage of moral reasoning?

Post-Conventional

If Marvin explains that he gave the patient the samples because "if the roles were reversed, he would want someone else to give him medicine that he needed but couldn't afford," how would this fit into the post-conventional stage of moral reasoning?

The Stages of Moral Reasoning are covered in:
Behavioral Sciences, Chapter 6: Identity and Personality

The High-Yield Science lessons for the next session begin on the following page ▶ ▶ ▶

CHEM/PHYS 2

High-Yield Science:

Reaction Rates

Solution Equilibria

Electric Potential Energy

REACTION RATES

In this lesson, you'll learn to:

- Identify the order and rate for elementary reactions within a reaction mechanism
- Calculate a rate law for a given reaction using a rate table

In 1940, Sir Christopher Ingold proposed the mechanism for the S_N1 reaction. He used experimentally determined rate laws for a great many S_N1 reactions to validate his theory that the S_N1 reaction follows a multi-step mechanism and that the rate-determining step is carbocation formation. Consider the following S_N1 substitution of *tert*-butyl bromide carried out in water and the accompanying experimental data about this reaction's rate:

$$H_3C-\underset{\underset{H_3C}{|}}{\overset{\overset{H_3C}{|}}{C}}-Br + CH_3OH + H_2O \longrightarrow H_3C-\underset{\underset{H_3C}{|}}{\overset{\overset{H_3C}{|}}{C}}-OCH_3 + Br^- + H_3O^+$$

	$[R_3CBr]$ (M)	$[CH_3OH]$ (M)	Initial Rate (M/s)
Trial 1	2.0×10^{-1}	4.0×10^{-2}	2.97×10^{-6}
Trial 2	2.0×10^{-1}	8.0×10^{-2}	2.78×10^{-6}
Trial 3	4.0×10^{-1}	8.0×10^{-2}	6.03×10^{-6}

Why do the experimental data prove that carbocation formation is the rate-determining step?

Any multi-step reaction mechanism—for example, S_N1—consists of at least two elementary reaction steps. What are the three possible elementary reactions and their rate laws?

	Reactants	Products	Rate Law
First Order	$\longrightarrow$		
Second Order	$\longrightarrow$		
	$\longrightarrow$		

Reaction Rates are covered in:
General Chemistry, Chapter 5: Chemical Kinetics

What are the specific elementary reactions in this S_N1 mechanism and what are their rate laws?

Step 1: Carbocation Formation

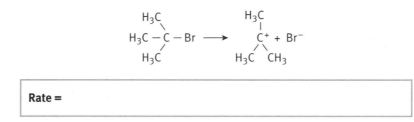

> Rate =

Step 2: Nucleophilic Attack

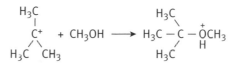

> Rate =

Step 3: Deprotonation

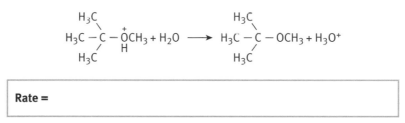

> Rate =

How does the experimental data in this question prove that carbocation formation is the rate-determining step in the S_N1 mechanism?

	[R$_3$CBr] (M)	[CH$_3$OH] (M)	Initial Rate (M/s)
Trial 1	2.0×10^{-1}	4.0×10^{-2}	2.97×10^{-6}
Trial 2	2.0×10^{-1}	8.0×10^{-2}	2.78×10^{-6}
Trial 3	4.0×10^{-1}	8.0×10^{-2}	6.03×10^{-6}

> Rate =

SOLUTION EQUILIBRIA

In this lesson, you'll learn to:

- Use key terms from molar solubility to make a plan for an MCAT question
- Recall and execute the steps to solving a molar solubility question
- Predict the impact of a common ion on the molar solubility of a compound

> The molar solubility of iron (III) hydroxide in pure water at 25°C is 9.94×10^{-10} M. How would the substance's molar solubility change if placed in aqueous solution with a pH of 10.0 at 25°C?

Solubility Product: The equilibrium constant for a dissolution reaction
Molar Solubility: The number of moles of a substance dissolved per liter of solution to reach equilibrium.

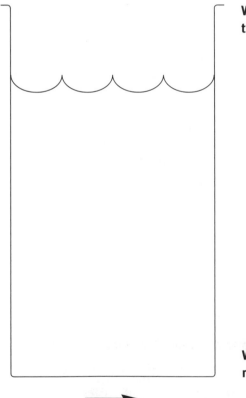

Why is the solubility product, K_{sp}, of this dissolution reaction less than the molar solubility of iron (III) hydroxide?

$$K_{eq} = \frac{[\text{Products}]}{[\text{Reactants}]}$$

$K_{sp} =$

Why does an increase in pH substantially decrease the molar solubility of iron (III) hydroxide?

Solution Equilibria is a topic covered in:
General Chemistry, Chapter 9: Solutions

This chapter continues on the next page. ▶ ▶ ▶

ELECTRIC POTENTIAL ENERGY

In this lesson, you'll learn to:

- Explain the usefulness of "charges separated by a great distance" to electrostatic work and energy
- Describe how input and output of work relate to positive and negative electrostatic potential energies
- Calculate the work done in moving charges relative to each other

> Three charges are lined up in a straight line at 1 mm intervals. Charge 1, in the center, has a charge of +1 μC. Charge 2, which is 1 mm to the right of Charge 1, has a charge of +2 μC. Charge 3, which is 1 mm to the left of Charge 1, has a charge of –3 μC. How much work was required to assemble this distribution of charges, assuming that the charges were initially separated by a distance of infinity? (Note: $k = 9 \times 10^9 \ \mathrm{Nm^2/C^2}$)

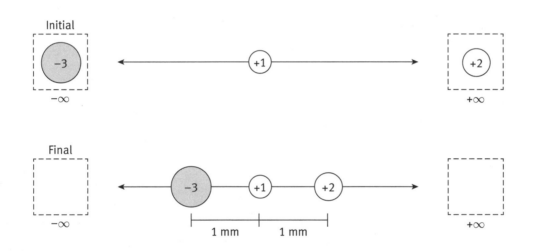

When physicists (or the MCAT test-makers) claim that, "Charges are initially separated by a distance of infinity," they mean that the charges are separated by a great enough distance that the electrostatic potential energy between the charges is practically zero. What distance would Charge 1 and Charge 2 need to be separated so that the energy of their interaction is less than 1 mJ?

Why would moving the second charge into position require positive work, and how much energy would be required?

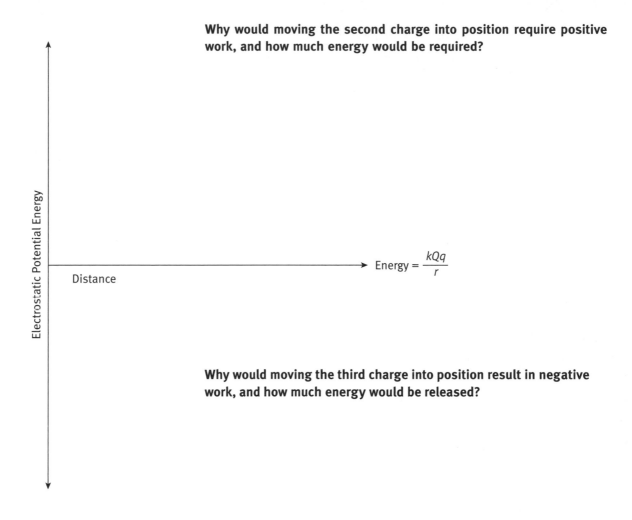

Electrostatic Potential Energy

Distance

$$\text{Energy} = \frac{kQq}{r}$$

Why would moving the third charge into position result in negative work, and how much energy would be released?

What is the net work done in arranging these charged particles?

Electric Potential Energy is a topic covered in:
Physics and Math, Chapter 5: Electrostatics and Magnetism

High-Yield Science:

The Menstrual Cycle

Action Potentials

THE MENSTRUAL CYCLE

In this lesson, you'll learn to:

- Recall the hormones of the hypothalamic–pituitary–gonadal hormone axis
- Describe estrogen's feedback mechanisms on the hypothalamic–pituitary–gonadal axis
- Contrast the roles of estrogen in the follicular phase of the menstrual cycle

Chronic anovulation, the consistent absence of ovulation in a reproductive-age woman, is one of the leading causes of female infertility. 70% of chronic anovulation cases are due to hormone imbalances, usually insufficient FSH or LH levels. In these cases, the drug clomiphene citrate, trade-name Clomid, is used to successfully and reliably induce ovulation. Clomid works by blocking estrogen receptors within the hypothalamus and the pituitary. Clomid is taken monthly in a five-day course. The timing of the dosing course is important: If "day 1" of the menstrual cycle is the first day of menstruation, Clomid should be taken from days 5–9 of the cycle. If Clomid is to be used to successfully induce ovulation, why should Clomid be taken during this part of the menstrual cycle?

One of estrogen's main roles during the follicular phase of the menstrual cycle is to influence the hypothalamic–pituitary–gonadal axis and its associated hormone cascade. Describe the hormones in this cascade and their ultimate effect on the ovaries.

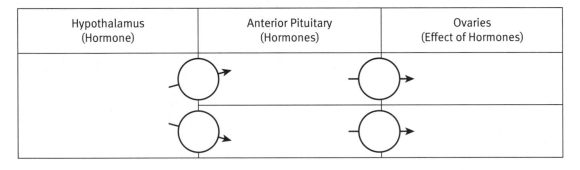

Hypothalamus (Hormone)	Anterior Pituitary (Hormones)	Ovaries (Effect of Hormones)

The Menstrual Cycle is a topic covered in:
Biology, Chapter 2: Reproduction

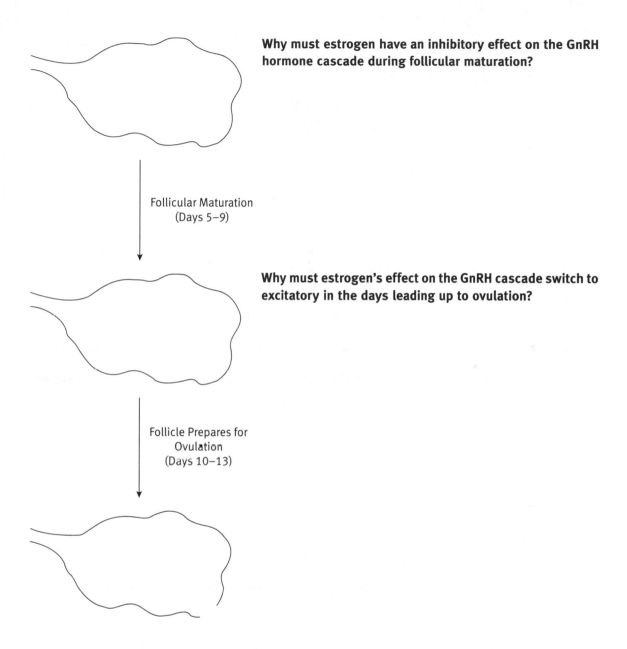

Why must estrogen have an inhibitory effect on the GnRH hormone cascade during follicular maturation?

Follicular Maturation
(Days 5–9)

Why must estrogen's effect on the GnRH cascade switch to excitatory in the days leading up to ovulation?

Follicle Prepares for
Ovulation
(Days 10–13)

In the case of a woman with chronic anovulation due to insufficient FSH and LH levels, why should she take Clomid during the period of follicular maturation, days 5–9? Why should she discontinue the medication during the days leading to ovulation, days 10–13?

ACTION POTENTIALS

In this lesson, you'll learn to:

- Graph the changes in membrane potential that occur during an action potential
- Explain how ion membrane potentials establish the resting potential of a neuron
- Predict the effects of ion imbalance on action potentials

Hyperkalemia is a condition characterized by elevated concentration of the electrolyte potassium in the blood, and consequently also in the extracellular fluid. Because of potassium's pivotal role both in establishing the resting potential and in controlling the action potential, hyperkalemia may disrupt nervous system activity. Hyperkalemia can arise as a possible complication due to the maltreatment of an athlete suffering from an imbalance of electrolytes. An athlete may lose large quantities of potassium through diaphoresis (sweating) during long periods of exercise. This potassium may be replaced using an intravenous administration of a KCl saline solution. However, if the KCl solution is administered too rapidly, the rapid influx of potassium ions into the athlete's circulatory system may cause hyperkalemia instead. If an athlete does begin to suffer from mild hyperkalemia, how would the resting potential and action potential be affected?

How does potassium efflux (and sodium influx) help establish the resting potential in a neuron?

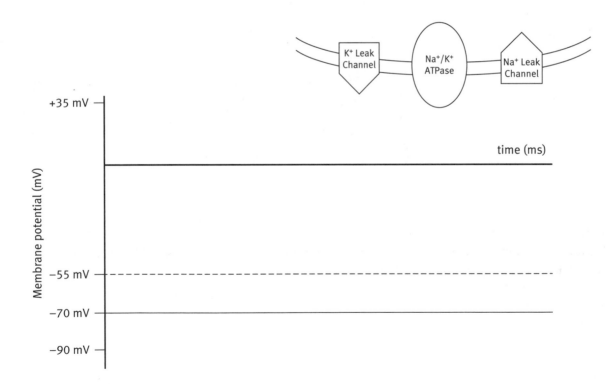

What role does potassium play in the action potential itself?

Why would hyperkalemia raise the resting potential?

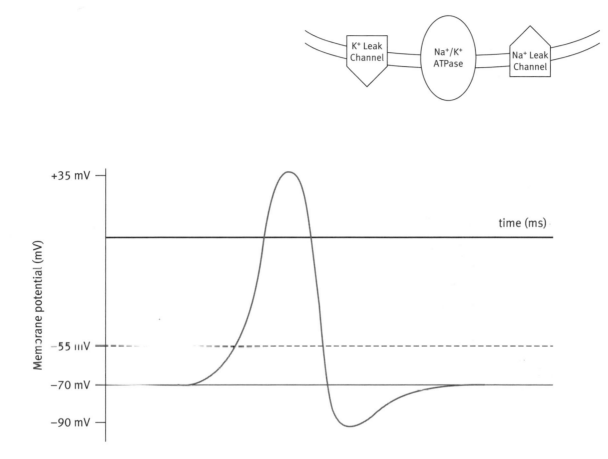

How would the period after depolarization be affected by hyperkalemia?

Action Potentials are covered in:
Biology, Chapter 4: The Nervous System

High-Yield Science:

Social Processes

Attribution Theory

The Endocrine System

SOCIAL PROCESSES

In this lesson, you'll learn to:

- Distinguish between the different behavioral changes classified as "social action"
- Predict how social actions are impacted by relevant variables
- Apply social action terminology to example scenarios

Social actions and social phenomena impact a huge proportion of life for all of humanity, regardless of culture or location. Some of the more notable effects of social situations on the behavior of individuals have been evaluated and characterized. Assess the following situations, evaluate how behavioral response is altered by size of group, and identify the relevant social phenomenon.

Predict how the following situations would respond to group dynamics, and identify the phenomenon.

Tyler is attending a concert and notices a stranger fall down several stairs.		
Alex was at a live event when some attendees (whom she had never met) became violent.		
Adam planned to play video games for the night, but his friends invite him to study instead.		
Isaac plays a trumpet piece he has been practicing in front of a live audience for the first time.		

Social Processes are covered in:
Behavioral Sciences, Chapter 8: Social Processes, Attitudes, and Behavior

This chapter continues on the next page. ▶ ▶ ▶

ATTRIBUTION THEORY

In this lesson, you'll learn to:

- Distinguish between situational and dispositional attributions
- Apply the fundamental attribution error to a given situation

You are chatting with your friend Carlton when a group walks by and one person casually mentions that they didn't get any studying done over the weekend for the upcoming biology midterm. Carlton shakes his head and says "Some people are just not made for pre-med courses. They procrastinate all the time and can't get things done." You point out to Carlton that he didn't get any studying done this weekend either. He says "Sure, but I studied all of last week and I'm doing great in class! Everyone was telling me I needed a break, and I'm definitely going to study tonight!" Why did Carlton use a different type of attribution for himself than he did for the stranger?

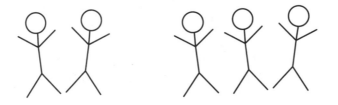

In attribution theory, why does it matter who the perceiver is (as opposed to the person(s)/thing(s) being perceived)?

Your friend makes one dispositional attribution and one situational attribution. Which attribution is which?

How does the fundamental attribution error apply to the given situation?

Suppose it had been you who had brought up the lack of studying this weekend. Would your friend be more likely to attribute your behavior to situation, or disposition?

Attribution Theory is a topic covered in:
Behavioral Sciences, Chapter 10: Social Thinking

This chapter continues on the next page. ▶ ▶ ▶

THE ENDOCRINE SYSTEM

In this lesson, you'll learn to:

- Recall the cause-and-effect relationships in the hypothalamic–pituitary–adrenal (HPA) axis
- Compare the effects of different diseases of the HPA axis

Depression is one symptom of a disease called Cushing syndrome. But where most cases of depression are treated over months using cognitive behavior therapy, depression in Cushing patients can be resolved in days using cortisol receptor blockers. Other classic symptoms of Cushing syndrome include acne, weakened muscles, and fatty deposits in the face and neck (called "moon facies" and "buffalo lumps"). Finally, in addition to these classic symptoms, some patients, though not all, may experience a darkening of the skin called hyperpigmentation. Interestingly, all of the symptoms of Cushing syndrome are resolved by cortisol receptor blockers, except hyperpigmentation.

Cushing syndrome is often caused by a hormone-secreting adenoma, which is a noncancerous tumor (tissue overgrowth) that is functionally similar to its gland of origin. Any one of the following three tumor types can cause Cushing syndrome: (1) A tumor in the anterior pituitary; (2) A tumor in the adrenal cortex; or (3) An "ectopic" ACTH-secreting tumor. This is a tumor that secretes ACTH, but is not found in an endocrine organ.

A physician can diagnose the tumor type using the results from two diagnostic measures. The physician will check for the presence or absence of hyperpigmentation. And also, the physician will administer dexamethasone, which is a cortisol analogue that acts on endocrine organs. The results of these diagnostics, plus well-developed critical thinking skills, allow the physician to make a diagnosis. Try it yourself: What is the likely cause of Cushing syndrome in a patient who exhibits hyperpigmentation, and who is unresponsive to dexamethasone?

How is it possible that three different types of tumors (indicated here by protrusions on the affected organ) can lead to the same set of classic Cushing syndrome symptoms?

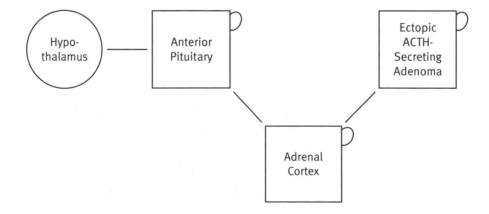

The Endocrine System is a topic covered in:
Biology, Chapter 5: The Endocrine System

Why would a lack of response to dexamethasone rule out a tumor of the anterior pituitary, but not a tumor of the adrenal cortex or an ectopic ACTH-secreting adenoma?

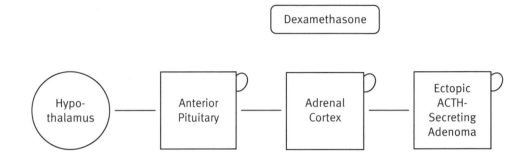

Why does the observation that the patient exhibits hyperpigmentation (the only symptom not resolved by cortisol receptor blockers) help rule out a tumor of the adrenal cortex?

Ectopic ACTH-secreting adenoma:

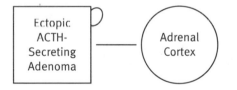

Adenoma of the adrenal cortex:

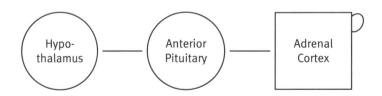

Diagnosis:

Anterior Pituitary Tumor

Adrenal Cortex Tumor

Ectopic ACTH-secreting Tumor

CHEM/PHYS 3

High-Yield Science:

Nucleophilic Acyl Substitution

Ideal Gases

Electrochemical Cells

Geometrical Optics

NUCLEOPHILIC ACYL SUBSTITUTION

In this lesson, you'll learn to:

- Distinguish between the carboxylic acid derivatives
- Recall each step of nucleophilic acyl substitution
- Recognize similarities and differences between transesterification, amide formation, and acid-catalyzed ester hydrolysis

Carboxylic acid derivatives are found in a vast array of organic molecules. Luckily, these can often be prepared from a few common intermediates. Take, for instance, the following reactions with methyl pivalate. Each of these produces a unique product. What are the products of each of these reactions?

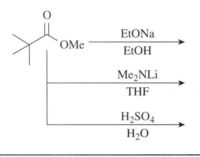

What functionality does each of the carboxylic acid derivatives have in common?

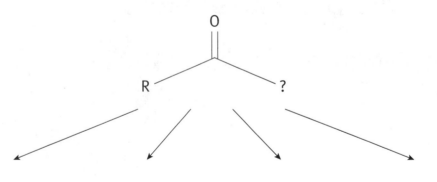

Carboxylic Acid   Ester   Amide   Acyl Halide

Nucleophilic Acyl Substitution is a topic covered in:
Organic Chemistry, Chapter 8: Carboxylic Acids

Using the general mechanism for nucleophilic acyl substitution, sketch the transesterification reaction.

How is the amide formation reaction similar to the transesterification reaction?

Why does hydrolysis require an acid catalyst?

IDEAL GASES

In this lesson, you'll learn to:

- Predict the impact of changing pressure, volume, and temperature in an ideal gas
- Identify how and when a gas may deviate from the ideal gas law

> The ideal gas law is used to characterize the behavior of theoretical gases that have no size or intermolecular effects. In the real world, this law is often confounded by additional effects, leading to the creation of the Van der Waals equation, which adjusts for some of the additional effects observed in real-world gases. Nitrous oxide (N_2O) is an anesthetic gas typically kept in small, pressurized canisters and administered via face mask. Even though the ideal gas law does allow for approximation of moles of compound (n), the ideal gas law cannot be used to correctly calculate the concentration of nitrous oxide gas. Why is it that nitrous oxide's behavior cannot be correctly characterized by the ideal gas law?

Using the ideal gas law, how are P, V, and T mathematically related to n?

How would P, V, and T affect each other in an ideal gas, using Boyle's and Charles's laws?

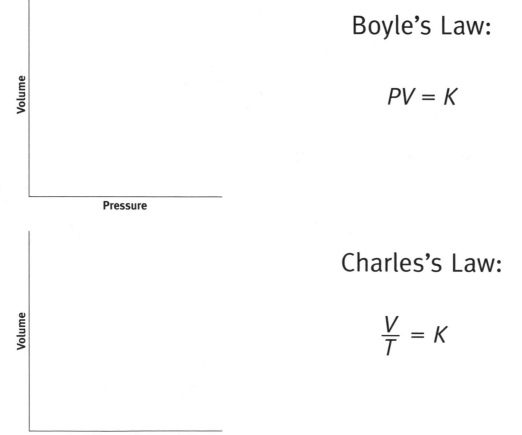

Boyle's Law:

$$PV = K$$

Charles's Law:

$$\frac{V}{T} = K$$

How would nitrous oxide deviate from the behavior of a more ideal gas, such as Helium?

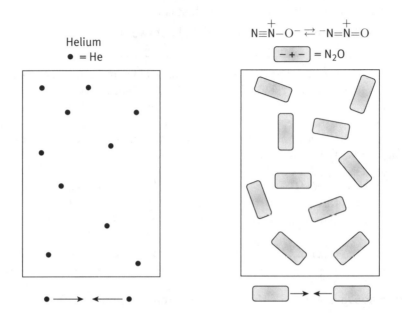

The measurement and dosing issues for nitrous oxide are resolved by its method of storage. Nitrous oxide is typically heavily pressurized (stored in an exceptionally small space) and kept at cool temperatures. How might NO_2 behave in these conditions?

Ideal Gases are covered in:
General Chemistry, Chapter 8: The Gas Phase

ELECTROCHEMICAL CELLS

In this lesson, you'll learn to:

- Contrast oxidation and reduction potentials
- Relate the mitochondrion to an electrochemical cell
- Calculate the EMF given the reduction potentials of two half reactions

---

The mitochondrion's electron transport chain (ETC) is a series of compounds that transfer electrons from electron donors to electron acceptors via redox reactions. Thus, this organelle can be thought of as an electrochemical cell. The ETC's first reaction is the oxidation of NADH, during which complex I catalyzes the transfer of electrons from NADH to CoQ10. The reduced ubiquinone (CoQ10) subsequently transports these electrons to the cytochrome b-c complex (part of complex III). Below are standard potentials for NADH, cytochrome b and cytochrome c.

$$NADH \rightarrow NAD^+ + 2\,e^- + H^+ \qquad\qquad E° = +0.320 \text{ V}$$
$$2 \text{ cytochrome } b_{(red)} \rightarrow 2 \text{ cytochrome } b_{(ox)} + 2\,e^- \qquad E° = -0.070 \text{ V}$$
$$2 \text{ cytochrome } c_{(ox)} + 2\,e^- \rightarrow 2 \text{ cytochrome } c_{(red)} \qquad E° = +0.254 \text{ V}$$

What is the chronological order in which the three compounds above are oxidized in the ETC?

Which half reaction above is given a different type of standard potential than the others?

How do you expect the reduction potentials of the following electron acceptors in the ETC (in chronological order, 1 → 2 → 3) to compare to that of cytochrome c?

1. $2 \text{ cytochrome } c_{(ox)} + 2\,e^- \rightarrow 2 \text{ cytochrome } c_{(red)}$
2. $2 \text{ cytochrome } a_{3(ox)} + 2\,e^- \rightarrow 2 \text{ cytochrome } a_{3(red)}$
3. $1/2\ O_2 + 2H^+ + 2\,e^- \rightarrow H_2O$

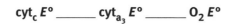

$$\text{cyt}_c\ E° \underline{\qquad} \text{cyt}_{a_3}\ E° \underline{\qquad} O_2\ E°$$

Conclusion:

A typical galvanic cell has two compartments linked by a metal wire that allows the transfer of electrons. What allows the mitochondrion to act as a galvanic cell without such a setup?

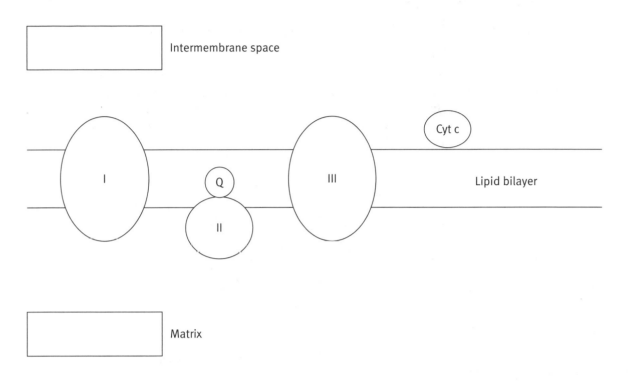

How can you calculate the EMF of the reaction below using two different equations?

$$2 \text{ cytochrome } c_{(ox)} + NADH \rightarrow 2 \text{ cytochrome } c_{(red)} + NAD^+ + H^+$$

$$2 \text{ cytochrome } c_{(ox)} + 2 \, e^- \rightarrow 2 \text{ cytochrome } c_{(red)} \quad E° = +0.254 \, V$$
$$NAD^+ + 2 \, e^- + H^+ \rightarrow NADH \qquad\qquad E° = -0.320 \, V$$

$$E°_{cell} = E°_{cathode} - E°_{anode} \qquad\qquad E°_{cell} = E°_{reduction} + E°_{oxidation}$$

$$E°_{cell} = \boxed{}\, 0.254 - (\boxed{}\, 0.320) \qquad E°_{cell} = \boxed{}\, 0.254 + (\boxed{}\, 0.320)$$

Electrochemical Cells are covered in:
General Chemistry, Chapter 12: Electrochemistry

GEOMETRICAL OPTICS

In this lesson, you'll learn to:

- Explain the role of the ocular media's refractive properties in normal vision
- Infer different causes of myopia and hyperopia

Cataracts are responsible for roughly half of blindness cases worldwide. Though this condition is marked by a clouding of the lens, cataracts may occasionally also lead to variation in the refractive index of the lens. This variation creates additional problems similar to those seen when the axial length of the eye is altered over time.

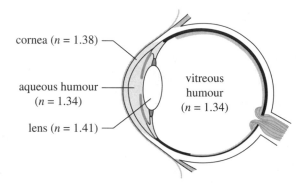

What condition might arise from the lens having a greater density than normal, and how might this condition be corrected?

How do variations in the axial length cause myopia and hyperopia? The rest of the eye is normal in these conditions.

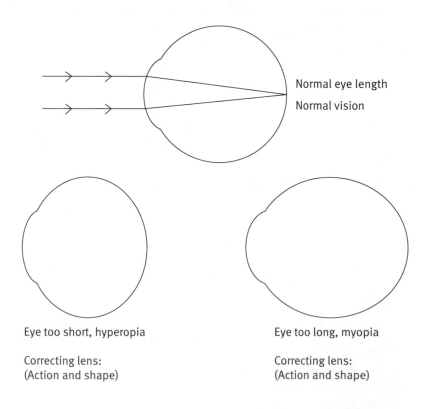

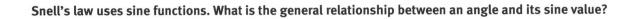

Snell's law uses sine functions. What is the general relationship between an angle and its sine value?

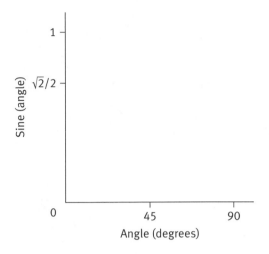

The lens' increased density confers it a slightly greater refractive index. How can Snell's law be used to determine the impact this has on where the image will form?

$$n_{aq.h.} \times \sin \theta_{aq.h.} = n_{lens} \times \sin \theta_{lens}$$

$$n_{lens} \times \sin \theta_{lens} = n_{vit.h.} \times \sin \theta_{vit.h.}$$

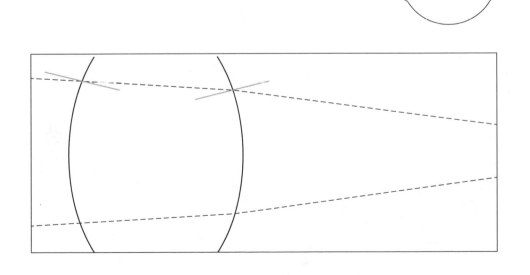

Geometrical Optics is a topic covered in:
Physics, Chapter 8: Light and Optics

55

BIO/BIOCHEM 3

High-Yield Science:

Hormonal Regulation of Metabolism

Oxyhemoglobin Dissociation

HORMONAL REGULATION OF METABOLISM

In this lesson, you'll learn to:

- Predict the mechanism of action of peptide and steroid hormones
- Contrast the anabolic effects of insulin and testosterone

Bodybuilders use a variety of anabolic substances to gain mass. Two such compounds are insulin and trenbolone. Insulin has significant anabolic and anti-catabolic properties and impacts the metabolism of various macromolecules, not just that of carbohydrates. Trenbolone binds the androgen receptor with an affinity five times higher than that of testosterone and is popular for its fat-burning and anabolic properties.

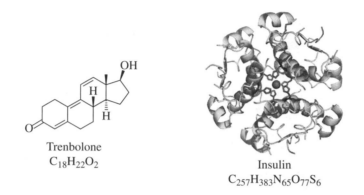

Trenbolone
$C_{18}H_{22}O_2$

Insulin
$C_{257}H_{383}N_{65}O_{77}S_6$

How do the different targets, mechanisms of action and durations of each drug ultimately lead to the same desired effect (increase in lean body mass)?

Why is trenbolone able to permeate the cell membrane?

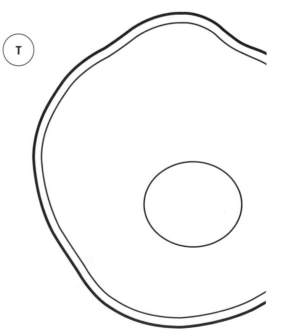

Once metabolized, trenbolone increases ammonium ion uptake in the muscle tissue. How does this promote mass gain?

Given insulin's structure, where is its target likely located?

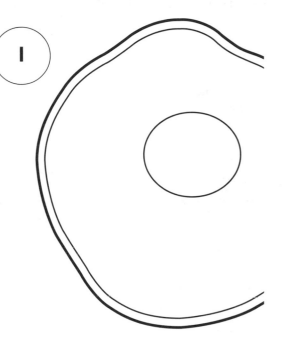

Insulin's adverse side effects include headache, nausea, hunger, confusion and weakness. What can these symptoms be attributed to?

Insulin has major effects on muscle and adipose tissue. It increases the rate of glucose transport across the cell membrane, decreases the rate of lipolysis, and increases uptake of triglycerides and some amino acids from the blood. In doing so, what metabolic processes does it favor?

Carbohydrates:

Lipids:

Proteins:

Hormonal Regulation of Metabolism is a topic covered in:
Biochemistry, Chapter 12: Bioenergetics and Regulation of Metabolism

OXYHEMOGLOBIN DISSOCIATION

In this lesson, you'll learn to:

- Plot the oxyhemoglobin dissociation curve
- Identify how changes in hemoglobin's binding affinity for oxygen will influence the curve

Carbon monoxide (CO) binding to hemoglobin occurs in competition with oxygen (O_2) binding to hemoglobin; hemoglobin's affinity for CO is over 200 times its affinity for O_2. However, the binding of CO at one site increases the affinity for O_2 at the remaining sites. Draw the oxyhemoglobin dissociation curve for CO poisoning, measuring hemoglobin oxygen content (in units of % hemoglobin saturation) on the vertical axis.

What two factors contribute to the sigmoidal shape of the oxyhemoglobin dissociation curve?

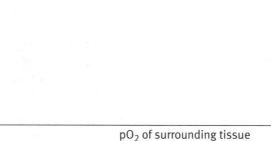

Why would carbon monoxide poisoning cause the curve to shift left while simultaneously flattening the top of the curve?

Oxyhemoglobin Dissociation is a topic covered in:
Biology, Chapter 7: The Cardiovascular System

SCIENCE CAPSTONE

High-Yield Science:

Acids and Bases

Solubility Based Separations

Amino Acid Electrophoresis

Central Dogma of Genetics

Hardy–Weinberg Equilibrium

ACIDS AND BASES

In this lesson, you'll learn to:

- Recall the properties of strong and weak acids and bases
- Compare the reactivity of an acid to the reactivity of its conjugate base
- Determine when a molecule is unreactive as either an acid or a base

Of the hydrogen halide series of acids (HF, HCl, HBr, and HI) only HF is classified as a "weak" acid; the other hydrogen halide acids—for example, HCl—are classified as "strong". Yet, HF is considerably more dangerous to human health than is HCl. According to the US Centers for Disease Control, "even small splashes of concentrated HF may be fatal." A patient exposed to concentrated HF will develop severe tissue damage at the exposure site, but this damage will develop slowly over a period of several hours. HF may even penetrate deeply enough to cause irreversible bone damage or, in fatal cases of exposure, HF will attack major organs, causing systemic organ failure. By contrast, exposure to HCl, even concentrated HCl, is rarely fatal. Concentrated HCl may cause immediate, often severe, chemical burns. However, these burns are usually superficial and may be immediately treated with running water, followed by a standard burn protocol. Finally, seemingly paradoxically: It is the very fact that HF is a "weak" acid that makes it so physiologically damaging. Resolve this apparent paradox using physiology and Brønsted-Lowry acid-base chemistry.

The K_a for HF is less than 1 and the K_a for HCl is greater than 1; how does this help explain the fact that HCl causes immediate chemical burns, while the tissue damage caused by HF is slower acting?

$$HF + H_2O \rightleftharpoons F^- + H_3O^+$$
$$K_a \approx 10^{-5}$$

$$HCl + H_2O \rightleftharpoons Cl^- + H_3O^+$$
$$K_a \approx 10^6$$

According to Brønsted–Lowry acid-base chemistry, how do the definitions of a "weak" acid and a "strong" acid correspond to the K-values of water and the hydronium cation?

$$H_3O^+ + H_2O \rightleftharpoons$$
$$K_a =$$

$$H_2O + H_2O \rightleftharpoons$$
$$K_w =$$

Acids and Bases are covered in:
General Chemistry, Chapter 10: Acids and Bases

Part of the physiological danger of HF stems from the reactivity of HF's "weak" conjugate base. According to Brønsted–Lowry acid-base chemistry, what makes a base "strong" or "weak"?

$$OH^- + H_2O \rightleftharpoons$$

$$K_b =$$

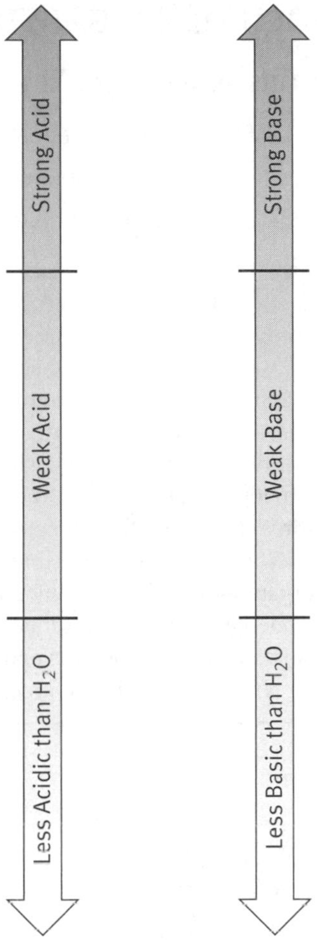

Use the relationship between the K_a of an acid and the K_b of its conjugate base to justify why the deprotonated form of HF is also dangerously reactive, while the deprotonated form of HCl is not.

HF vs. F⁻

$$K_a \times K_b = K_w$$

HCl vs. Cl⁻

$$K_a \times K_b = K_w$$

Why does the fact that HF only weakly dissociates allow it to penetrate physiological membranes and cause deep tissue damage?

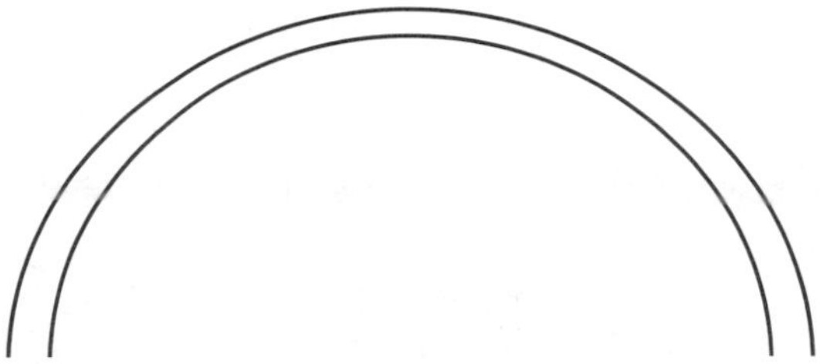

Strong Acid

Weak Acid

Less Acidic than H_2O

Strong Base

Weak Base

Less Basic than H_2O

SOLUBILITY BASED SEPARATIONS

In this lesson, you'll learn to:

- Explain how a separatory funnel accomplishes extraction
- Predict which phase compounds will resolve into during a given extraction
- Describe how chemical properties can influence physical properties

A student studying electrophilic aromatic substitution synthesizes several substituted aromatic compounds from benzene. Following the series of synthesis reactions, the student is left with a mixture of two products, benzoic acid and 4-nitroaniline. However this mixture is also contaminated with unreacted benzene and unreacted small electrophiles that were used in the synthesis. The student next wishes to separate this mixture. To perform the separation, the liquid mixture is dissolved in 500 mL dichloromethane (density = 1.33 g/mL). The solution is washed with water three times and the aqueous layer (**A**) is collected. The remaining organic layer is then washed with 20% aqueous NaOH three times, and the aqueous layer (**B**) is collected. Next, the remaining organic layer is washed with 10% aqueous HCl three times and the aqueous layer (**C**) is once again collected, leaving behind the organic layer (**D**). The student discards the two layers containing unreacted contaminants. Finally, the student removes the purified benzoic acid and the purified 4-nitroaniline products from their respective solvents using a rotary evaporator. However, the student observes that the yield of benzoic acid is significantly lower than predicted. What are the contents of layers (**A**), (**B**), (**C**), and (**D**)?

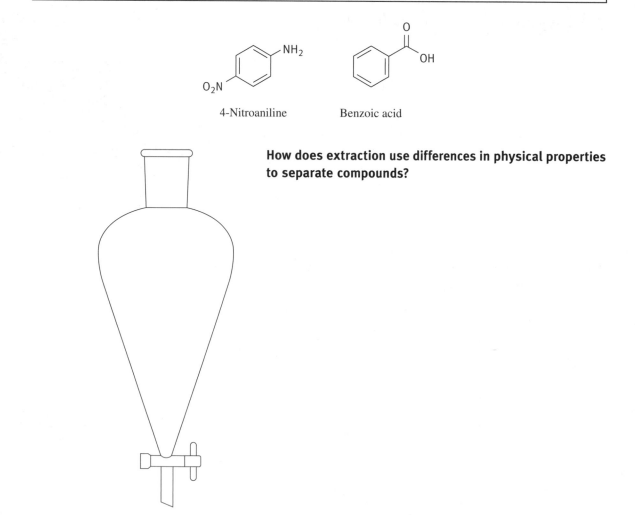

4-Nitroaniline

Benzoic acid

How does extraction use differences in physical properties to separate compounds?

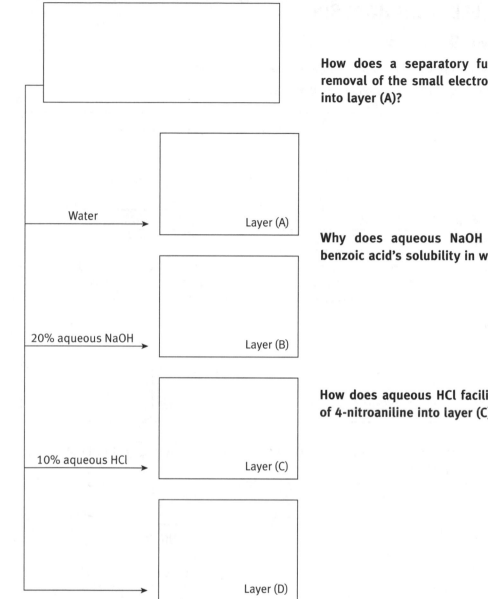

How does a separatory funnel facilitate the removal of the small electrophile contaminants into layer (A)?

Why does aqueous NaOH radically increase benzoic acid's solubility in water?

How does aqueous HCl facilitate the extraction of 4-nitroaniline into layer (C)?

Extraction is a topic covered in:
Organic Chemistry, Chapter 12: Separations and Purifications

AMINO ACID ELECTROPHORESIS

In this lesson, you'll learn to:

- Describe how pH affects the ratio of conjugate base to conjugate acid
- Determine the net charge of an amino acid at a given pH

A biochemist is trying to separate a mixture of glycine, glutamic acid and lysine given the following information:

	pK_a, COOH group	pK_a, NH_3^+ group	pK_a, R group
Glycine	2.34	9.60	–
Glutamic acid	2.19	9.67	4.25
Lysine	2.18	8.95	10.53

The mixture of amino acids is loaded onto the center of a polyacrylamide gel. The gel has a pH of 6. An electric potential difference of 220 V is applied for forty five minutes and the three points below indicate the three final locations of the amino acids within the gel. Which point corresponds to which amino acid?

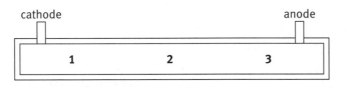

Glycine's isoelectric point is about 6. What is the conjugate base to conjugate acid ratio of its two functional groups at this pH?

COO⁻ : COOH ratio

$$pH = pK_a + \log\left(\frac{[COO^-]}{[COOH]}\right)$$

NH_2 : NH_3^+ ratio

$$pH = pK_a + \log\left(\frac{[NH_2]}{[NH_3^+]}\right)$$

Conclusion:

Amino Acid Electrophoresis is a topic covered in:
Biochemistry, Chapter 3: Nonenzymatic Protein Function and Protein Analysis

In what proportion do glycine's three ionizable states exist when the pH of the surrounding solution is equal to glycine's pI?

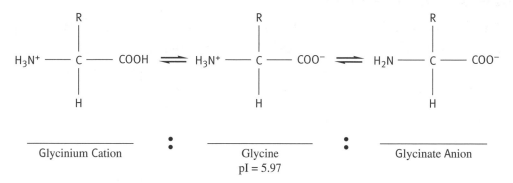

Glycinium Cation   Glycine   Glycinate Anion
                           pI = 5.97

What net charges do glutamic acid and lysine carry at a pH of 6?

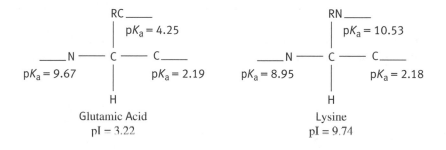

Glutamic Acid   Lysine
pI = 3.22   pI = 9.74

Electrophoresis is always run using an electrolytic cell. This means the negative terminal of a power source is connected to the cathode and the positive terminal is connected to the anode. To which point does each amino acid migrate?

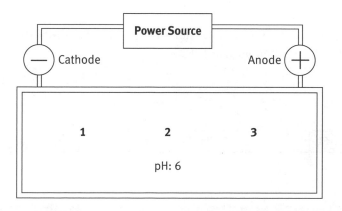

CENTRAL DOGMA OF GENETICS

In this lesson, you'll learn to:

- Predict the implications of malfunction of proteins associated with DNA synthesis
- State the purposes of different steps in biochemical techniques

Werner Syndrome is a form of adult onset progeria caused by a mutation to a single protein, the WRN protein, a helicase used in single- and double-strand break repair. There are many types of mutations that can potentially affect the WRN protein. To characterize the specific type of mutation in a given subpopulation of Werner patients, researchers run the following tests:

- A Northern blot reveals that while Werner patients do produce mRNA transcripts of the WRN gene, these transcripts are found to run at a lower than normal molecular weight.
- WRN protein is extracted from an affected patient and is found to function normally.
- A Western blot finds lower than normal concentrations of WRN protein in affected patient cells.

Using these data, what is the impact of the WRN mutation affecting this patient subpopulation?

WRN protein is a helicase, but has its major function in repair machinery. Without that information, what would have been the expected function of WRN helicase, given its protein class?

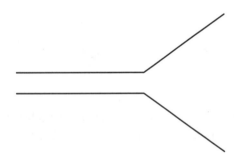

What type(s) of mutations are implicated by the Northern blot data that the mRNA is at the correct concentration, but at a lower than normal MW?

Cap	5' UTR	Coding Sequence	3' UTR	Poly-A Tail

If the protein produced is able to function, why might Werner's patients still be experiencing symptoms?

Consider the following Western blot, which shows the effective concentration of WRN protein. What must this mutation be impacting?

Blot for WRN helicase:

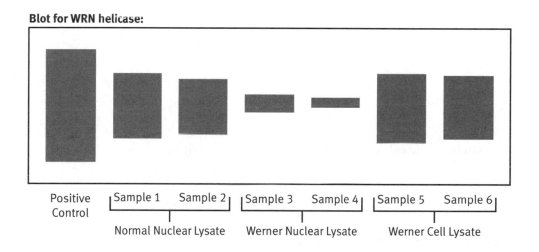

Positive Control	Sample 1	Sample 2	Sample 3	Sample 4	Sample 5	Sample 6
	Normal Nuclear Lysate		Werner Nuclear Lysate		Werner Cell Lysate	

Why might this mutation have this functional impact?

The Central Dogma of Genetics is a topic covered in:
Biochemistry, Chapter 6: DNA Replication

HARDY–WEINBERG EQUILIBRIUM

In this lesson, you'll learn to:

- Recognize and solve for terms in Hardy–Weinberg equilibrium expressions
- Use population-level data to resolve allele, genotype, and phenotype frequency questions

> Gigantism is coded for by a recessive allele. The dominant allele for the same gene codes for the normal phenotype. In an isolated geographic area, 9 people out of a sample of 10,000 were found to have gigantism, whereas the rest had normal phenotypes. Assuming Hardy–Weinberg equilibrium, calculate the frequency of the recessive and dominant alleles as well as the number of heterozygotes in the population.

Hardy–Weinberg Equilibrium: $\quad p^2 + 2pq + q^2 = 1$ $\qquad\qquad p + q = 1$

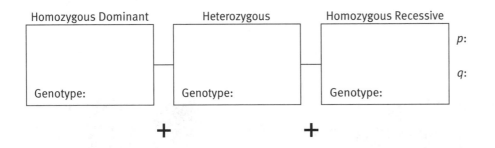

Homozygous Dominant	Heterozygous	Homozygous Recessive	
			p:
			q:
Genotype:	Genotype:	Genotype:	

$+$ $\qquad\qquad$ $+$

How can we successfully calculate the frequency of the recessive allele to be 3%?

Why is the frequency of the dominant allele 97%?

Why must 2pq be used to solve for heterozygote frequency?

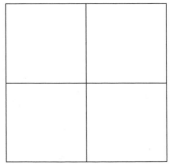

Genotypic Frequency Derivation

Hardy–Weinberg Equilibrium is a topic covered in:
Biology, Chapter 12: Genetics

The High-Yield Science lessons for the next session begin on the following page ▶ ▶ ▶

High-Yield Science:

Kidney Function

Aerobic Metabolism

Lipid Metabolism

KIDNEY FUNCTION

In this lesson, you'll learn to:

- Explain the three major functions of the nephron and their impact on urine volume and concentration
- Describe the effects of ADH, aldosterone, and filtrate osmolarity on urine production

Acesulfame potassium is a calorie-free artificial sweetener, used to sweeten many popular diet sodas. Within the GI tract, acesulfame potassium is rapidly and completely absorbed; however, it is neither stored nor metabolized within the body, and is instead filtered and excreted by the kidney. A student discovers that drinking diet caffeinated soda, sweetened with acesulfame potassium, results in a significant increase in urine volume and frequency. What are the physiological factors driving this phenomenon?

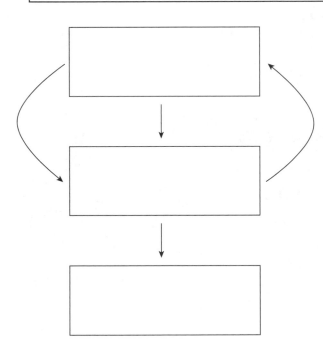

Why might a reduction in reabsorption or an increase in secretion increase urinary output?

Why does caffeine's inhibition of antidiuretic hormone increase urine volume?

By what mechanism does ingesting a large volume of soda increase urine volume?

Acesulfame potassium is not actively reabsorbed by the nephron. Why does this factor also increase urine volume?

Kidney Function is a topic covered in:
Biology, Chapter 10: Homeostasis

This chapter continues on the next page. ▶ ▶ ▶

AEROBIC METABOLISM

In this lesson, you'll learn to:

- Describe the effects of "uncoupling" the electron transport chain and oxidative phosphorylation
- Use molecular shape to help explain the physiological effects of a biologically active molecule

2,4-Dinitrophenol, also known as DNP, is a molecule that was once marketed as a weight loss "miracle" drug. DNP works by "uncoupling" oxidative phosphorylation from the electron transport chain, causing rapid weight loss. However, DNP also causes unpleasant, sometimes even fatal side effects, including tachypnea (elevated breathing rate) and hyperthermia. DNP was quickly pulled from the market as doctors realized that a fatal dose of DNP might be as little as twice the effective dose for weight loss. How does DNP cause weight loss and why might this mechanism explain the potentially fatal side effects of this drug?

In spite of the fact that hydroxyl groups are normally only very weakly acidic, 2,4-dinitrophenol (DNP) will mostly be deprotonated at physiological pH. Why?

2,4-DInitrophenolate
$pK_a = 4$

Why can DNP cross physiological membranes, despite being a charged compound at normal physiological pH?

Aerobic Metabolism is a topic covered in:
Biochemistry, Chapter 10: Carbohydrate Metabolism II Aerobic Respiration

What does it mean to say that ATP production depends on "coupling" the electron transport chain and oxidative phosphorylation? What is oxygen's role in this process?

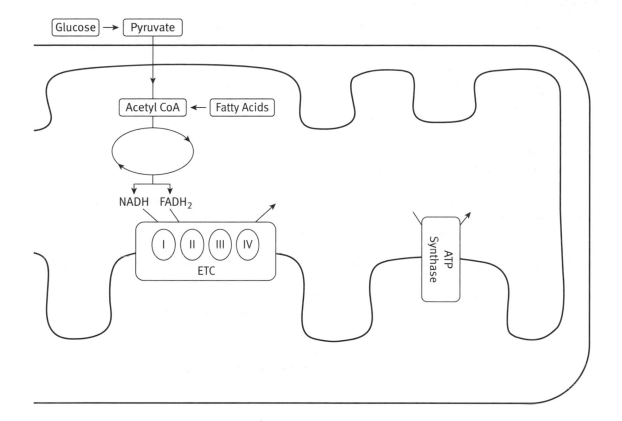

Why does protonating DNP within the intermembrane space disrupt chemiosmosis?

Why does disrupting chemiosmosis cause weight loss? How does this mechanism explain DNP's potentially fatal side effects?

LIPID METABOLISM

In this lesson, you'll learn to:

- Use MCAT-level science to explain aspects of complex modern medical techniques
- Describe the difference in energy density between fats and sugars

---

Thermogenin is a protein that newborn humans use to generate heat through the oxidation of fatty acids by uncoupling the electron transport chain and oxidative phosphorylation within specialized fat cells. Because thermogenin activity leads to fatty acid metabolism, it also causes weight loss. Recently, researchers discovered that adult humans also express small amounts of thermogenin, and that lean adults tend to express more thermogenin, and obese adults less. One possible conclusion from this observation is that inducing thermogenin expression may be a treatment for obesity.

One group of researchers hypothesizes that thermogenin expression in adults is blocked by a suppressor protein. This group has filed a patent protecting their as-yet-unfinished method of inducing thermogenin expression using exogenous microRNAs, which are small segments of RNA complementary to a target gene. However, even if this group can successfully induce thermogenin expression using microRNA, they must also determine a method to make these microRNA molecules target only adipose tissue. Explain this group's plan to use microRNA to induce thermogenin expression. Why must thermogenin expression be limited to adipose tissue?

The question stem describes a microRNA as being "complementary to a target gene." By what mechanism would such a molecule prevent the suppressor protein from suppressing thermogenin?

Why would researchers seek to induce thermogenin expression only in adipose tissue and not in tissues that rely primarily on carbohydrates for energy?

Decanoic Acid
MW = 172 g/mol

Glucose
MW = 180 g/mol

ß-Oxidation is a topic covered in:
Biochemistry, Chapter 11: Lipid and Amino Acid Metabolism

SECTION II

MCAT Skills

CHAPTER 1

Science Skill 1: Science Knowledge

Skill 1 (Science Knowledge) Basics

In this lesson, you'll learn to:

- Recognize and recall scientific principles when mentioned in a question
- Recognize and recall scientific principles when given a specific example in a question
- Recognize and recall correct scientific principles when a question seems to be indicating another topic

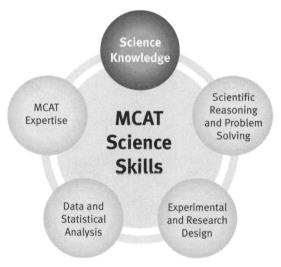

Science Topics:

- Stoichiometry
- Organic Chemistry Nomenclature
- Thermodynamics
- Fluids

MCAT STRATEGY—SCIENCE KNOWLEDGE QUESTIONS

ASSESS THE QUESTION
Read the question, looking for clues to the science topic.

PLAN YOUR ATTACK
Recall what you know about the topic being tested.

EXECUTE THE PLAN
Figure out the correct answer.

ANSWER BY MATCHING, ELIMINATING, OR GUESSING
Find the right answer in the answer choices.

LESSON 1.1, LEARNING GOAL 1:

• Recognize and recall scientific principles when mentioned in a question

CHEM/PHYS CONCEPT MAP

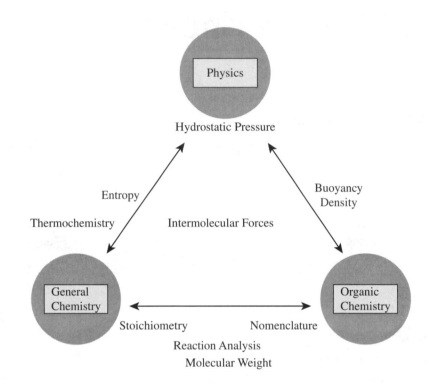

*Biochemistry is also a subject within the Chem/Phys section on the MCAT.

Sample Questions

1. What type of heat transfer is the primary way the sun's heat reaches Earth?

What do you know about heat transfer?

2. What is the correct IUPAC name for the following compound?

$$CH_3CHCHCOOCHCl_2$$

What factors influence the name of an organic compound?

3. Which of the following is true of liquids, but NOT true of gases?

What are the general properties of fluids (liquids and gases)?

4. How would the plot of hydrostatic pressure versus depth change for a vessel filled with liquid and exposed to the environment if it were transported to the moon?

What do you know about hydrostatic pressure?

KAPLAN TIP

The MCAT will demand that you recall science knowledge to solve Skill 1 questions. If you quickly and confidently bring your knowledge of the content to these questions, you can pick up points.

Answer the Questions:

1. What type of heat transfer is the primary way the sun's heat reaches Earth?

   A. Convection
   B. Radioactivity
   C. Conduction
   D. Radiation

2. What is the correct IUPAC name for the following compound?

   $$CH_3CHCHCOOCHCl_2$$

   A. Chloromethyl-2-butenoate
   B. Dichloromethyl-2-butenoate
   C. 2-Butene-chloromethanoate
   D. 2-Butene-dicholoromethanoate

3. Which of the following is true of liquids, but NOT true of gases?

   A. They will conform to fit the shape of their container.
   B. They are essentially incompressible.
   C. Larger constituent molecules will move at lower velocities, given equal temperatures.
   D. They exert pressure on objects contained within them.

4. How would the plot of hydrostatic pressure versus depth change for a vessel filled with liquid and exposed to the environment if it were transported to the moon?

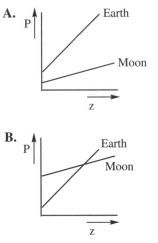

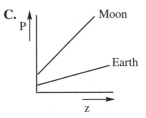

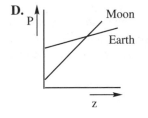

LESSON 1.1, LEARNING GOAL 2:

- Recognize and recall scientific principles when given a specific example in a question

Sample Questions

5. A sample of monatomic ideal gas is taken through an adiabatic expansion and is then isothermally compressed until the gas returns to its original pressure. Which of the following is true of this process?

What topic is being tested?

What do you know about this topic?

6. A student reacts 28 grams of iron with 24 grams of sulfur to produce iron(II) sulfide (FeS), but has some unreacted chemicals left over at the end of the reaction. How much of which chemicals are left over and why?

What topic is being tested?

What do you know about this topic?

7. A child plays with a toy in which a small, air- and liquid-filled balloon floats within a bottle that is closed and completely filled with water (see diagram below). The bottle is flexible such that when the child squeezes it, the bottle can just slightly compress. Upon squeezing the bottle, the balloon sinks. Why does this happen?

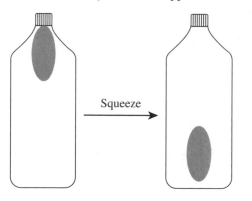

Squeeze

What topic is being tested?

What do you know about this topic?

Answer the Questions:

5. A sample of monatomic ideal gas is taken through an adiabatic expansion and is then isothermally compressed until the gas returns to its original pressure. Which of the following is true of this process?

    A. The net heat input into the gas is zero.
    B. The net work done by the gas is zero.
    C. The final state of the gas has a lower total internal energy than the initial state.
    D. The final state of the gas has a higher average temperature than the initial state.

Process	Definition
Isothermal	no change in temperature
Isobaric	no change in pressure
Isovolumetric / Isochoric	no change in volume
Adiabatic	no heat in or out of system

$$PV = nRT$$
$$\Delta U = Q - W_{\text{by system}}$$
$$U = \frac{3}{2} PV = \frac{3}{2} nRT$$

6. A student reacts 28 grams of iron with 24 grams of sulfur to produce iron(II) sulfide (FeS), but has some unreacted chemicals left over at the end of the reaction. How much of which chemicals are left over and why?

    A. Iron is left over because there are fewer moles of it present initially. There are 8 grams of it left.
    B. Sulfur is left over because there are more moles of it present initially. There are 8 grams of it left.
    C. Sulfur is left over because there is less mass of it present initially. There are 8 grams of it left.
    D. Both chemicals are left over because neither is the limiting reagent. There are 8 grams of each left.

7. A child plays with a toy in which a small, air- and liquid-filled balloon floats within a bottle that is closed and completely filled with water (see diagram below). The bottle is flexible such that when the child squeezes it, the bottle can just slightly compress. Upon squeezing the bottle, the balloon sinks. Why does this happen?

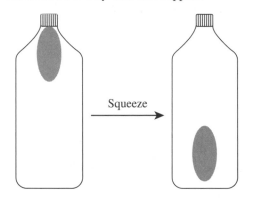

Squeeze

A. The balloon is compressed upon squeezing, thus increasing its density.

B. The water in the bottle is compressed, increasing its density and, thus, the buoyant force on the balloon.

C. Atmospheric pressure increases upon squeezing, forcing the balloon to sink.

D. As the balloon sinks, the depth decreases the hydrostatic pressure, causing the balloon to sink further.

LESSON 1.1, LEARNING GOAL 3:

• Recognize and recall correct scientific principles when a question seems to be indicating another topic

Sample Questions

8. A cube of solid ice is floating in a glass of water. After the ice melts into the liquid phase, the level of water in the glass:

   A. is higher.
   B. is lower.
   C. remains the same.
   D. cannot be determined with the information provided.

What topic is directly mentioned?

What topic is related and necessary to answer the question?

What do you already know about this related topic?

9. A student reads that mixing a strong acid and a strong base is a neutralization reaction and should produce a solution with a neutral pH. So the student mixes equal volumes of equally concentrated sulfuric acid and sodium hydroxide. Rather than a neutral pH, however, the pH of the resulting solution is acidic. Why is this? (Assume the neutralization reaction goes to completion.)

   A. Sulfuric acid is sufficiently strong as an acid so as not to react at all but still neutralize the sodium hydroxide.
   B. There are more moles of sulfuric acid than sodium hydroxide, so there is sulfuric acid left over at the end of the reaction.
   C. There are more hydrogen ions from the sulfuric acid than there are hydroxide ions from the sodium hydroxide, so there are hydrogen ions left over at the end of the reaction.
   D. There are fewer hydrogen ions from the sulfuric acid than there are hydroxide ions from the sodium hydroxide, so there are hydroxide ions left over at the end of the reaction.

What topic is directly mentioned?

What topic is related and necessary to answer the question?

What do you already know about this related topic?

10. Compound E reacts with semicarbazide to form the semicarbazone F according to the following equation:

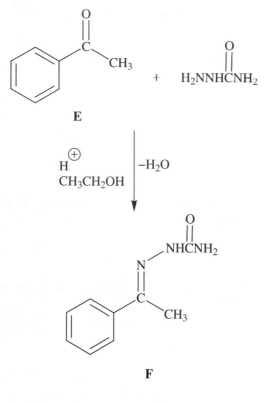

Compound F contains what functional groups?

A. Imine, amine, amide
B. Imine, amine, carbonyl
C. Amine, amide, hydroxyl
D. Phenyl, amide, imine

What topic is directly mentioned?

What topic is related and necessary to answer the question?

What do you already know about this related topic?

KAPLAN TIP

Questions like these can be some of the hardest Skill 1 questions on the MCAT. You'll answer these questions correctly, though, if you're careful to identify exactly what each one is asking.

LESSON 1.1 REVIEW

MCAT Strategy—Science Questions

Assess the question by reading it and looking for clues to the science topic.

Recall what you know about scientific principles when you read them in a question:

When the scientific principle is directly mentioned

When given a specific example of a scientific principle in a question

Recall correct scientific principles when a question seems to be indicating another topic.

Math on the MCAT

In this lesson, you'll learn to:

- Solve MCAT math problems using minimal calculation
- Identify when math is needed to solve a problem

Science Topics:

- Fluids
- Translational Motion
- Energy
- Intermolecular Forces

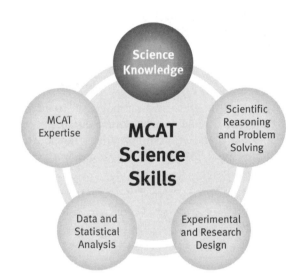

MCAT STRATEGY—SCIENCE QUESTIONS WITH CALCULATIONS

ASSESS THE QUESTION
Read the question and decide if calculations are necessary to solve it.

PLAN YOUR ATTACK
Recall what formulas you need and plan how to set up the math.

EXECUTE THE PLAN
Implement the plan to figure out the correct answer.

ANSWER BY MATCHING, ELIMINATING, OR GUESSING
Find the right answer using the choices to guide you if necessary.

LESSON 1.2, LEARNING GOAL 1:

• Solve MCAT problems using minimal calculation

Sample Questions:

1. Decelerating uniformly, a car traveling north at 25 m/s takes 10 seconds to come to a complete stop. What is the magnitude and direction of the car's acceleration as it slows down?

   A. North, at 2.5 m/s²
   B. South, at 2.5 m/s²
   C. North, at 9.8 m/s²
   D. South, at 25 m/s²

2. In a head-on collision, a car moving at 10 m/s is uniformly brought to a halt over a distance of 0.5 m, the size of the car's crumple zone. How much time does it take for the car to come to a complete stop?

   A. 0.05 s
   B. 0.1 s
   C. 0.2 s
   D. 0.5 s

3. Blood moves toward a dialysis machine according to the equation Flow = 100^x, where x is the pressure at which the filtration system is set. To what pressure must the filtration system be set to ensure that blood flows evenly through the filtration system with no backup or vacuum created, if flow must equal 1,000 upon exiting the filtration system?

   A. 0.66
   B. 1.33
   C. 1.5
   D. 2.5

KAPLAN TIP

You can minimize calculation—saving time and reducing errors on Test Day—by using "close enough" numbers and eliminating answer choices aggressively.

LESSON 1.2, LEARNING GOAL 2:

- Identify when math is needed to solve a problem

Sample Questions:

4. If a car moving at 15 m/s suffers a collision, causing it to decelerate uniformly at 2 m/s^2, approximately how far does the car travel during time t?

    A. $15t + t^2$ m
    B. $15\left(\dfrac{t}{3}\right) - \left(\dfrac{t}{3}\right)^2$ m
    C. $15t$ m
    D. $15t - t^2$ m

Is it necessary to use calculations to solve this problem?

If so, what calculations are necessary?

5. What is the distance a 75 kg patient can be pushed upward using a downward force of 20 N over 15 m (accomplished through several foot pumps) on a hydraulically powered surgical bed?

    A. 0.4 m
    B. 0.8 m
    C. 2 m
    D. 4 m

Is it necessary to use calculations to solve this problem?

If so, what calculations are necessary?

6. When an external uniform electric field, E, is applied to an atom, the nucleus and the electron cloud shift, moving in opposite directions and forming an induced dipole moment $p = qd$. The induced dipole moment is directly proportional to the external field $p = \alpha E$, where α is the atomic polarizability. The atomic polarizability has the SI units:

A. $\dfrac{C^2 \cdot s^2 \cdot m^3}{kg}$

B. $\dfrac{C^2 \cdot s^2}{kg}$

C. $\dfrac{C^2 \cdot s^2}{kg \cdot m^3}$

D. $\dfrac{kg \cdot s^2}{C^2}$

Is it necessary to use calculations to solve this problem?

If so, what calculations are necessary?

KAPLAN TIP

Knowing when to perform calculations, and especially when *not* to, is a key MCAT skill!

LESSON 1.2 REVIEW

MCAT Strategy—Science Questions with Calculations

ASSESS THE QUESTION

Read the question and decide if calculations are necessary to solve it.

PLAN YOUR ATTACK

Recall what formulas you need and plan how to set up the math.

EXECUTE THE PLAN

Implement the plan to figure out the correct answer.

ANSWER BY MATCHING, ELIMINATING, OR GUESSING

Find the right answer using the choices to guide you if necessary.

Concepts in Multiple Forms

In this lesson, you'll learn to:

- Identify the same science concept presented across multiple disciplines
- Recognize and apply ideas regardless of their presentation format

Science Topics:

- Oxidation and Reduction
- Gene Regulation

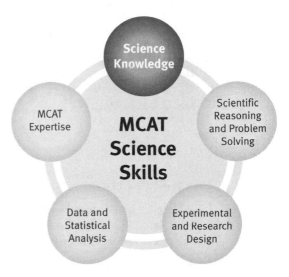

LESSON 1.3, LEARNING GOAL 1:

• Identify the same science concept presented across multiple disciplines

Oxidation and Reduction

In General Chemistry

1. The formation of rust occurs via the reaction below.

$$4\,Fe + 3\,O_2 \rightarrow 2\,Fe_2O_3$$

During the formation of rust, iron:

A. acts as an oxidizing agent.
B. gains electrons.
C. is oxidized.
D. is the oxidant.

In Biology

3. In the lungs, deoxyhemoglobin is converted to oxyhemoglobin. As a part of this process:

A. the oxidation state of iron in hemoglobin decreases.
B. the hemoglobin becomes more efficient at absorbing red light.
C. hemoglobin conforms such that it has decreased affinity for oxygen.
D. hemoglobin binds to an oxidizing agent.

In Organic Chemistry

2. Aldoses can be reduced with lithium aluminum hydride to compounds known as alditols. What is the product of the reduction reaction of D-glucose?

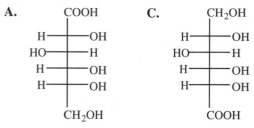

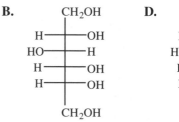
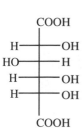

Regulation Mechanisms

The *trp* operon:

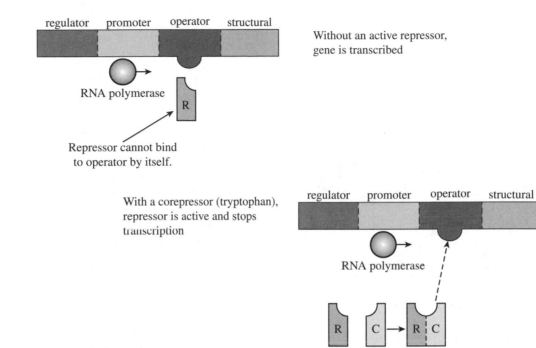

Without an active repressor, gene is transcribed

Repressor cannot bind to operator by itself.

With a corepressor (tryptophan), repressor is active and stops transcription

corepressor (end product)

In Biochemistry

4. If transcription of the gene that codes for the repressor (R) in the figure above is repressed, the production of tryptophan synthetase, an enzyme coded for by the *trp* structural genes, will most likely occur:

   A. only in the presence of tryptophan.
   B. only in the absence of tryptophan.
   C. in the presence and absence of tryptophan.
   D. neither in the presence nor absence of tryptophan.

In Biology

5. Normally, dexamethasone (a synthetic glucocorticoid) inhibits ACTH secretion and, consequently, cortisol secretion. A patient with low ACTH and elevated cortisol levels after dexamethasone administration most likely has:

   A. an adrenal cortical tumor.
   B. a hypothalamic tumor.
   C. an anterior pituitary tumor.
   D. no pathology in endogenous cortisol production.

KAPLAN TIP

Questions 4 and 5 involve two systems that are different on the surface, but both systems incorporate the same regulatory mechanism: negative feedback.

LESSON 1.3, LEARNING GOAL 2:

- Recognize and apply ideas regardless of their presentation format

Practice Questions:

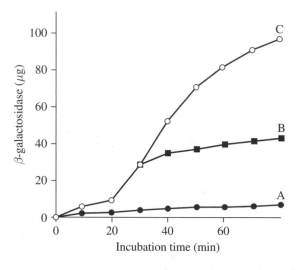

6. The protein β-galactosidase is encoded by the *lacZ* structural gene of the *lac* operon. The figure above shows β-galactosidase levels for three *E. coli* cultures grown on a substrate containing lactose. Sample A was given glucose at 0 mins, Sample B at 30 mins, and Sample C was not given any glucose. The data most strongly suggest:

   A. glucose decreases expression of the *lac* operon regulatory gene.
   B. lactose is sufficient to cause an increase in β-galactosidase.
   C. glucose decreases expression of the *lac* operon in the presence of lactose.
   D. glucose is necessary for β-galactosidase production.

7. In order for *E. coli* to utilize lactose as a carbon and energy source, the *lacZ* structural gene of the *lac* operon must be transcribed, which allows the protein β-galactosidase to be translated. In the presence of both lactose and glucose, *E. coli* will preferentially utilize glucose, conserving the resources necessary to produce β-galactosidase. However, when glucose is absent, lactose will functionally induce the expression of β-galactosidase. This most strongly suggests:

   A. glucose decreases expression of the *lac* operon regulatory gene.
   B. lactose is sufficient to cause an increase in β-galactosidase.
   C. glucose decreases expression of the *lac* operon in the presence of lactose.
   D. glucose is necessary for β-galactosidase production.

8. The protein β-galactosidase is encoded by the *lacZ* structural gene of the *lac* operon. In order to test regulation of this gene, scientists created mutant strains of *E. coli*. Each haploid mutant contained one mutant sequence of DNA. Trials were conducted with and without glucose and lactose, and the plates were tested for the presence of β-galactosidase. The results are shown below.

		Substrate		
		Glucose	Lactose	Glucose and Lactose
Mutated sequence	*lacZ* (β-galactosidase)	–	–	–
	lac o (operator)	+	+	+
	lacI (repressor)	+	+	+
	wild type	–	+	–

The data most strongly suggest:

A. glucose decreases expression of the *lac* operon repressor gene.
B. lactose is sufficient to increase β-galactosidase production.
C. glucose decreases expression of *lacZ* in the presence of lactose.
D. glucose is necessary for β-galactosidase production.

LESSON 1.3 REVIEW

Remember to ...

Be flexible when a basic scientific concept comes up in any question in any science section.

Remember that science concepts can be represented as:

• Text
• Data Tables
• Graphs of Results
• Equations
• Figures

Skill 1 (Science Knowledge) in Action

In this lesson, you'll learn to:

- Identify the content needed to solve Skill 1 questions
- Solve Skill 1 questions
- Prioritize your content study by depth of knowledge

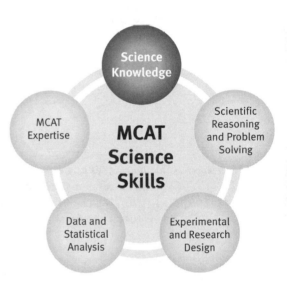

Science Topics:

- Periodic Trends
- Acid/Base Chemistry
- Electrostatics
- Circuits
- Electron Transport Chain
- Theories of Emotion

From the AAMC*:

"The questions in this skill category will ask you to demonstrate your knowledge of the foundational concepts that you are responsible for knowing when you take the MCAT exam. These questions will ask you to recognize, recall, or define basic concepts in the sciences as well as their relationship with one another. The concepts and scientific principles may be represented by words, graphs, tables, diagrams, or formulas."

*The Official Guide to the MCAT Exam (MCAT2017), Fifth Edition

LESSON 1.4, LEARNING GOALS 1 AND 2:

- Identify the content needed to solve Skill 1 questions
- Solve Skill 1 questions

Example Questions

1. Which one of the following is the most electro-negative element?

    A. C
    B. I
    C. N
    D. P

What content underlies this question?

2. A student observes that nitroacetic acid ($pK_a = 1.68$) is significantly more acidic than acetic acid ($pK_a = 4.76$). Which of the following statements accounts for this observation?

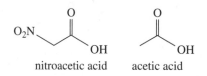
nitroacetic acid   acetic acid

    A. Nitroacetic acid has a greater molecular mass.
    B. The nitro group on nitroacetic acid is strongly electron withdrawing.
    C. The nitro group on nitroacetic acid is a poor leaving group.
    D. The conjugate base of acetic acid is not resonance stabilized.

What content underlies this question?

3. Which of the following will undergo ester hydrolysis most rapidly?

What content underlies this question?

A.

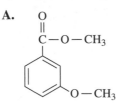

B.

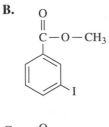

C.

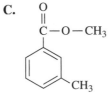

D.

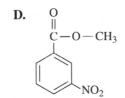

KAPLAN TIP

Skill 1 questions can directly mention a science topic, give a specific illustration or example involving a science topic, or even seem to mislead you about the topic being tested. In every case, you should first determine what topic the question is actually testing.

LESSON 1.4, LEARNING GOAL 3:

- Prioritize your content study by depth of knowledge

Physics Example—Meters

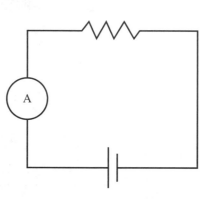

Ammeter (A) in series

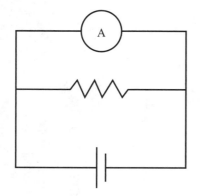

Ammeter (A) in parallel

What does an ammeter do?

Should an ammeter be wired in series or in parallel?

How will an ammeter behave differently when it has non-negligible resistance?

Biochemistry Example—The Electron Transport Chain

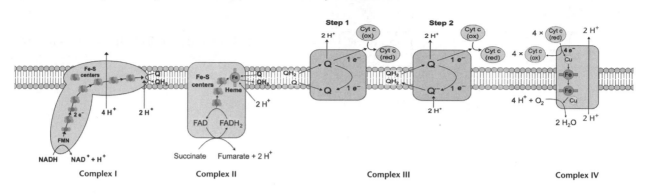

What does FADH$_2$ contribute to the electron transport chain?

In what way does Complex II interact with the citric acid cycle?

What is true of the reduction potential of coenzyme Q compared to the reduction potential of FAD?

Behavioral Sciences Example—Theories of Emotion

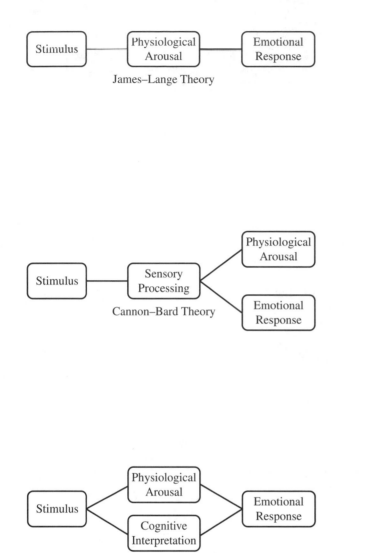

James–Lange Theory

Cannon–Bard Theory

Schachter–Singer Theory

What is the Cannon–Bard theory of emotion?

In what ways is the Cannon–Bard theory of emotion similar to and different from the Schachter–Singer theory of emotion?

According to the Cannon–Bard theory of emotion, what should happen to an individual's emotions if he is unable to perceive his own physiological responses?

KAPLAN TIP

Success on the MCAT does not mean recalling every granular content detail. Though studying content almost always helps, it is better to know something about every topic area than to know everything about a few topic areas and nothing about others.

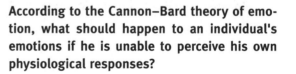

LESSON 1.4 REVIEW

Chapter 1 Learning Goals

1.1 Skill 1 (Knowledge) Basics

- Recognize and recall scientific principles when mentioned in a question
- Recognize and recall scientific principles when given a specific example in a question
- Recognize and recall correct scientific principles when a question seems to be indicating another topic

1.2 Math on the MCAT

- Solve MCAT math problems using minimal calculation
- Identify when math is needed to solve a problem

1.3 Concepts in Multiple Forms

- Identify the same science concept presented across multiple disciplines
- Recognize and apply ideas regardless of their presentation format

CHAPTER 2

Science Skill 2: Critical Thinking

Skill 2 (Critical Thinking) Basics

In this lesson, you'll learn to:

- Recall relevant scientific concepts with limited or no clues in the question stem or answer choices
- Apply known scientific principles to novel and/or complicated situations

Science Topics

- Electrostatics
- Thermochemistry (General Chemistry)
- Thermodynamics (General Chemistry)

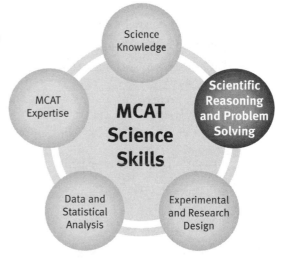

LESSON 2.1, LEARNING GOALS 1 AND 2:

- Recall relevant scientific concepts with limited or no clues in the question stem or answer choices
- Apply known scientific principles to novel and/or complicated situations

The Question Behind the Question

1. The Haber process for the production of ammonia is represented by the equation below:

$$N_2(g) + 3 H_2(g) \leftrightarrow 2 NH_3(g) + 22 \text{ kcal}$$

Which of the following will decrease the yield of ammonia?

   A. A decrease in temperature and an increase in pressure
   B. A decrease in temperature and a decrease in pressure
   C. An increase in temperature and an increase in pressure
   D. An increase in temperature and a decrease in pressure

What is the relevant science concept?

2. Which of the following statements is true regarding the diagram below?

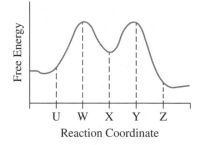

   A. Going from U to W requires less energy than going from X to Y.
   B. Going from U to X occurs more readily than going from X to Z.
   C. X will be more easily isolated in solution than Y or W.
   D. The reaction U to X releases energy while the reaction X to Z would absorb it.

What is the relevant science concept?

The Question Behind the Question

3. Which of the following statements is NOT true of melting ice?

    A. The reaction happens spontaneously at 298 K.
    B. The molecules become more ordered.
    C. The reaction requires energy.
    D. The volume of the substance decreases.

What is the relevant science concept?

4. The distance separating the two strands that make up DNA is about 1 nm. The magnitude of the force between the hydrogen-bonded bases would hypothetically:

    A. decrease as the distance decreases to 0.3 nm.
    B. exhibit no change as the distance decreases.
    C. increase as the distance increases to 2 nm.
    D. decrease as the distance increases to 2 nm.

What is the relevant science concept?

5. A certain biological reaction requires two ATP (adenosine triphosphate) molecules to work within close proximity. Which of the following is true?

    A. Work needs to be done on the molecules by an external force to bring them close because they repel each other.
    B. No external force is needed in order to bring the two molecules together because they attract each other.
    C. Work needs to be done on the molecules by an external force to bring them close because they attract each other.
    D. The potential energy of the molecules is unaffected by bringing them close together.

What is the relevant science concept?

KAPLAN TIP

Clues or "buzzwords" in the question stem *or* the answer choices can help you identify the relevant science topic and get closer to points on Test Day.

LESSON 2.1 REVIEW

Critical Thinking Basics

The question and the answer choices

- Contain valuable clues
- Are linked conceptually
- Will indicate the relevant science concepts, if sometimes indirectly

Critical Thinking on the MCAT

- Is imperative for making an effective plan to attack the question
- Makes a multistep problem more manageable
- Helps identify where to look for information when answering a question:

  ◦ Your knowledge base
  ◦ The passage
  ◦ The question
  ◦ Combinations of the above

MCAT Scientific Reasoning

In this lesson, you'll learn to:

- Determine the likelihood of a scientific phenomenon or a given explanation for a phenomenon
- Determine the likely cause or effect of a phenomenon
- Determine how observations influence scientific theories or models
- Gather information from various sources to draw conclusions

Science Topics:

- Chemical Kinetics and Equilibrium
- Solubility
- Acids and Bases and Titrations

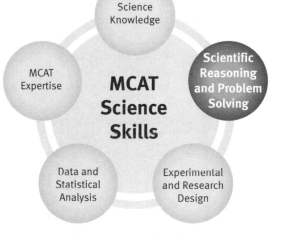

LESSON 2.2, LEARNING GOAL 1:

- Determine the likelihood of a scientific phenomenon or a given explanation for a phenomenon

Example Questions

1. In the following chemical mechanism, is acid acting as a catalyst?

    $$H_2O_2 + H^+ \rightleftharpoons H_3O_2^+ \qquad \textbf{Step 1}$$

    $$I^- + H_3O_2^+ \longrightarrow HOI + H_2O \qquad \textbf{Step 2}$$

    $$I^- + HOI \longrightarrow I_2 + OH^- \qquad \textbf{Step 3}$$

    $$H^+ + OH^- \longrightarrow H_2O \qquad \textbf{Step 4}$$

    A. Yes, because it lowers the activation energy of the reaction.
    B. Yes, because it makes the reaction proceed faster.
    C. No, because in the absence of nitric acid, the same reaction would occur at the same rate.
    D. No, because the H^+ is not regenerated.

    What is the phenomenon in this question?

2. If 0.5 L of a 1.0×10^{-5} M NaBr solution is added to 0.5 L of a 1.0×10^{-5} M AgCl solution, will there be any precipitate? (The K_{sp} of AgBr is 5.4×10^{-13}.)

    A. No, both NaBr and AgCl are completely soluble.
    B. No, all ion concentrations are at or below saturation levels.
    C. Yes, both AgBr and NaCl are completely insoluble.
    D. Yes, Ag^+ and Br^- concentrations are above saturation levels.

    What is the phenomenon in this question?

LESSON 2.2, LEARNING GOAL 2:

- Determine the likely cause or effect of a phenomenon

Example Questions

3. In a reaction at equilibrium, it is concluded that helium gas behaves more ideally than carbon dioxide. Which of the following accurately explains why this is so?

    I. CO_2 exerts a greater pressure because its molecules have lesser volume.
    II. The intermolecular forces between CO_2 molecules are stronger than those in He.
    III. He molecules have greater kinetic energy, and therefore behave more ideally.

    A. I only
    B. II only
    C. II and III only
    D. I, II, and III

What is the phenomenon in this question?

4. A researcher dissolves 385.43 mg of an acid solid in water to make a standard solution of acid. He then titrates the acid using NaOH of unknown concentration. Despite not knowing how much water the acid was dissolved in, the calculated concentration of NaOH is unaffected. Why?

    A. The volume of acid determines the volume of base added, not the concentration of that base.
    B. The concentration of the base is determined solely by how many liters of acid are required to neutralize the base.
    C. The concentration of the base is determined solely by how many moles of acid are required to neutralize the base.
    D. The concentration of NaOH could not have actually been calculated due to the volume of the acid being unknown.

What is the phenomenon in this question?

KAPLAN TIP

Thinking through the scientific phenomena at hand and using your critical reasoning skills will help answer Skill 2 questions on Test Day!

LESSON 2.2, LEARNING GOAL 3:

- Determine how observations influence scientific theories or models

Passage Excerpt (Questions 5–6)

Phosphatidylcholine (PC) is an important component of the lipid bilayer and is also involved in membrane-mediated cell signalling. The first step in PC synthesis involves the transfer of a phosphate group from ATP to choline to produce phosphocholine, a reaction catalyzed by the enzyme choline kinase (CK) (Figure 1). A researcher is interested in determining the reaction mechanism for CK, and hypothesizes that choline needs to bind the active site before ATP binds.

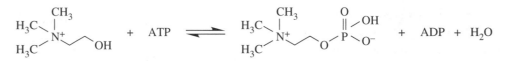

Figure 1. Phosphorylation of choline catalyzed by CK

The researcher purifies CK and induces supersaturation to form crystals in order to determine the 3-D structure of CK using x-ray crystallography. Crystals of pure protein are exposed to x-rays, and the ordered arrangement of protein molecules in a crystal lattice will cause the x-ray beams to diffract in a predictable pattern. Mathematical interpretation of the constructive interference of x-rays diffracting from ordered electrons will give an electron density map, and threading the amino acid sequence of CK into the map will allow the 3-D placement of the atoms.

Using x-ray crystallography, the researcher determines the 3-D structure of CK to a 2 angstrom resolution (1 Å = 10^{-10} m). Resolution describes how accurately the distance between atoms can be measured. For reference, a typical carbon-carbon bond would be 1.5 Å in length. The results indicate the structure of the crystalline CK to be a homodimer, with each monomer composed of an N-terminal domain, and a larger C-terminal domain. Interestingly, evidence shows that CK does not function as a dimer *in vivo*. Electrostatic mapping of the surface of the 3-D structure of CK shows a negatively charged pocket.

Passage Excerpt Questions

5. A student replicates the researcher's procedure and finds that a 20 micron crystal diffracts to 5 Å resolution, but a 200 micron crystal has 1.8 Å resolution. Based on the passage, what is the most plausible reason for this difference? (1 micron = 10^{-6} m)

    A. The 200 micron crystal contains more molecules of CK, and additional CK molecules contribute to increased constructive interference.
    B. The 200 micron crystal had molecules of CK that were disordered, and therefore contributed to the overall poor resolution of the crystal.
    C. The 20 micron crystal did not achieve sufficient supersaturation.
    D. The 20 micron crystal can resolve atoms in the sidechains of critical amino acids.

What is the new observation in this question?

6. Suppose that an in-depth analysis of CK *in vivo* reveals a single active site with the ATP binding site deep within and the choline binding site near the surface. How does this affect the researcher's hypothesis?

    A. It weakens the researcher's hypothesis because the observation would suggest that the ATP needs to bind before choline.
    B. It weakens the researcher's hypothesis because the positive charge on choline would interact with the negative charge on the phosphates.
    C. It strengthens the researcher's hypothesis because the active site is in the interface of the dimer.
    D. It strengthens the researcher's hypothesis because resolution of the data is sufficient to monitor the real-time movement of the substrates in the active site.

What is the new observation in this question?

LESSON 2.2, LEARNING GOAL 4:

- Gather information from various sources to draw conclusions

Practice Passage (Questions 7–10)

Lactic acidosis is a form of metabolic acidosis characterized by a blood pH lower than 7.35 and heightened lactate levels in the blood. This condition may arise either through excess lactate production by the tissues, limited hepatic metabolism, or a combination of these factors. In healthy individuals, the liver acts as a blood pH regulator. Two mechanisms by which the liver can regulate pH are as follows:

Mechanism 1: Increasing or decreasing metabolism of acid anions, such as lactate, citrate, gluconate, and acetate, will increase or decrease blood pH, respectively. In the case of lactate, two pathways by which lactate is metabolized are illustrated below:

Reaction 1: Lactate + $3O_2 \rightarrow HCO_3^- + 2CO_2 + 2H_2O$

Reaction 2: 2 Lactate + $2CO_2 + 2H_2O \rightarrow 2HCO_3^- +$ glucose

Mechanism 2: Production of plasma proteins, such as albumin, that can buffer H^+.

An anesthesiologist conducted an experiment to investigate the effects of Hartmann's solution on lactic acidosis. Hartmann's solution is isotonic with blood and consists of $NaCl$, $NaC_3H_5O_3$ (sodium lactate), $CaCl_2$, and KCl. In the experiment, patients suffering from lactic acidosis received intravenous Hartmann's solution. In order to determine the outcome of the treatment, each patient had his or her anion gap measured before and after treatment. After the experiment, the anesthesiologist concluded that Hartmann's solution failed to treat the lactic acidosis in all cases.

Anion gap is calculated as follows: anion gap = $[Na^+] - ([Cl^-] + [HCO_3^-])$. Table 1 illustrates the significance of anion gap measurements. Typically, a low anion gap occurs due to hypoalbuminemia (low blood albumin levels) and a high anion gap is the result of lactic acidosis.

Physiological Condition	Anion Gap (mEq/L)
Abnormally low	Less than 6
Normal	6–12
Abnormally high	Greater than 12

Table 1. Anion gap measurements comparison.

Passage Outline

P1.

    M1.

    R1.

    R2.

    M2.

P2.

P3.

    T1.

7. Why is the anion gap generally greater in patients suffering from lactic acidosis?

    A. Hepatic function is limited, so endogenous bicarbonate production is reduced.

    B. Serum albumin levels are too high, displacing the anions used to calculate anion gap.

    C. Urine volume increases to remove bicarbonate from the body and Na^+ follows.

    D. Citrate and gluconate cannot be properly metabolized, so H^+ is abundant.

8. Typically, serum lactate level is measured to determine the severity of lactic acidosis. Why is this not the ideal approach in the experiment with Hartmann's solution from the passage?

    A. Acid anions other than lactate are also relevant in causing lactic acidosis.

    B. Hypoalbuminemia may be masking the effects of a heightened lactate concentration.

    C. Hartmann's solution will confound the measurement of serum lactate.

    D. It is not clear whether each patient's lactic acidosis is caused by Hartmann's solution or exercise.

9. A 20 mL blood sample is taken from a patient with lactic acidosis. The pH is measured and found to be below physiological pH. What must be true of the $[OH^-]$ of the sample?

    A. It is less than the $[H^+]$ in the sample.

    B. It has a minimum value of approximately 4.5×10^{-8} mmol/mL.

    C. It has maximum value of approximately 2.3×10^{-7} mmol/mL.

    D. It is impossible to make any judgments on $[OH^-]$ with this information.

10. The patients in the study have developed lactic acidosis due to hypoxia. The lactate dehydrogenase reaction is:

$$Pyruvate + NADH + H^+ \leftrightarrow Lactate + NAD^+$$

The ratio of lactate to pyruvate is 10:1 in cells of a healthy individual. If the cells of patients in the study have an average ratio of 20:1, which of the following is most likely to also be true?

    A. The high levels of lactate are driven by a buildup of NADH.

    B. The low levels of pyruvate are driven by reduced rates of glycolysis.

    C. Their ratio of lactate to H^+ must be less than the ratio in a healthy individual.

    D. Their ratio of NAD^+ to pyruvate must be less than the ratio in a healthy individual.

KAPLAN TIP

Don't forget to use the whole passage to answer questions, especially Skill 2 questions.

K

LESSON 2.2 REVIEW

MCAT Skill 2 Questions

Scientific Reasoning and Problem Solving

Reasoning about scientific principles, theories, and models

Analyzing and evaluating scientific explanations and predictions

To answer these types of questions:

Determine the likely cause or effect of a phenomenon and determine how observations influence scientific theories or models.

Determine the validity of an explanation of a phenomenon.

Formulas on the MCAT

In this lesson, you'll learn to:

- Select the right formula to use in solving a quantitative question

Science Topics:

- Sound
- Thermochemistry and Thermodynamics
- Acids and Bases and Titrations
- Circuit Elements
- Electrostatics

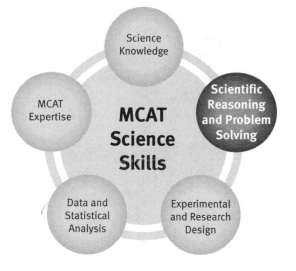

LESSON 2.3, LEARNING GOAL 1:

- Select the right formula to use in solving a quantitative question

Equation Recall

1. The human circulatory system can be thought of as an electric circuit with the heart as the voltage source and the flow of blood as the current. Given this, what is the flow rate if the heart is supplying a potential difference of 5 units and the resistance is at 61 units?

    A. 4.1×10^{-3} units
    B. 8.2×10^{-2} units
    C. 4.1×10^{-1} units
    D. 8.2×10^{1} units

    Which variables are given?

    Which variable needs to be solved for?

    Which equation should you use?

2. Given the following data, at what temperature is the system at equilibrium?

    $x(l) \rightarrow x(g)$

    $\Delta H = 44 \text{ kJ}$

    $\Delta S = 118 \text{ J/K}$

    A. 53°C
    B. 86°C
    C. 100°C
    D. 119°C

    Which variables are given?

    Which variable needs to be solved for?

    Which equation should you use?

3. A train is moving at 80 mph. A car in front of it is moving in the same direction at 50 mph. If the frequency of a whistle on the train is f, what is the frequency heard by a passenger riding in the car? (v = speed of sound in air in mph)

    A. $f\dfrac{(v+50)}{(v+80)}$
    B. $f\dfrac{(v-50)}{(v+80)}$
    C. $f\dfrac{(v+50)}{(v-80)}$
    D. $f\dfrac{(v-50)}{(v-80)}$

    Which variables are given?

    Which variable needs to be solved for?

    Which equation should you use?

Connecting Equations

4. The K_a of methyl red is 8.1×10^{-6}. At 25°C, the concentration of the conjugate base is 10 times that of the acid form of methyl red. What is the pH of the solution?

   A. 4.1
   B. 5.1
   C. 6.1
   D. 7.1

Which variables are given?

Which variable needs to be solved for?

Which variable connects the given variables to the variables in the answer choices?

Which equations should you use?

5. The two plates of a capacitor are 0.45 m apart and experience an instantaneous electrostatic force of 11 N. If the instantaneous charge on one of these plates is 0.005 C, what is the potential difference between the plates?

   A. 990 V
   B. 1,595 V
   C. 2,080 V
   D. 10,045 V

Which variables are given?

Which variable needs to be solved for?

Which variable connects the given variables to the variables in the answer choices?

Which equations should you use?

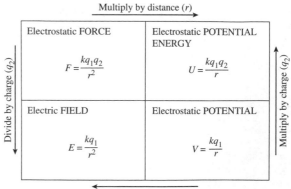

KAPLAN TIP

Flashcards are a great way to keep track of all the equations you'll need for Test Day!

LESSON 2.3 REVIEW

Study Skills

Make use of equation flashcards

Solving MCAT Problems Using Equations

Determine which variables are given

Determine which variable needs to be solved for

Think of any potential equations to connect given variables to unknown variables

Recall the correct equations

Skill 2 (Critical Thinking) in Action

In this lesson, you'll learn to:

- Identify and solve Skill 2 questions
- Determine whether missed Skill 2 questions were due to content or critical thinking mistakes

Science Topics:

- Sound and Waves
- Electrostatics
- Electrochemistry

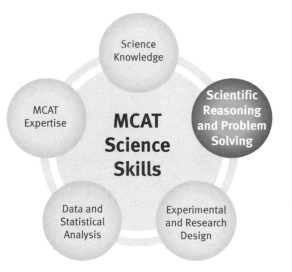

From the AAMC[*]:

"Questions that test scientific reasoning and problem-solving skills differ from questions that test skill 1 by asking you to use your scientific knowledge to solve problems in the natural, behavioral, and social sciences.

As you work on questions that test this skill, you may be asked to use scientific theories to explain observations or make predictions about natural or social phenomena. Questions may ask you to judge the credibility of scientific explanations or to evaluate arguments about cause and effect. Or they may ask you to use scientific models and observations to draw conclusions. They may ask you to recognize scientific findings that call a theory or model into question. Questions in this category may ask you to look at pictures or diagrams and draw conclusions from them. Or they may ask you to determine and then use scientific formulas to solve problems."

---

*The Official Guide to the MCAT Exam (MCAT2017), Fifth Edition

LESSON 2.4, LEARNING GOALS 1 AND 2:

- Identify and solve Skill 2 questions
- Determine whether missed Skill 2 questions were due to content or critical thinking mistakes

Example Questions

1. The net charge of a particular amino acid is x. If three copies of this amino acid are equidistant from point A, what is the electric potential at A?

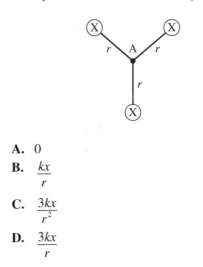

A. 0

B. $\dfrac{kx}{r}$

C. $\dfrac{3kx}{r^2}$

D. $\dfrac{3kx}{r}$

What content (Skill 1) does this question test?

Why is this ultimately a critical thinking (Skill 2) question?

How does the relevant equation help you?

What mistake might lead a student to choose...	
Choice A?	
Choice B?	
Choice C?	
Choice D?	

2. A person standing at the top of a hill hears a loud explosion followed by a tremor of the ground beneath his feet. What is the most likely explanation for this phenomenon?

   A. The sound waves produced from the explosion traveled faster through the air than they did through the ground.

   B. The temperature of the air is greater than the temperature of the ground.

   C. The bulk modulus of the ground is less than the bulk modulus of the air.

   D. The explosion and the tremor did not simultaneously originate from the same source.

What content (Skill 1) does this question test?

Why is this ultimately a critical thinking (Skill 2) question?

How do facts about the speed of sound help reason through this question?

What mistake might lead a student to choose...	
Choice A?	
Choice B?	
Choice C?	
Choice D?	

KAPLAN TIP

If your review reveals that you are missing many questions due to content errors, identify your weak content areas and then study and practice them.

K

3. Which of the following sets of graphs accurately represents the relationship between standard cell potential (E°_{cell}) and standard Gibbs free energy (ΔG°), and between equilibrium constant (K_{eq}) and standard cell potential (E°_{cell}), respectively?

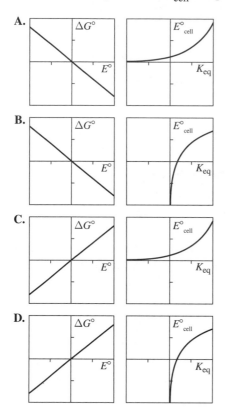

What content (Skill 1) does this question test?

Why is this ultimately a critical thinking (Skill 2) question?

How do the shapes of the plots help answer this question?

What mistake might lead a student to choose...	
Choice A?	
Choice B?	
Choice C?	
Choice D?	

KAPLAN TIP

If reviewing your tests reveals that you are missing questions due to critical thinking errors, compile data about specific critical thinking trends that are costing you points. Knowing your flaws is the first step to correcting your flaws!

LESSON 2.4 REVIEW

Chapter 2 Learning Goals

2.1 Skill 2 (Critical Thinking) Basics

- Recall relevant scientific concepts with limited or no clues in the question stem or answer choices
- Apply known scientific principles to novel and/or complicated situations

2.2 MCAT Scientific Reasoning

- Determine the likelihood of a scientific phenomenon or a given explanation for a phenomenon
- Determine the likely cause or effect of a phenomenon
- Determine how observations influence scientific theories or models
- Gather information from various sources to draw conclusions

2.3 Formulas on the MCAT

- Select the right formula to use in solving a quantitative question

CHAPTER 3

Science Skill 3: Experimental & Research Design

Skill 3 (Research Design) Basics

In this lesson, you'll learn to:

- Recognize the application of the scientific method
- Distinguish between testable and untestable hypotheses
- Identify the independent and dependent variables in an experiment

Science Topics:

- Biological Bases of Behavior
- Sensory Processing

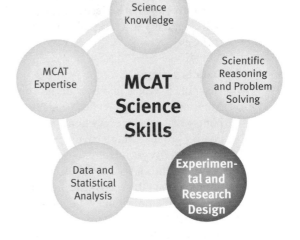

LESSON 3.1, LEARNING GOAL 1:

- Recognize the application of the scientific method

The Scientific Method—An Archetypal Experiment

Dave is **fascinated** by how his friend Rose, who works at a restaurant, is able to hold and carry hot plates that he can't stand to touch. He **does some research** on the subject, learns about sensory thresholds and adaptation, and receives permission from his lab to run a small experiment. **His hypothesis is** that laboratory mice exposed to uncomfortably hot surfaces over a period of time will eventually react less adversely to those hot surfaces.

What question is Dave trying to answer with his experiment?

Data is gathered over the next few weeks. He splits the mice into two groups: one—the experimental group—whose cage floor is made hot for one minute every hour, and the other—the control group—whose cage is left alone and who otherwise live identically to the experimental group. At the end of one week, Dave exposes all mice (in both groups) to a hot surface and monitors their reactions. Upon **analysis of the data**, he immediately sees that mice in the experimental group react less visibly to the hot surface, and some seem to not be affected at all. He therefore **concludes** that his hypothesis was correct, and that his friend Rose is in some ways like the mice in the experimental group: acclimated to hot surfaces.

Why is the second group of mice (the control group) included in the study?

Finally, Dave attempts to **publish** his findings so that others can see his procedure, duplicate the experiment, and see if they yield the same results. If this process also confirms the hypothesis a sufficient number of times, the results are considered **verified**.

Why are these last two steps important to the scientific method?

KAPLAN TIP

The scientific method on this page, which includes publishing and verification as explicit steps, is a more "institutionalized" version of the method. In a formal sense, studies that are not published can still be called "scientific."

LESSON 3.1, LEARNING GOAL 2:

• Distinguish between testable and untestable hypotheses

Sample Hypotheses

(Circle one)

Hypothesis		
"If someone experiences an increase in inter-neuron dopamine levels, he or she reports an increase in positive affect."	**Testable**	**Untestable**
"More brain activity occurs in Broca's area during speech than at other times."	**Testable**	**Untestable**
"The brain processes visual images by using a spatial map on the occipital lobe."	**Testable**	**Untestable**
"People with nasal congestion who take this medicine will normally feel better the next day."	**Testable**	**Untestable**
"If I take this medicine now, I will feel better in the morning."	**Testable**	**Untestable**

The FINER Method

Proposed Study Hypothesis	What's Wrong with It?
Individuals born before 1800, because of pre-industrial air quality, will score higher than today's adults on a modern intelligence test.	
Neurons placed in one brand of carbonated soft drink will have higher conductance than those placed in other brands of soft drink.	
Rhythmic vibrations at higher frequencies are perceived by humans as higher-pitched sounds.	.
When ordered to do so by an authority, test subjects will willingly harm another human being.	
Pure gold, when aggregated in weights of more than one metric ton, can act as a moderately effective magnet.	

KAPLAN TIP
Remember that most testable hypotheses either are, or can be rephrased as, "if-then" statements.

LESSON 3.1, LEARNING GOAL 3:

- Identify the independent and dependent variables in an experiment

Experiment 1

... Data is gathered over the next few weeks. He splits the mice into two groups: one—the experimental group—whose cage floor is made hot for one minute every hour, and the other—the control group—whose cage is left alone and who otherwise live identically to the experimental group. At the end of one week, Dave exposes all mice (in both groups) to a hot surface and monitors their reactions ...

What is the independent variable in this study?

What is the dependent variable in this study?

Experiment 2

... Running the rat through the same maze multiple times gives a learning curve. The experience variable is the number of times the rat has gone through the maze and the learning variable is the number of mistakes that it has made ...

What is the independent variable in this study?

What is the dependent variable in this study?

Experiment 3

... The experimenters compared the relative athletic skill (as measured by sprinting speed, strength, and agility) of identical twins raised together, identical twins raised apart, and fraternal twins raised together. They then set their data next to the variability in athletic skill present in the general population ...

What are the independent variables in this study?

What is the dependent variable in this study?

KAPLAN TIP

Certain types of studies are more commonly used in certain experimental fields. For instance, twin studies are used often in behavioral genetics and Stroop tests are often used in studies of working memory and cognitive load. Being familiar with these common types of studies is advantageous on Test Day, but the MCAT won't expect you to know all the details at a single mention of the class of study.

LESSON 3.1 REVIEW

The Scientific Method

1. Generate a testable question
2. Gather data and resources
3. Form a hypothesis
4. Collect new data
5. Analyze the data
6. Interpret the data and existing hypothesis
7. Publish
8. Verify results

The FINER Method for Testable Hypotheses

Is the study you'd like to conduct ...

- **F**easible?
- **I**nteresting?
- **N**ovel?
- **E**thical?
- **R**elevant?

Independent and Dependent Variables

- **Independent variables** are manipulated by the experimenter in a controlled setting
  - In graphical representations, independent variables are generally placed on the *x-axis*
  - When a hypothesis is stated as an "if-then" statement, the independent variable is generally the "*if*" part of the statement

- **Dependent variables** are monitored for change by the experimenter
  - In graphical representations, dependent variables are generally placed on the *y-axis*
  - When a hypothesis is stated as an "if-then" statement, the dependent variable is generally the "*then*" part of the statement

- The *purpose of an experiment* is generally to see if, and by how much, the independent variable has an effect on the dependent variable

Critique of Studies and Conclusions

In this lesson, you'll learn to:

- Define and distinguish between samples and populations
- Judge the appropriateness of generalizations, based on facts about the sample and population of a study
- Use aspects of a study to determine the likelihood of true associations between variables
- Recognize research ethics principles in MCAT questions

Science Topics:

- Psychological Disorders
- Emotion

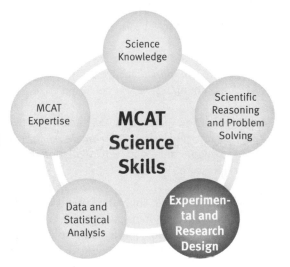

LESSON 3.2, LEARNING GOALS 1 AND 2:

- Define and distinguish between samples and populations
- Judge the appropriateness of generalizations, based on facts about the sample and population of a study

Samples and Populations

(Circle one)

… *Study participants* were divided into two groups: a control group and an intervention group …	**Sample**	**Population**
… Researchers devised a study to determine whether a causal link existed between income level and psychosis in *urban communities* …	**Sample**	**Population**
… After devising the hypothesis, *randomly selected individuals* from different religious communities were invited to the lab …	**Sample**	**Population**
… The experiment's conclusion was that *individuals with borderline personality disorder* struggle more with self-regulation under high-pressure situations …	**Sample**	**Population**

… In order to study the familiarity of the universal emotions, the professor's students were asked to choose the most likely caption for pictures of faces displaying different emotions…

What is this study's sample?

What is this study's population?

Samples and Populations in Context

Practice Passage 1 (Questions 1–2)

Although the origin of clinical depression is still in large part a mystery, one possible explanation is monoamine theory. Monoamines are neurotransmitters such as dopamine, serotonin, and norepinephrine. According to the theory, reduced activity of monoamines in the brain is linked to depression. This theory was proposed following the accidental discovery that monoamine oxidase (MAO) inhibitors could successfully treat some cases of depression. Monoamine oxidase is an enzyme that catalyzes the breakdown of monoamines to corresponding aldehydes and ammonia. If monoamine oxidase activity is inhibited, monoamine levels will rise in the brain.

Experiment 1

Despite successful treatment of certain patients with MAO inhibitors, depression is only partially explained by the monoamine hypothesis. A study was done to analyze the effects of monoamine intervention in healthy persons. Researchers handpicked ten patients to use in the study. After being split into a control group and an experimental group, patients were told which group they were in and informed that the study was designed to reveal the root cause of clinical depression. Using pharmacological agents, the experimental group's monoamine levels were raised by 35% and maintained at this level for three months. At the start of each day, patients in both groups were asked to record their mood in a journal. After the data collection period ended, it was determined that increased monoamine concentrations did not significantly impact mood in healthy individuals.

1. Experiment 1 suffers from several flaws that could cast doubt on its conclusions. Based on the information in the passage, which of the following is NOT one of these flaws?

   A. Temporal ambiguity
   B. Selection bias
   C. The Hawthorne effect
   D. Lack of blinding

2. If the conclusion of Experiment 1 is further proven in future experiments, to which of the following groups would the findings most apply?

   A. People with depression who record their mood in a journal at least once each day
   B. People without depression who take MAO inhibitors for Parkinson's Disease
   C. People who are misdiagnosed with depression and are prescribed MAO inhibitors
   D. People who display depressive symptoms when their monoamine levels drop by 35%

KAPLAN TIP

Even though the MCAT will test flaws in the design and execution of research, it will rarely completely discredit a study in a passage. More likely, the MCAT will ask you to see the positives and the negatives of a study by asking about its potential conclusions and its flaws.

K

LESSON 3.2, LEARNING GOALS 3 AND 4:

- Use aspects of a study to determine the likelihood of true associations between variables
- Recognize research ethics principles in MCAT questions

Research Design Flaws in Context

Practice Passage 1 (Questions 3–6)

Although the origin of clinical depression is still in large part a mystery, one possible explanation is monoamine theory. Monoamines are neurotransmitters such as dopamine, serotonin, and norepinephrine. According to the theory, reduced activity of monoamines in the brain is linked to depression. This theory was proposed following the accidental discovery that monoamine oxidase (MAO) inhibitors could successfully treat some cases of depression. Monoamine oxidase is an enzyme that catalyzes the breakdown of monoamines to corresponding aldehydes and ammonia. If monoamine oxidase activity is inhibited, monoamine levels will rise in the brain.

Experiment 2

Brunner syndrome occurs due to a mutation in the MAO-A gene. Individuals with this genetic condition suffer from dramatically increased aggression due to heightened monoamine levels. Researchers hypothesized that norepinephrine is the primary contributor to this behavioral phenomenon. To test this hypothesis, 25 transgenic mice had their MAO-A gene knocked out. It was calculated that in the knockout mice, serotonin levels were approximately ten times greater and norepinephrine levels were about three times greater than in normal mice. When compared to baseline levels, the knockout mice exhibited fearfulness and increased aggression if threatened. The behavioral effects of the gene knockout were reversed by administration of parachlorophenylalanine, a potent inhibitor of serotonin synthesis. The researchers concluded that increased serotonin concentration is to blame for the aggressive behavior associated with Brunner syndrome and rejected their original hypothesis.

Causality

3. What would be the most appropriate conclusion to draw if, in Experiment 2, dopamine levels were also measured upon administration of parachlorophenylalanine and were found to be similar to baseline levels?

   A. Dopamine levels likely contribute in some way to the symptoms of Brunner syndrome.
   B. Dopamine is not likely to contribute to the symptoms of Brunner syndrome.
   C. Dopamine may or may not contribute to the symptoms of Brunner syndrome.
   D. Dopamine contributes to the symptoms of Brunner syndrome when levels match those of other monoamines.

Plausibility

4. In a retrospective analysis of Experiment 2, the following four external conditions were also found to correlate with aggressive and fearful behavior in the mice being studied. Which one is most likely to be a true causative relationship?

    A. A similar study on monoamines began in a neighboring lab shortly after high aggression was first measured.
    B. The chairs in the lab's lobby changed shortly before the gene knockout was reversed.
    C. The highest measures of aggression tended to be measured during waxing moon phases.
    D. The technician who handles the mice was changed near the times when monoamine concentrations changed sharply.

Alternative Explanations

5. Which of the following is true of Experiment 2 and reveals a flaw in the researchers' reasoning?

    A. Increased serotonin has other proven effects besides those stated in the passage.
    B. Male mice in the study reacted with more aggression than female mice.
    C. The study did not produce sufficient evidence to reject the researchers' original hypothesis.
    D. Monoamine concentrations have not been linked to mood in studies other than this one.

Research Ethics

6. Suppose there is a two-year study on human participants studying a new drug for Brunner syndrome. After one year, researchers have sufficient evidence to conclude that the drug is dramatically more effective than any current treatment. Which of the following actions should be taken by the researchers?

    A. Begin offering the new drug, instead of a placebo, to the control group.
    B. End the study and withdraw treatment from all participants.
    C. Begin charging participants for the drugs they are receiving.
    D. Inform participants of the results and continue the study as before.

KAPLAN TIP

The most important lesson about critiquing studies is simply to see and identify research flaws in the first place. Don't take the experiments in MCAT passages at face value—notice their problems, too!

LESSON 3.2 REVIEW

Samples and Populations

- A sample is the group of individuals that an experiment is conducted on. These are often called subjects, participants, volunteers, or patients.

- A population is the group of people or other beings to whom the conclusion of a study applies.

- A study's conclusion can only fairly be applied to a population if certain criteria are satisfied, including representativeness of the sample and the avoidance of possible flaws, such as those described below.

Possible Flaws in Experimental Design

Temporality
- The independent variable of a study (sometimes known as the "intervention") must occur temporally prior to the dependent variable.

Plausibility
- When proposing a connection between variables, there must be some scientifically plausible way that one affects the other.

Alternative Explanations
- Attention must be paid to other explanations for a phenomenon besides the one hypothesized by a study.

- If alternative explanations are ruled out, remaining explanations become more likely.

Other Criteria/Possible Flaws in Study Design

- Causality
- Random assignment
- Selection bias
- Blinding (and double-blinding)
- The Hawthorne effect
- Sample size
- Representative samples
- Consistency
- External validity
- Confounding variables
- Correlation *vs.* causation
- Ethics (e.g., beneficence, justice, equipoise, respect for persons, informed consent)

Advanced Experimental Design

In this lesson, you'll learn to:

- Make and identify valid conclusions that can be drawn from research results
- Relate the results of a study to real-world situations

Science Topics

- The Excretory System
- The Immune System
- The Lymphatic System
- The Circulatory System
- The Digestive System
- DNA as Genetic Material/Genetic Analysis
- Mendelian Concepts

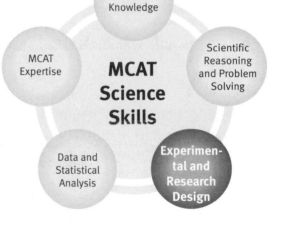

LESSON 3.3, LEARNING GOAL 1:

- Identify and make valid conclusions that can be drawn from research results

Questioning the Validity of Conclusions

Study 1

Cholecystitis, or inflammation of the gall bladder, occurs when there is an obstruction of the cystic duct. One treatment is surgical removal of the gallbladder, or cholecystectomy. There are two options for surgical intervention: 1) an open exploratory surgery or 2) a closed laparoscopic surgery facilitated by the use of a camera. A group of gastroenterologists conduct a series of randomized controlled trials to examine the effectiveness of the two interventions in the general population. A total of 448 patients were asked to participate in the study. A total of 322 were randomized into one of the two intervention groups. Those that were not randomized were either too frail to undergo an open surgical procedure or displayed advanced gall bladder disease, both of which required laparoscopic intervention. After gathering postoperative outcome data, the doctors found that laparoscopic surgery—the intervention utilizing the camera—is the preferred treatment method for cholecystitis in the general population.

Looking at the table below, what concerns you about their conclusion?

	Men (n)	Women (n)	Age (average)
Randomized Group	41	281	43
Non-Randomized Group	60	66	58

Table 1. Demographics of cholecystectomy study.

Study 2

Huntington's disease is a neurodegenerative disease that is transmitted through autosomal dominant inheritance. Patients do not exhibit symptoms until age 35–44 years. Given these facts and the chance that 50 to 100 percent of affected patients' offspring will have the trait, genetic screening is recommended for the children of affected patients. A neurologist tests the effectiveness of a digital intervention to encourage genetic testing by gathering the email addresses of affected patients who visit as well as those of their adult children. Patients and their children were randomized into either a control group that received a letter about genetic screening, or an intervention group that received an email from their physician about genetic testing. Of the 34 patients in the intervention group, eight viewed the email and two set up appointments to discuss genetic testing. Only one of the seven adult children of affected patients viewed the email, and none signed up for genetic testing. Given these results, the neurologist concluded that email intervention is not an effective method for raising awareness about genetic testing.

What aspect of the findings might lead us to question the neurologist's conclusion?

This lesson continues on the next page ▶ ▶ ▶

Making Valid Conclusions—Practice Passage (Questions 1–4)

Type 1 diabetics lose the ability to synthesize insulin, so regular insulin injections become necessary. The active form of insulin is a monomer, but insulin is usually stored as a more stable hexamer. Porcine insulin has a similar structure to human insulin, and has been used to treat diabetes since the 1920s. However, in 1978 a method was developed to make human insulin in *E. coli* using recombinant DNA techniques.

A researcher conducts a similar experiment to the one that originally produced recombinant insulin. She uses the plasmid pUC18 as a vector for the human insulin gene (Figure 1). This plasmid contains a gene, *bla,* for resistance to the antibiotic ampicillin. This plasmid also contains a *lac* operon to allow for the induction and transcription of the insulin gene. After amplifying and isolating the insulin gene, the researcher performs two experiments to optimize expression of recombinant insulin.

Experiment 1

The researcher first treats the pUC18 plasmid and the human insulin gene with different restriction enzymes to optimize plasmid splice sites. The researcher combines the digested gene and plasmid with DNA ligase to permanently recombine the plasmid with the human gene. A small volume of the plasmid solution is added to 50 µL of competent *E. coli* cell culture to transform the bacteria. The culture is then plated onto a nutrient-complex media that contains ampicillin. The researcher incubates the plates at 37°C for 24 hours.

	(–) control plates	pUC18 plates
ScaI and HindIII	–	–
BamHI and HindIII	–	+++

Table 1: Results of Experiment 1

Experiment 2

After 24 hours, successful transformants are selected from the plates and grown in large cultures. The researcher tests different methods of induction of insulin expression by adding lactose, isopropyl-ß-D-thiogalactoside (IPTG, a lactose analogue), and maltose. Results are shown in Figure 2.

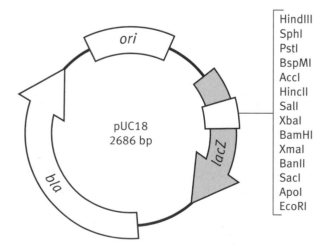

Figure 1. pUC18 plasmid map with known lacZ restriction sites

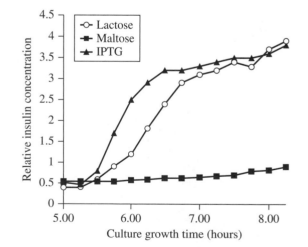

Figure 2. Results of Experiment 2. Cultures were induced after five hours of growth.

Passage Outline

P1.

P2.

E1.

T1.

E2.

F1.

F2.

1. Based on the researcher's results, which of the following best explains the outcome of experiment 1?

    A. HindIII cuts the *bla* gene, rendering it nonfunctional.
    B. HindIII cuts the *lac* operon, rendering it nonfunctional.
    C. ScaI cuts the *bla* gene, rendering it nonfunctional.
    D. BamHI cuts the *lac* operon, rendering it nonfunctional.

2. The most probable explanation for the results of experiment 2 is that:

    A. IPTG can be used to effectively induce expression of the *lac* operon and maltose is not effective to induce expression of the *lac* operon.
    B. maltose triggers proteases to degrade the expressed insulin, while IPTG does not trigger proteases to degrade the expressed insulin.
    C. maltose acts as an uncompetitive inhibitor of insulin synthesis, while IPTG acts as a competitive inhibitor.
    D. Both IPTG and maltose are not as effective for inducing protein synthesis as lactose.

3. A student replicates experiment 1 with a pET28a plasmid that does not contain the *bla* gene. How will this affect her research results?

    A. The results would mimic those of experiment 1.
    B. The plasmid containing the insulin gene would fail to transform into the *E. coli*.
    C. Her plates will be susceptible to bacterial infection.
    D. She will not be able to determine if any of the *E. coli* were successfully transformed.

4. What is the structural difference between the active form of insulin and the form when stored in the body?

    A. Stored insulin is a steroid hormone and active insulin is a peptide hormone.
    B. Active insulin is a peptide with quaternary structure and stored insulin is only a tertiary structure.
    C. Stored insulin is a peptide with quaternary structure and active insulin is only a tertiary structure.
    D. The primary structure of porcine insulin differs from human insulin by a single amino acid.

KAPLAN TIP
Always remember to look at study design with a critical eye on Test Day, because incorrect execution of a study will hurt its validity.

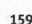

LESSON 3.3, LEARNING GOAL 2:

- Relate the results of a study to real-world situations

Real-World Implications—Practice Passage (Questions 5–7)

Diabetes mellitus is a common disorder caused by either a lack of or an insensitivity to insulin, and results in patients having excess glucose in their blood. This excess glucose causes unwanted glycosylation reactions in some of the smallest and most vulnerable blood vessels in the body, including those of the eyes, feet, and kidney. A common measure of kidney function, and a marker of the extent to which the vasa recta have been glycosylated, is creatinine levels in the blood (normal values 0.6–1.2 mg/dL), since damaged renal vessels will fail to filter waste products such as creatinine.

An endocrinologist wants to learn more about one of the renal complications of diabetes, diabetic nephropathy, in her practice and conducts the following two studies:

Study 1
First, the doctor surveys patient data from her two separate office locations and charts the data comparing creatinine levels and age.

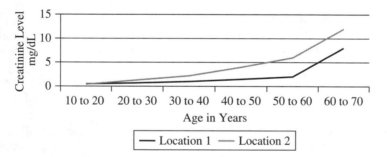

Figure 1. Creatinine levels *vs.* age for the two locations.

Study 2
Second, the doctor studies the effect of administering an ACE (angiotensin-converting enzyme) inhibitor, captopril, on creatinine levels in patients with diabetic nephropathy. The results are shown below:

	Month 1	Month 2	Month 3	Month 4	Month 5	Month 6
Diabetic NO Captopril	3 mg/dL	3.5 mg/dL	4.2 mg/dL	4.8 mg/dL	5.0 mg/dL	5.3 mg/dL
Diabetic WITH Captopril	2.8 mg/dL	3.0 mg/dL	3.1 mg/dL	3.1 mg/dL	3.0 mg/dL	3.1 mg/dL

Table 1. Concentration of creatinine in patients with and without captopril treatment.

5. Based on the results of Study 1, which of the following interventions makes the most sense for the doctor to implement?

   A. A new policy lessening the number of required checkups at location 1.
   B. Diabetic nephropathy counseling at location 1 for patients who are 20–40 years old.
   C. Decreasing the glucose-controlling medications given to patients at location 2.
   D. Diabetic nephropathy counseling at location 2 for patients who are 30–50 years old.

6. How can the doctor use the results of Study 2 to help the patients included in Study 1?

   A. Treat only patients at location 2 with captopril.
   B. Treat patients with a creatinine level of 2 mg/dL or higher with captopril.
   C. Treat patients with a creatinine level of 1 mg/dL or lower with captopril.
   D. The doctor cannot use the results of Study 2 to help the patients in Study 1.

7. Patients with diabetes are advised to limit their salt intake as one way to decrease the progression of diabetic nephropathy. This recommendation mirrors the findings in which one of the studies run by the endocrinologist? Why?

   A. Study 1, because as time goes on, patients lose the ability to process salt.
   B. Study 2, because the patients not receiving captopril have lower blood sugar.
   C. Study 2, because the patients receiving captopril are also lowering their blood pressure.
   D. Study 1, because the patients at location 1 have lower blood pressure.

KAPLAN TIP

Relevancy is an important reason to conduct research, and the more relevant the research, the more applicable it will be to real-world situations.

LESSON 3.3 REVIEW

Making Valid Conclusions

Internal Validity

- Measures the degree to which a study answers the question it set out to answer.
- Factors affecting internal validity include anything that causes flaws in the design or data collection process (i.e., subject variability, attrition, sample size, and instrument sensitivity).

External Validity

- Measures the extent to which the study findings can be generalized.
- Factors affecting external validity include population characteristics, subject selection, the effect of time, and the effect of the research environment.

Once Validated

- One can feel comfortable about the conclusions reported.
- The findings can be applied to real-world situations in order to improve results in a given area.

Skill 3 (Research Design) in Action

In this lesson, you'll learn to:

- Identify the key components of a complicated experimental procedure
- Recognize limitations of the experimental procedure that is described
- Infer conclusions based on the design and limitations of an experimental procedure

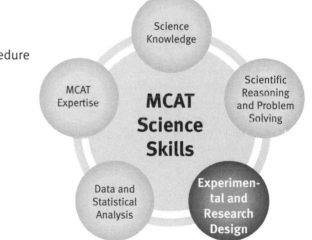

Science Topics:

- Molecular Genetics
- The Cell Cycle
- Gene Regulation

From the AAMC*:

"Questions that test reasoning about the design and execution of research will ask you to demonstrate your scientific inquiry skills by showing that you can 'do' science. They will ask you to demonstrate your understanding of important components of scientific methodology. These questions will ask you to demonstrate your knowledge of the ways in which natural, behavioral, and social sciences conduct research to test and extend scientific knowledge."

---

*The Official Guide to the MCAT Exam (MCAT2017), Fifth Edition

LESSON 3.4, LEARNING GOAL 1:

- Identify the key components of a complicated experimental procedure

Practice Passage (Questions 1–6)

Throughout the cell cycle, many proteins bind and release chromatin. One example is the protein cohesin, expressed in both *S. cerevisiae* (baker's yeast) and humans. Cohesin helps hold sister chromatids together from S phase through metaphase. The cohesin protein is made of four subunits that, together, form a closed loop. Scientists hypothesize that during S phase, cohesin proteins loop around sister chromatids at many sites along the chromosome and then, in metaphase, these cohesin loops open, allowing the sister chromatids to separate.

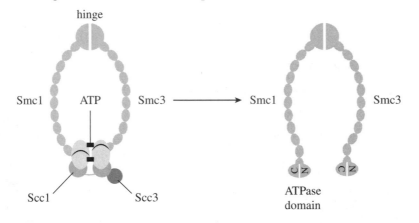

Figure 1. The cohesin ring structure, closed and open.

In *S. cerevisiae*, scientists study these time- and location-based interactions between DNA and cohesin using a technique called chromatin immunoprecipitation assay, or ChIP assay. A ChIP assay measures the relative amount of cohesin bound to a chromosome at varying locations on the chromosome and at varying points of the cell cycle.

A typical ChIP assay occurs in the following steps:

1. A yeast culture is frozen in G_1 by exposing the cells to alpha mating factor.
2. A protease degrades alpha mating factor, releasing the cells synchronously into the cell cycle.
3. At periodic time points, samples of the culture are isolated and formaldehyde is used to permanently bind DNA to any associated cohesin proteins. This step also freezes the sample's cell cycle.
4. Sonication is used to shear the chromatin into short fragments, 300–500 nucleotides in length. Importantly, cohesin proteins remain bound to these DNA fragments.
5. Anti-cohesin antibodies are used to isolate cohesin molecules, which remain bound to their respective DNA fragments.
6. Proteases are used to degrade the cohesin protein, releasing bound fragments of DNA.

Results are generated by isolating and sequencing these DNA fragments. Each fragment type corresponds to a unique site on the chromosome, indicating where cohesin binds the chromosome, and the relative number of each fragment type indicates the relative number of cohesin molecules bound to each site.

Identify the...	
Independent Variable	
Dependent Variable	

Practice Passage Questions

1. In a typical ChIP assay, what is the purpose of adding alpha mating factor to the yeast culture?

   A. Alpha mating factor induces cohesin to bind DNA.
   B. Alpha mating factor release sets the zero time point in the experiment.
   C. Rapid growth of the yeast culture is caused by alpha mating factor.
   D. Synchronous release into the cell cycle minimizes intercellular signalling between yeast cells.

   Which of the experimental variables does alpha mating factor influence?

2. In a ChIP assay for cohesin, what is the purpose of the sequencing step?

   A. Sequencing reveals the structure of the gene coding for cohesin.
   B. Sequenced fragments of DNA can be re-joined to reconstruct the original chromosome.
   C. Sequencing fragments of the yeast chromosome helps build the yeast genomic map.
   D. Sequencing DNA fragments isolated in a ChIP assay reveals the chromosomal location of DNA-bound cohesin.

   Which of the experimental variables does sequencing influence?

LESSON 3.4, LEARNING GOAL 2:

- Recognize limitations of the experimental procedure that is described.

Practice Passage (Questions 1–6)

Throughout the cell cycle, many proteins bind and release chromatin. One example is the protein cohesin, expressed in both *S. cerevisiae* (baker's yeast) and humans. Cohesin helps hold sister chromatids together from S phase through metaphase. The cohesin protein is made of four subunits that, together, form a closed loop. Scientists hypothesize that during S phase, cohesin proteins loop around sister chromatids at many sites along the chromosome and then, in metaphase, these cohesin loops open, allowing the sister chromatids to separate.

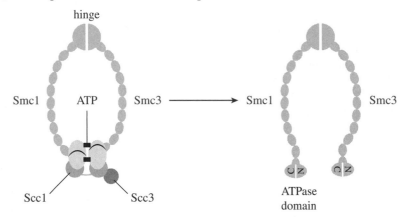

Figure 1. The cohesin ring structure, closed and open.

In *S. cerevisiae*, scientists study these time- and location-based interactions between DNA and cohesin using a technique called chromatin immunoprecipitation assay, or ChIP assay. A ChIP assay measures the relative amount of cohesin bound to a chromosome at varying locations on the chromosome and at varying points of the cell cycle.

A typical ChIP assay occurs in the following steps:

1. A yeast culture is frozen in G_1 by exposing the cells to alpha mating factor.
2. A protease degrades alpha mating factor, releasing the cells synchronously into the cell cycle.
3. At periodic time points, samples of the culture are isolated and formaldehyde is used to permanently bind DNA to any associated cohesin proteins. This step also freezes the sample's cell cycle.
4. Sonication is used to shear the chromatin into short fragments, 300–500 nucleotides in length. Importantly, cohesin proteins remain bound to these DNA fragments.
5. Anti-cohesin antibodies are used to isolate cohesin molecules, which remain bound to their respective DNA fragments.
6. Proteases are used to degrade the cohesin protein, releasing bound fragments of DNA.

Results are generated by isolating and sequencing these DNA fragments. Each fragment type corresponds to a unique site on the chromosome, indicating where cohesin binds the chromosome, and the relative number of each fragment type indicates the relative number of cohesin molecules bound to each site.

	Identify the...
Sample	
Population	

Practice Passage Questions

3. Which of the following weakens the choice of *S. cerevisiae*, baker's yeast, as a model organism for the study of cohesin?

   A. The human cohesin complex is built using a different subunit than the *S. cerevisiae* cohesin complex.
   B. *S. cerevisiae* chromosomes are linear.
   C. Human cells have 21 unique chromosomes, whereas *S. cerevisiae* cells have 16 unique chromosomes.
   D. *S. cerevisiae* is susceptible to alpha mating factor where human cells are not.

What factors help link the study of yeast cells to the study of human cells?

4. Which of the following factors, if true, would NOT cast doubt on the results of a cohesin ChIP assay, as described in the passage?

   A. Some yeast cells are not susceptible to alpha mating factor.
   B. Yeast cells do not all progress through the cell cycle at the same rate.
   C. Formaldehyde will permanently bind many proteins to the DNA, meaning other proteins than cohesin will be bound to DNA fragments.
   D. Sonication produces DNA fragments ranging in length, meaning it is hard to tell exactly where on a fragment cohesin originally bound.

What factors can cast doubt on the veracity of experimental conclusions?

LESSON 3.4, LEARNING GOAL 3:

- Infer conclusions based on the design and limitations of an experimental procedure.

Practice Passage (Questions 1–6)

Throughout the cell cycle, many proteins bind and release chromatin. One example is the protein cohesin, expressed in both *S. cerevisiae* (baker's yeast) and humans. Cohesin helps hold sister chromatids together from S phase through metaphase. The cohesin protein is made of four subunits that, together, form a closed loop. Scientists hypothesize that during S phase, cohesin proteins loop around sister chromatids at many sites along the chromosome and then, in metaphase, these cohesin loops open, allowing the sister chromatids to separate.

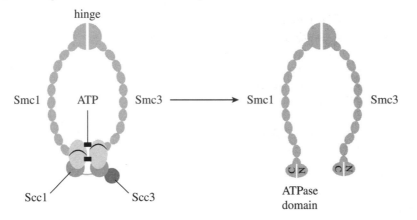

Figure 1. The cohesin ring structure, closed and open.

In *S. cerevisiae*, scientists study these time- and location-based interactions between DNA and cohesin using a technique called chromatin immunoprecipitation assay, or ChIP assay. A ChIP assay measures the relative amount of cohesin bound to a chromosome at varying locations on the chromosome and at varying points of the cell cycle.

A typical ChIP assay occurs in the following steps:

1. A yeast culture is frozen in G_1 by exposing the cells to alpha mating factor.
2. A protease degrades alpha mating factor, releasing the cells synchronously into the cell cycle.
3. At periodic time points, samples of the culture are isolated and formaldehyde is used to permanently bind DNA to any associated cohesin proteins. This step also freezes the sample's cell cycle.
4. Sonication is used to shear the chromatin into short fragments, 300–500 nucleotides in length. Importantly, cohesin proteins remain bound to these DNA fragments.
5. Anti-cohesin antibodies are used to isolate cohesin molecules, which remain bound to their respective DNA fragments.
6. Proteases are used to degrade the cohesin protein, releasing bound fragments of DNA.

Results are generated by isolating and sequencing these DNA fragments. Each fragment type corresponds to a unique site on the chromosome, indicating where cohesin binds the chromosome, and the relative number of each fragment type indicates the relative number of cohesin molecules bound to each site.

	Identify the...
Hypothesis	
Conclusion	

Practice Passage Questions

5. The following are four proposed supplemental functions of cohesin. Suppose a ChIP assay reveals cohesin bound to *S. cerevisiae* chromosomes during G_1. Which proposed cohesin function would this observation support?

    A. Cohesin facilitates spindle attachment onto chromosomal kinetochores.
    B. Cohesin helps direct DNA polymerase during replication.
    C. Cohesin plays a role in transcriptional regulation.
    D. Cohesin helps protect chromosomal structure during genetic recombination.

What is distinct about the new observation in this question stem?

6. Suppose a researcher is troubleshooting a flawed ChIP assay protocol. All the steps of the protocol are followed correctly, and yet the protocol fails to isolate cohesin bound fragments. Which possible conclusion does this observation support?

    A. The anti-cohesin antibody is defective.
    B. The sequencing step improperly sequenced the DNA.
    C. The yeast cells did not respond to alpha mating factor.
    D. The formaldehyde permanently bound cohesin to DNA.

In what way is this question testing your understanding of the experimental procedure?

LESSON 3.4 REVIEW

Chapter 3 Learning Goals

3.1 Skill 3 (Research) Basics

- Recognize the application of the scientific method
- Distinguish between testable and untestable hypotheses
- Identify the independent and dependent variables in an experiment

3.2 Critique of Studies and Conclusions

- Define and distinguish between samples and populations
- Judge the appropriateness of generalizations, based on facts about the sample and population of a study
- Use aspects of a study to determine the likelihood of true associations between variables
- Recognize research ethics principles in MCAT questions

3.3 Advanced Experimental Design

- Make and identify valid conclusions that can be drawn from research results
- Relate the results of a study to real-world situations

CHAPTER 4

Science Skill 4: Data & Statistical Analysis

Skill 4 (Data Analysis) Basics

In this lesson, you'll learn to:

- Analyze and interpret visual representations of data
- Use data to identify and explain relationships between variables, and match these relationships to visual representations
- Use data to determine a study's conclusions and make predictions about the likelihood of future events

Science Topics:

- Sensory Processing
- Biological Bases of Behavior

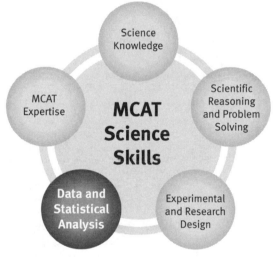

LESSON 4.1, LEARNING GOAL 1:

- Analyze and interpret visual representations of data

Data Interpretation

Experiment 1

A neuropsychologist is interested in finding out how a specific type of lesion in the reticular formation of the brain stem would affect how long a patient remains in a specific sleep stage. In order to test this, he invited six people with this type of lesion to participate in a simple sleep study.

The results of the study for all six participants are shown in Table 1.

Person	Hours spent in: NREM-1	Hours spent in: NREM-2	Hours spent in: NREM-3	Hours spent in: NREM-4	Hours spent in: REM	Hours spent in: Total
1	1.0	1.4	1.4	2.0	4.4	10.1
2	1.3	1.1	2.0	1.5	4.0	9.5
3	2.0	1.0	2.1	1.0	3.4	9.5
4	1.2	2.0	1.1	1.5	3.6	9.4
5	2.1	1.0	1.1	3.1	3.5	10.7
6	1.4	1.3	1.2	2.0	3.4	9.3

Table 1. Hours spent in sleep stages in patients with a lesion in the reticular formation.

1. Looking at the results, in which stage of sleep did participants spend the most time?

   A. NREM-1
   B. NREM-3
   C. NREM-4
   D. REM

The researcher then compared the time that each participant spent in REM sleep with that of their control counterparts (participants with no lesion in the reticular formation of the brain stem). The results are shown in Figure 1.

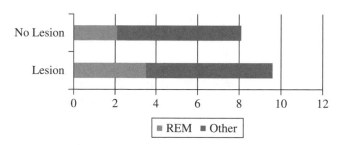

Figure 1. Comparison of REM and NREM sleep times.

2. On average, how do the patients with the lesion compare with their unaffected counterparts?

A. The unaffected control participants slept more and spent more time in REM sleep than the affected counterparts.

B. The unaffected control participants slept less and spent more time in REM sleep than the affected counterparts.

C. The affected participants slept more and spent more time in REM sleep than their unaffected counterparts.

D. The affected participants slept less and spent more time in REM sleep than their unaffected counterparts.

The neuropsychologist partnered with a neurobiologist during the study in order to study the levels of specific neurotransmitters present throughout the different stages of sleep. The results for two of the neurotransmitters are shown in Figure 2.

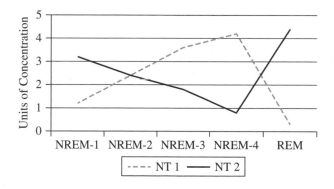

Figure 2. Levels of NT 1 and NT 2 in each sleep stage.

3. Given the information in the graph, during which stage of sleep is the difference between the two neurotransmitter levels the greatest?

A. NREM-1
B. NREM-3
C. NREM-4
D. REM

LESSON 4.1, LEARNING GOAL 2:

- Use data to identify and explain relationships between variables, and match these relationships to visual representations

Study 1
A scientist conducts a study to test how levels of interneuron dopamine levels change with an individual's mood. He finds that an improved mood state corresponds with increasing levels of interneuron dopamine over time.

4. Which of the following is the most appropriate representation of the scientist's findings?

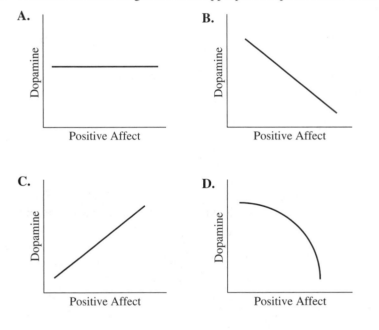

Study 2

In order to study the severity of unilateral sensorineural hearing loss in her patients, a researcher performs audiograms to document their deficits. She finds that patients with this type of hearing loss have a higher threshold for all frequencies than patients without it.

5. Which of the following is the appropriate representation for the scientist's findings if the solid line represents patients with hearing loss and the dotted line represents patients without it?

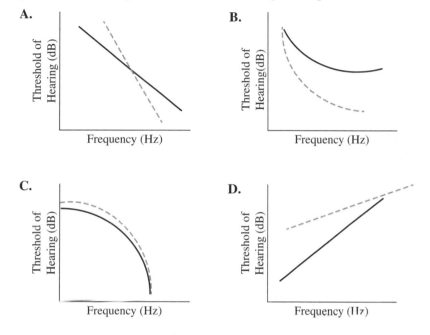

KAPLAN TIP

Determining which visual representation is best for your data set requires an understanding of the goal of the study in the first place.

Study 3

In order to replicate Weber's law for contrast perception, a researcher plots contrast units *vs.* intensity. Results are shown in Figure 3 below.

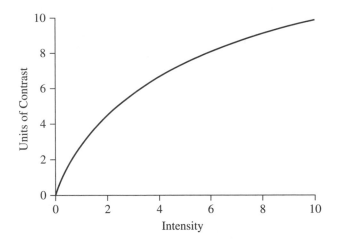

Figure 3. Contrast *vs.* intensity in brightness.

6. Given that "perceived contrast" can be calculated by taking the difference between two points on this line, the most reasonable interpretation of the data in Figure 3 is:

    A. The perceived contrast doubles with every twofold increase in intensity.
    B. In order to perceive the same contrast, a larger increase in intensity is needed at higher intensities
    C. No interpretation can be made, since the axes of the graph necessitate a semilog plot.
    D. Intensity is directly proportional to perceived contrast.

LESSON 4.1, LEARNING GOAL 3:

- Use data to determine a study's conclusions and make predictions about the likelihood of future events

Conclusions and Predictions

Experiment 1

A researcher conducts an experiment to study reflex times and the integration of several sensory processes. In the study, participants have to catch a ball that has been dropped. As an approximation for reflex "speed," researchers measure how far the ball falls before the participant catches it. The data in Table 1 is obtained.

Participant	Age	Trial 1	Trial 2	Trial 3
1	25	13.3 cm	12.9 cm	11.6 cm
2	21	13.9 cm	13.6 cm	13.1 cm
3	24	13.6 cm	13.0 cm	12.1 cm
4	30	13.2 cm	13.0 cm	10.3 cm

Table 1. Results of three trials showing distances before participants caught the ball.

7. What can be concluded from this data?

   A. Reaction time is positively correlated with age and positively correlated with attempt number.
   B. Reaction time is positively correlated with age and negatively correlated with attempt number.
   C. Reaction time is negatively correlated with age and positively correlated with attempt number.
   D. Reaction time is negatively correlated with age and negatively correlated with attempt number.

8. The researcher repeats the reflex study above with a 17-year-old, Participant 5, and adds another trial. What should the researcher expect to be true about the value of the fourth trial of Participant 5?

   A. The result of a fourth trial of Participant 5 is difficult to predict with the data given.
   B. The result of Trial 4 should be a longer reaction time compared to other participants and previous trials.
   C. The result should be a shorter reaction time compared to the other participants.
   D. The reaction time would be unchanged from Trial 3 to Trial 4.

KAPLAN TIP

As you can see, data interpretation on Test Day is not just about the data; it's also about your ability to think critically about the data in front of you.

Experiment 2

A neuropsychologist is interested in finding out how a specific type of lesion in the reticular formation of the brain stem would affect how long a patient remained in a specific sleep stage. In order to test this, he invited six people with this type of lesion to participate in a simple sleep study. The researcher compared the time that each participant spent in different stages of sleep with that of their control counterparts. Results are shown in Figure 4.

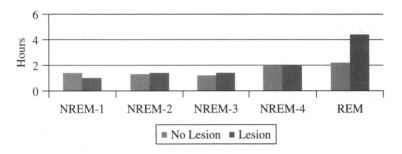

Figure 4. Time spent in stages of sleep for participants with and without the lesion.

9. Given the data above, what can you conclude about the sleep patterns in the two patient populations?

    A. The patients with lesions spend more time in each NREM stage of sleep compared to the REM stage.
    B. The patients without lesions spend an equal amount of time in each of the NREM sleep stages and double that time in the REM stage.
    C. The patients with lesions showed no difference in their sleep patterns compared to their unaffected counterparts.
    D. The patients with lesions spend about the same amount of time as unaffected patients in the NREM stages of sleep.

The neuropsychologist partnered with a neurobiologist during the study in order to measure the levels of specific neurotransmitters present throughout the different stages of sleep. The results for two of the neurotransmitters are shown in Figure 5.

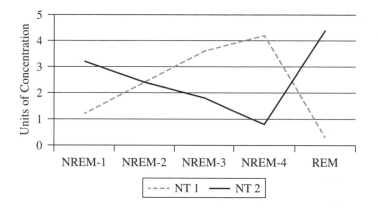

Figure 5. Levels of NT 1 and NT 2 in each sleep stage.

10. Assuming that the neurobiologist was able to measure and depict levels of glutamate, which of the existing neurotransmitter patterns would it mirror?

   A. NT 1, because it is an excitatory neurotransmitter that will be increased in the REM stage.
   B. NT 1, because it is an inhibitory neurotransmitter that will be decreased in the REM stage.
   C. NT 2, because it is an inhibitory neurotransmitter that will be decreased in the REM stage.
   D. NT 2, because it is an excitatory neurotransmitter that will be increased in the REM stage.

LESSON 4.1 REVIEW

When Interpreting Data

- Look for overall trends
  - Are the data points increasing? decreasing? scattered?
- If asked to compare
  - Look for the widest gaps
  - Pay attention to axes and variables

Representation of Data

- A data set can be represented in more than one way.
- The representation of the data can be a clue to the questions that will be asked.
  - Table: Specific comparison/calculation
  - Line Graph: Progress of a variable over time
  - Bar Graph: Comparison of variables
  - Pie Chart: Part of a whole

Possible Relationship Between Variables

- Correlational
  - Positive: a linear relationship where the independent variable increases as the dependent variable increases (and when one decreases, the other also decreases).
  - Negative: a linear relationship where independent variable decreases as dependent variable increases (or vice versa)
  - None: Independent
- Causation
  - Rare, and requires a lot of experimental confirmation
- Curvilinear
  - Exponential: Growth rate accelerates quickly as independent variable increases
  - Logarithmic: Growth rate decelerates as independent variable increases; tends to "level off"

Data Distributions

In this lesson, you'll learn to:

- Use common measures of central tendency and dispersion to describe data
- Recognize anomalous data, given background information on the study in question

Science Topics:

- Associative Learning
- Memory

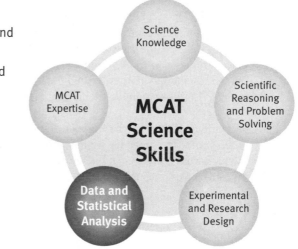

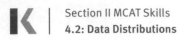

LESSON 4.2, LEARNING GOALS 1 AND 2:

- Use common measures of central tendency and dispersion to describe data
- Recognize anomalous data, given background information on the study in question

Data Distributions in Context—Practice Passage (Questions 1–7)

In studies of learning curves, the dependent variable is measured, while the independent variable is the experience of the learner. Experience is easily quantifiable; it can be measured in quantities such as hours studied or times through a maze. These values represent the amount of work done to enhance learning. To measure the effect of this experience, there must also be tests that show what effects the experience has on the skills of the subject.

One of the classical examples of quantifying learning and creating learning curves is running rats through a maze. Animal maze experiments began in the late 19th century, and by the early 20th century rats became the standard model for animal testing. The design of animal mazes is simple: place a rat at an entrance point and allow it to find the exit point. Because some rats are faster than others, researchers normally keep track of how many dead ends ("mistakes") a rat runs into on its way to the exit, rather than the exact time taken for completion.

Running a rat through the same maze multiple times gives a learning curve. The experience variable is the number of times the rat has gone through the maze and the learning variable is the number of mistakes that it has made: the fewer mistakes, the more the rat has learned. A simple equation can be given to make the curve positive:

$$L = \frac{1}{(n+1)}$$

where n is the number of mistakes made in a given trial of the maze. Table 1 shows the number of mistakes made by each of five rats in an animal maze experiment.

Rat	Trial 1	Trial 2	Trial 3	Trial 4	Trial 5	Trial 6	Trial 7	Trial 8
1	11	11	8	9	7	5	4	3
2	13	9	7	4	5	4	3	2
3	15	11	11	9	7	5	5	4
4	10	11	10	9	8	7	6	2
5	15	13	11	9	7	6	11	4

Table 1. Results of eight trials in a maze-running experiment.

Passage Outline

P1.

P2.

P3.

> **Equation 1.**
>
> **Table 1.**

1. In the study described in the passage, what is the mean L for rats running through the maze for the fourth time?

    A. $\frac{1}{10}$
    B. $\frac{3}{25}$
    C. 8
    D. 9

2. If the data in Table 1 is standardized by removing the most mistake-filled run for each rat, how many modes does the full set of standardized data have?

    A. 0 modes
    B. 1 mode
    C. 2 modes
    D. 3 or more modes

3. How does the standard deviation of mistakes per maze run change from Trial 1 to Trial 8?

    A. There is less deviation and the standard deviation decreases from approximately 13 to approximately 3.
    B. There is more deviation and the standard deviation increases from approximately 3 to approximately 13.
    C. There is less deviation and the standard deviation decreases from approximately 2 to approximately 1.
    D. There is more deviation and the standard deviation decreases from approximately 5 to approximately 2.

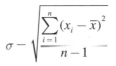

$$\sigma = \sqrt{\frac{\sum_{i=1}^{n}(x_i - \bar{x})^2}{n-1}}$$

Standard Deviation Formula

KAPLAN TIP

Exact calculations of the more complicated statistical variables, like standard deviation, will almost certainly NOT be necessary on the test. So if those calculations seem necessary, look for a better way!

Data Distributions in Context—Practice Passage (Questions 1–7)

In studies of learning curves, the dependent variable is measured, while the independent variable is the experience of the learner. Experience is easily quantifiable; it can be measured in quantities such as hours studied or times through a maze, These values represent the amount of work done to enhance learning. To measure the effect of this experience, there must also be tests that show what effects the experience has on the skills of the subject.

One of the classical examples of quantifying learning and creating learning curves is running rats through a maze. Animal maze experiments began in the late 19th century, and by the early 20th century rats became the standard model for animal testing. The design of animal mazes is simple: place a rat at an entrance point and allow it to find the exit point. Because some rats are faster than others, researchers normally keep track of how many dead ends ("mistakes") a rat runs into on its way to the exit, rather than the exact time taken for completion.

Running a rat through the same maze multiple times gives a learning curve. The experience variable is the number of times the rat has gone through the maze and the learning variable is the number of mistakes that it has made: the fewer mistakes, the more the rat has learned. A simple equation can be given to make the curve positive:

$$L = \frac{1}{(n+1)}$$

where n is the number of mistakes made in a given trial of the maze. Table 1 represents the data of an animal maze experiment with five rats, each of which had eight trials in the maze.

Rat	Trial 1	Trial 2	Trial 3	Trial 4	Trial 5	Trial 6	Trial 7	Trial 8
1	11	11	8	9	7	5	4	3
2	13	9	7	4	5	4	3	2
3	15	11	11	9	7	5	5	4
4	10	11	10	9	8	7	6	2
5	15	13	11	9	7	6	11	4

Table 1. Results of trials in a maze-running experiment.

4. How would the average slope of the learning curve for a longer, more complicated maze most likely differ from that of the curve for a shorter, less complicated maze? (Assume each rat stops running the maze once it has a trial with zero mistakes.)

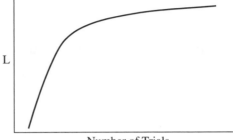

Number of Trials

   A. It would be less steep, but L would have the same maximum value.
   B. It would be steeper, but L would have a larger maximum value.
   C. It would be less steep, but L would have a larger maximum value.
   D. It would be steeper, but L would have a smaller maximum value.

5. Which rat has the lowest median for number of mistakes made throughout all eight trials?

   A. Rat 1
   B. Rat 2
   C. Rat 3
   D. Rat 4

6. What is the interquartile range for Rat 4's mistakes made?

   A. 3.5
   B. 5.6
   C. 8
   D. 11

7. Which of the following trials includes a potential significant outlier?

   I. Trial 2
   II. Trial 4
   III. Trial 6
   IV. Trial 7

   A. I and II only
   B. II and III only
   C. II and IV only
   D. II, III, and IV only

KAPLAN TIP

On Test Day, Skill 4 questions like this will be distributed across each science section, usually with one every passage or two.

LESSON 4.2 REVIEW

Key Concepts in Distributions (Centrality and Variance)

Mean

- Equals the sum of the values in a set divided by the number of values
- Often called the *"average"*

Median

- Equals the middle value in a set, when the items are ordered from least to greatest (or greatest to least)
- In sets with an even number of items, the median is the average of the middle *two* items

Mode

- The most commonly appearing value in a set
- *Bimodal* distributions have two "spikes" of common values

Standard Deviation

- Larger standard deviation means values are more spread out
- Standard deviation is the square root of the *variance* of a set

Quartiles

- Q_1, Q_2, Q_3, and Q_4 are the top ends of the first, second, third, and fourth quarter of a data set when the data is organized from least to greatest
- The *interquartile range* is the range between Q_1 and Q_3

Outliers

- Outliers are data points that are much larger or smaller than the other points in a data set, and are, by definition, not representative of the whole distribution
- Two common measures of outliers:
  - 1.5 × (Interquartile Range) or more below or above Q_1 or Q_3, respectively
  - 3 or more standard deviations below or above the mean value of the set

Experimental Error and Uncertainty

In this lesson, you'll learn to:

- Identify random and systematic error
- Compare and contrast random and systematic error
- Explain the statistical significance and uncertainty of a data set

Science Topics:

- Psychological Disorders
- Emotion

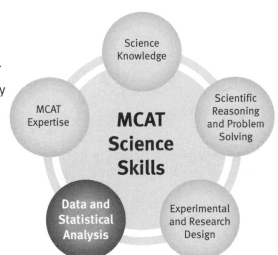

LESSON 4.3, LEARNING GOALS 1 AND 2:

- Identify random and systematic error
- Compare and contrast random and systematic error

Sources of Experimental Uncertainty

Study 1

In order to test physiological responses to emotion, a psychologist measures several parameters of the sympathetic response (heart rate, breathing rate, blood pressure) while participants watch a clip of a horror movie with three previously identified suspenseful moments. She also measures the same parameters in a control group who don't receive any stimulation. A sample of the findings is shown in Table 1.

	Heart Rate		Respiratory Rate		Blood Pressure	
	Expt	Control	Expt	Control	Expt	Control
Moment 1	140 bpm	76 bpm	21	10	150/100	120/80
Moment 2	148 bpm	81 bpm	17	12	140/90	115/65
Moment 3	135 bpm	66 bpm	20	11	155/108	125/70

Table 1. Measures of sympathetic response at three predetermined moments.

The psychologist wants to use her data to generalize to a larger population. How might random error in the study limit this?

Study 2

A local health center measures the one-year prevalence rates for psychological disorders in its community by surveying the health records of patients who seek out medical assistance at their facility. Results of the survey are shown in Table 2.

Disorder	% affected	Number
Any	26	81
Major Depressive Disorder	7	21
Generalized Anxiety Disorder	3	9
Obsessive Compulsive Disorder	1	3

Table 2. Prevalence and number of psychological disorders at the local health center.

The health center wants to use its data to generalize to a larger population. How will systematic error in the study limit this?

Practice Passage 1 (Questions 1–3)

Although the origin of clinical depression is still in large part a mystery, one possible explanation is monoamine theory. Monoamines are neurotransmitters such as dopamine, serotonin, and norepinephrine. According to the theory, reduced activity of monoamines in the brain is linked to depression. This theory was proposed following the accidental discovery that monoamine oxidase (MAO) inhibitors could successfully treat some cases of depression. Monoamine oxidase is an enzyme that catalyzes the breakdown of monoamines to corresponding aldehydes and ammonia. If monoamine oxidase activity is inhibited, monoamine levels will rise in the brain.

Experiment 3
Previous research indicates that oral MAO inhibitors limit bodily tyramine breakdown. Tyramine is a primary ingredient in aged cheese and acts as a vasoconstrictor. Due to this dietary limitation, oral MAO inhibitors were removed from the market and replaced with the selegiline transdermal system, another form of MAO inhibition. Six patients diagnosed with clinical depression were treated with the selegiline transdermal system; a dosage of 8 mg/day was delivered to each patient. To determine the precise impact that diet, or the consumption of aged cheese, has on blood pressure using this treatment, the patients were asked to eat cheese in measured increments until they experienced an increase in blood pressure of 30 mmHg; the total amount of cheese eaten (in ounces) was recorded in each case. The procedure was repeated three times and the results are indicated in Table 1.

	Trial 1	Trial 2	Trial 3
Patient 1	3.3	2.5	1.2
Patient 2	3.6	4.4	2.7
Patient 3	2.5	4.8	2.9
Patient 4	1.6	2.7	3.6
Patient 5	4.7	2.9	3.8
Patient 6	1.8	2.7	3.6

Table 1. Number of ounces of cheese consumed to elevate blood pressure by 30 mmHg.

1. The results provided in Table 1 indicate that Experiment 3 is subject to what type of error?

    A. Systematic error because the selegiline transdermal dosage varied for each patient.
    B. Random error because the amount of cheese consumed varied from one trial to another.
    C. Neither random nor systematic error because it is unethical to ask patients to eat unhealthy foods.
    D. Both random and systematic error because there are only 6 patients enrolled in the study.

2. Which of the following scenarios could potentially be a source of systematic error in Experiment 3?

    A. Varying the type of lotion each patient used prior to administration of the selegiline transdermal system.
    B. Measuring the patients' blood pressure while sitting in different rooms.
    C. Weighing the cheese consumed on a scale that reads 0.25 ounces less than it should.
    D. Giving the patients all the same brand of cheese.

3. The experimental uncertainty in Experiment 3 could be reduced or minimized by

    I.   enrolling more patients into the study.
    II. standardizing the sphygmomanometers used to measure blood pressure.
    III. having the patients measure their cheese consumption using their own scales.

    A. I, II, III   C. II, III only
    B. I, III only   D. I, II only

LESSON 4.3, LEARNING GOAL 3:

- Explain the statistical significance and uncertainty of a data set

The Null Hypothesis and Significance

Study 1

In order to test physiological responses to emotion, a psychologist measures several parameters of the sympathetic response (heart rate, breathing rate, blood pressure) while participants watch a clip of a horror movie with 3 previously identified suspenseful moments. She also measures the same parameters in a control group who don't receive any stimulation.

What is the null hypothesis for this study?

What results would allow the researchers to reject the null hypothesis?

Study 2

A psychiatrist wants to compare the efficacy of treating the positive symptoms of schizophrenia (delusions and hallucinations) with psychotherapy versus antipsychotic drugs such as Haldol. He randomized patients into two study groups, one receiving 2 hours of psychotherapy daily and the other receiving Haldol daily, and measured the number of positive symptoms at the end of the study period. The results are shown in the graph below:

What is the null hypothesis for this study?

Can this researcher reject the null hypothesis?

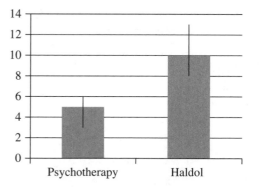

Figure 1. Total # of positive symptoms reported ($p < 0.05$).

KAPLAN TIP

Statistical significance signals the degree to which study results can be explained by chance, while the confidence interval indicates the certainty with which the values are representative of the population.

Practice Passage 1 (Questions 4–5)

Although the origin of clinical depression is still in large part a mystery, one possible explanation is monoamine theory. Monoamines are neurotransmitters such as dopamine, serotonin, and norepinephrine. According to the theory, reduced activity of monoamines in the brain is linked to depression. This theory was proposed following the accidental discovery that monoamine oxidase (MAO) inhibitors could successfully treat some cases of depression. Monoamine oxidase is an enzyme that catalyzes the breakdown of monoamines to corresponding aldehydes and ammonia. If monoamine oxidase activity is inhibited, monoamine levels will rise in the brain.

Experiment 4

Some researchers argue that genetic influence on depressive behavior is less significant than environmental factors. A study was carried out to verify the legitimacy of this claim. At present, there are two known variants of the MAO-A gene, the high activity variant (normal) and the mutated limited activity variant. Four hundred adolescent males with different variants of the MAO-A gene were observed over the course of five years; 39 percent of these individuals were maltreated during their pre-adolescent years. Data analysis indicated that the individuals with a low activity variant of the MAO-A gene were 7 percent more likely to develop adolescent conduct disorder ($p = 0.18$). In addition, the maltreated individuals were 67 percent more likely to be diagnosed with adolescent conduct disorder than the normal individuals ($p < 0.05$). Researchers concluded that both the low activity variant of the MAO-A gene and maltreatment significantly impacted behavior.

4. Critics of the researchers' conclusion might argue which of the following?

   A. Only maltreatment can be statistically correlated to adolescent conduct disorder.
   B. The low activity variant and maltreatment are negatively correlated with respect to the disorder.
   C. Neither the low activity variant nor maltreatment data is statistically significant.
   D. No valid conclusions can be made, since there aren't any confidence intervals provided.

5. Given their analysis of significance and uncertainty, what can the researchers most reasonably conclude?

   A. There is at least a 95 percent likelihood that maltreated individuals will be diagnosed with adolescent conduct disorder at some point.
   B. There is less than a 5 percent likelihood that the increased incidence of adolescent conduct disorder in maltreated individuals is a result of chance.
   C. It is at least 95 percent likely that the average incidence of adolescent conduct disorder in maltreated individuals is the same as that of non-maltreated individuals.
   D. It is at most 5 percent likely that the average incidence of adolescent conduct disorder in maltreated individuals from the study is the same as that of non-maltreated individuals.

LESSON 4.3 REVIEW

Experimental Uncertainty

1. Random Error

   - Statistical fluctuations in measured data due to the precision limitations of the measurement device
   - Can be in either direction
   - Affects variance
   - Can be overcome by increasing the number of data points
     - For example, getting a different result when performing the same task over several trials

2. Systematic Error

   - A consistent inaccuracy in measured data
   - Often in the same direction and throughout all of the collected data
   - Cannot be overcome by increasing data points
   - Affects the mean
     - For example, using a measuring tool that is not calibrated correctly

Statistical Significance

1. *p*-value

   - Refers to the probability that a given result occurred by chance
   - Significance indicates the ability to reject the null hypothesis
   - Desired *p*-value for significance should be set before a study begins
   - In most studies, $p < .05$ (5%) is necessary for significance

2. Confidence Intervals

   - Allow researchers to estimate population data based on sample findings
   - Calculation is similar to that of *p*-values, but usage is different
   - Expressed as a range, with minimum and maximum values
   - Says, essentially, "We are *x* percent certain that the true value lies between these two values."
   - Percentage can be any value, but usually 95% or above

3. Type 1 (False Positive) and Type 2 (False Negative) Errors

Skill 4 (Data Analysis) in Action

In this lesson, you'll learn to:

- Apply common measures of central tendency and dispersion to data sets
- Organize and interpret data
- Compare and contrast error types

Science Topics:

- Molecular Genetics
- The Cell Cycle

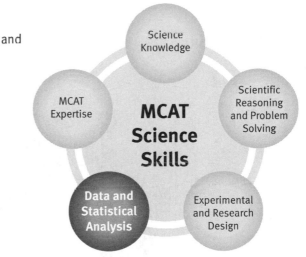

From the AAMC[*]:

"Like questions about the third science skill, questions that test the fourth skill will ask you to show that you can 'do' science, this time by demonstrating your data-based and statistical reasoning skills. Questions that test this skill will ask you to reason with data. They will ask you to read and interpret results using tables, graphs, and charts. These questions will ask you to demonstrate that you can identify patterns in data and draw conclusions."

---

*The Official Guide to the MCAT Exam (MCAT2017), Fifth Edition

LESSON 4.4, LEARNING GOAL 1:

- Apply common measures of central tendency and dispersion to data sets

Practice Passage (Questions 1–6)

Cohesin is a molecule that binds to DNA in order to mediate sister chromatid cohesion, the process by which sister chromatids are held together. Cohesin binding patterns can be measured using a technique called chromatin immunoprecipitation assay, or ChIP assay. A scientist uses a ChIP assay to investigate cohesin binding patterns at three potential cohesin binding regions on an *S. cerevisiae* (baker's yeast) chromosome throughout the cell cycle. To generate more reliable data, she runs her assay three times. Her results are compiled in Figure 1.

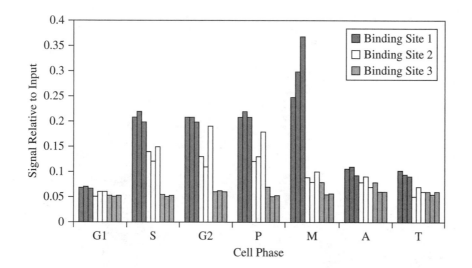

Figure 1. Relative cohesin binding amounts at three chromosomal sites and at different phases of the cell cycle.

Furthermore, at each stage of the cell cycle, the scientist looks at the total abundance of unique gene signatures in the ChIP data. This information is related to the total number of cohesin binding locations across the entire chromosome. These data are summarized in Table 1.

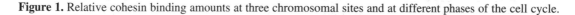

	G_1	S	G_2	P	M	A	T
Trial 1	10	115	120	63	8	3	4
Trial 2	15	117	127	50	7	5	2
Trial 3	13	102	113	49	8	7	5

Table 1. Total abundance of gene signatures throughout the cell cycle.

Practice Passage Questions

1. According to Table 1, how do the mean and median number of binding sites in prophase compare?

   A. The mean is greater than the median.
   B. The mean is less than the median.
   C. The mean and the median are equal.
   D. There is not enough data to compare the two quantities.

Which measure of central tendency is more sensitive to "extreme" data points?

2. For Table 1, which phase has the highest standard deviation?

   A. S phase
   B. Telophase
   C. G_1
   D. Metaphase

What, qualitatively, does standard deviation tell us about a sample?

LESSON 4.4, LEARNING GOAL 2:

- Organize and interpret data

Practice Passage (Questions 1–6)

Cohesin is a molecule that binds to DNA in order to mediate sister chromatid cohesion, the process by which sister chromatids are held together. Cohesin binding patterns can be measured using a technique called chromatin immunoprecipitation assay, or ChIP assay. A scientist uses a ChIP assay to investigate cohesin binding patterns at three potential cohesin binding regions on an *S. cerevisiae* (baker's yeast) chromosome throughout the cell cycle. To generate more reliable data, she runs her assay three times. Her results are compiled in Figure 1.

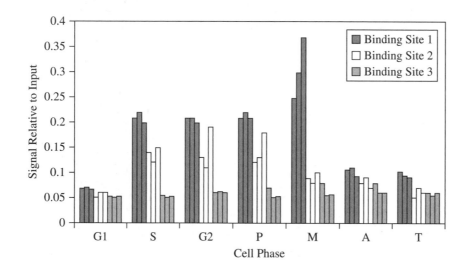

Figure 1. Relative cohesin binding amounts at three chromosomal sites and at different phases of the cell cycle.

Furthermore, at each stage of the cell cycle, the scientist looks at the total abundance of unique gene signatures in the ChIP data. This information is related to the total number of cohesin binding locations across the entire chromosome. These data are summarized in Table 1.

	G_1	S	G_2	P	M	A	T
Trial 1	10	115	120	63	8	3	4
Trial 2	15	117	127	50	7	5	2
Trial 3	13	102	113	49	8	7	5

Table 1. Total abundance of gene signatures throughout the cell cycle.

Practice Passage Questions

3. Which graph accurately represents the data in Table 1?

What trends are present in the data in Table 1?

A.

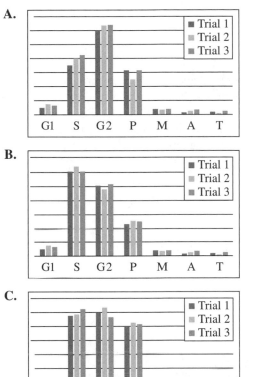

B.

C.

D.

4. Which of the following conclusions is supported by the data shown for binding region 1 in the experiment?

What trend does the data show for binding region 1?

A. Cohesin molecules bind to DNA during G_1 to help facilitate sister chromatid cohesion.
B. Trial 3 should be considered an outlier, because the data in the table contradicts the figure.
C. Region 2 is the complimentary strand to region 1 since its signal is always slightly below the signal of region 1.
D. Sister chromatids detach at the transition from metaphase to anaphase.

LESSON 4.4, LEARNING GOAL 3:

- Compare and contrast error types

Practice Passage (Questions 1–6)

Cohesin is a molecule that binds to DNA in order to mediate sister chromatid cohesion, the process by which sister chromatids are held together. Cohesin binding patterns can be measured using a technique called chromatin immunoprecipitation assay, or ChIP assay. A scientist uses a ChIP assay to investigate cohesin binding patterns at three potential cohesin binding regions on an *S. cerevisiae* (baker's yeast) chromosome throughout the cell cycle. To generate more reliable data, she runs her assay three times. Her results are compiled in Figure 1.

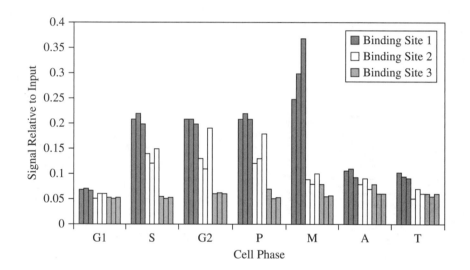

Figure 1. Relative cohesin binding amounts at three chromosomal sites and at different phases of the cell cycle.

Furthermore, at each stage of the cell cycle, the scientist looks at the total abundance of unique gene signatures in the ChIP data. This information is related to the total number of cohesin binding locations across the entire chromosome. These data are summarized in Table 1.

	G_1	S	G_2	P	M	A	T
Trial 1	10	115	120	63	8	3	4
Trial 2	15	117	127	50	7	5	2
Trial 3	13	102	113	49	8	7	5

Table 1. Total abundance of gene signatures throughout the cell cycle.

Practice Passage Questions

5. For a population of *S. cerevisiae* growing in optimal conditions, the time per cell cycle is distributed normally around the mode; some *S. cerevisiae* cells will progress through the cell cycle faster than average, while others will progress slower than average. Which of the following will NOT reduce the error introduced by this asynchronous growth?

   A. Increasing the number of ChIP assay trials run at each stage.
   B. Increasing the size of the yeast culture for each trial.
   C. Increasing the sensitivity of the sequencing device.
   D. Increasing yield of measureable sample produced by the experimental protocol.

What kind of error is being described in this question stem?

6. Suppose the sequencing device used to generate data consistently underreports the signal for binding site 1 and consistently overreports the signal for binding site 2. This would be an example of:

   A. random error.
   B. systematic error.
   C. selection bias.
   D. the Hawthorne effect.

What kind of error is being described in this question stem?

LESSON 4.4 REVIEW

Chapter 4 Learning Goals

4.1 Skill 4 (Data Analysis) Basics

- Analyze and interpret visual representations of data
- Choose the appropriate representation for a given data set
- Use data to identify and explain relationships between variables
- Use data to determine a study's conclusions and make predictions about the likelihood of future events

4.2 Data Distributions

- Use common measures of central tendency and dispersion to describe data
- Recognize anomalous data, given background information on the study in question

4.3 Experimental Error and Uncertainty

- Identify random and systematic error
- Compare and contrast random and systematic error
- Explain the statistical significance and uncertainty of a data set

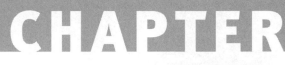

CHAPTER

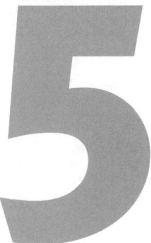

5

Science Skill 5:
MCAT Expertise

Science Passage Strategy

In this lesson, you'll learn to:

* Preview a science passage at a glance, determining likely topics and difficulty
* Identify the most question-relevant information in a science passage
* Create efficient and useful passage outlines

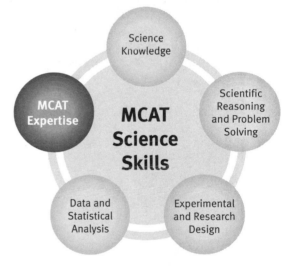

Science Topics:

* Intermolecular Forces
* Organic Chemistry Reaction Analysis
* Translational Motion

MCAT STRATEGY—SCIENCE PASSAGES

SCAN FOR STRUCTURE
Determine your "gut feeling" about the passage with a quick preview

READ STRATEGICALLY
Read the passage, focusing your attention on the more test-worthy details

LABEL EACH COMPONENT
Write down a short label or summary for each paragraph and figure as you read

REFLECT ON YOUR OUTLINE
Make a full passage summary for yourself before moving to the questions

LESSON 5.1, LEARNING GOAL 1:

- Preview a science passage at a glance, determining likely topics and difficulty

The Previewing Process

Practice Passage 1

The cell's cytoplasm includes all the liquid and solutes in the cell as well as all the organelles, excluding the nucleus. Also included are sodium, calcium, potassium, and all other ions as well as all the proteins in the cell. This "cell soup" provides the basis for cellular micro-processes that eventually lead to the macro-processes that we see as organismal activity. Many of these processes are derived from intermolecular forces between different parts of the cytoplasm.

The water basis of the cytoplasm helps to dissolve these solutes in the substrate. Around larger solutes, water forms solvation layers. These layers have water arranged in specific ways that use the partial charges of water to stabilize the ions and dipoles of the solutes. Depending on the species, water can hydrogen bond to the solutes for a stronger bond.

Important molecules, such as **ATP**, use intermolecular forces to make sure proper reactions occur. **ATP**, when binding to proteins, also binds to a divalent cation, usually magnesium. Without magnesium, the dissociation constant between the **ATP** and protein is increased.

A biochemist performs an experiment to determine the effects of **Mg** on hexokinase enzyme activity and **ATP-Mg** dissociation, where K_{ATP-Mg} is the dissociation constant for **ATP-Mg** and k_{cat} is proportional to V_{max} of the enzyme. The results are displayed in Table 1.

What do you notice in the first sentence?

What stands out in the rest of the passage text?

What kinds of figures are present?

Free [Mg⁺⁺]	[Mg-ATP]	[Peptide]	$K_{\text{ATP-Mg}}$	k_{cat}
0.5 mM	0.3 mM	1 mM	3.50	12.9 s⁻¹
3 mM	0.3 mM	1 mM	2.50	13.3 s⁻¹
7 mM	0.3 mM	1 mM	0.95	13.3 s⁻¹
10 mM	0.3 mM	1 mM	0.20	13.3 s⁻¹

Table 1. Effect of free magnesium on various quantities.

Practice Passage 2

Van der Waals forces are also important in the cell membrane. Although hydrophobic interactions bring a cell membrane together, the membrane is stabilized by van der Waals forces. These are usually transient, but in certain cases, as with cholesterol and sphingolipids such as sphingomyelin, they form lipid rafts that are thicker than the cell membrane and a stable place for certain membrane proteins to accumulate. Sphingomyelin's structure is shown in Figure 1.

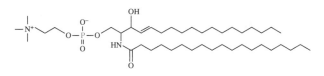

Figure 1. Structure of sphingomyelin.

What science topic is being tested in the passage?

How hard do you think this passage (and its questions) will be for you?

Would you skip this passage on Test Day?

KAPLAN TIP

The grayed-out text on this page is meant to represent that during preview, only certain parts of a passage—figures, numbers, formulas, and the like—will stand out to you. The blocked-out text *doesn't* mean that you should be "skimming" passages when you decide to dive in; once you've committed to reading a passage, it's important to read every word.

The Previewing Process

Practice Passage 3

When evaluating automobile safety, there are three major factors to consider: the vehicle, the operator, and the driving conditions.

Vehicles have become much safer over the last few decades due to innovations in passenger safety. The seatbelt restrains the wearer against sharp forward motion and distributes the force of impact over the rider's chest and pelvis. Riders wearing a seatbelt have a good chance of surviving a collision, as long as their deceleration doesn't exceed $30g$. Airbags, installed in the center of the steering wheel, inflate quickly after impact, forming a cushion for the driver. Crumple zones in the front and rear of a car are designed to absorb a large fraction of the energy during a collision.

Human factors—such as the driver's behavior, visual and auditory acuity, decision-making ability, and reaction time—also contribute to the incidence of accidents. A driver's reaction time, $t_{reaction}$, is the time elapsed between observing a dangerous situation and acting on it. For a car traveling at speed v, the minimum safe distance, d, between the car and the hazard is:

$$d = vt_{reaction} + \frac{v^2}{2a},$$

where a is the maximum rate of deceleration of the car, which is largely dependent upon the frictional force between the tires and the roadway.

What do you notice in the first sentence?

What stands out in the rest of the passage text?

What kinds of figures are present?

Crash tests are routinely conducted by manufacturers and regulating government agencies in order to assess the safety of automobiles. Sophisticated anthropomorphic test devices (**ATDs**) are often employed to replace human passengers. These mannequins are constructed from materials with properties similar to those of the human body. Accelerometers, force transducers, and displacement sensors within **ATDs** collect data during a crash. Figure 1 shows data from two head-on collisions at 40 km/hr.

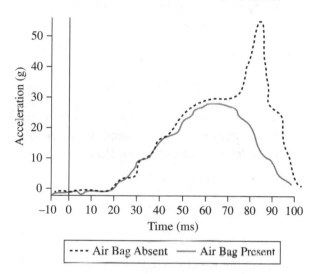

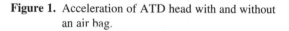

Figure 1. Acceleration of ATD head with and without an air bag.

What science topic is being tested in the passage?

How hard do you think this passage (and its questions) will be for you?

Would you skip this passage on Test Day?

KAPLAN TIP

Don't overcomplicate the preview process; it's supposed to be very quick and lead to snap decisions. As long as previewing isn't taking you more than 5–10 seconds per passage and you get a good "first impression," then you're doing it right!

LESSON 5.1, LEARNING GOAL 2:

- Identify the most question-relevant information in a science passage

Biochemistry Passage Sample

The water basis of the cytoplasm helps to dissolve these solutes in the substrate. Around larger solutes, water forms solvation layers. These layers have water arranged in specific ways that use the partial charges of water to stabilize the ions and dipoles of the solutes. Depending on the species, water can hydrogen bond to the solutes for a stronger bond.

What outside science knowledge will most likely be required to answer questions based on this passage?

Important molecules, such as ATP, use intermolecular forces to make sure proper reactions occur. ATP, when binding to proteins, also binds to a divalent cation, usually magnesium. Without magnesium, the dissociation constant between the ATP and protein is increased.

What information in this sample would be *likely* material for MCAT-style questions?

A biochemist performs an experiment to determine the effects of Mg on hexokinase enzyme activity and ATP-Mg dissociation, where K_{ATP-Mg} is the dissociation constant for ATP-Mg and k_{cat} is proportional to V_{max} of the enzyme. The results are displayed in Table 1.

What information in this sample would be *unlikely* material for MCAT-style questions?

Free [Mg^{++}]	[Mg-ATP]	[Peptide]	K_{ATP-Mg}	k_{cat}
0.5 mM	0.3 mM	1 mM	3.50	12.9 s^{-1}
3 mM	0.3 mM	1 mM	2.50	13.3 s^{-1}
7 mM	0.3 mM	1 mM	0.95	13.3 s^{-1}
10 mM	0.3 mM	1 mM	0.20	13.3 s^{-1}

Table 1. Effect of free magnesium on various quantities.

Organic Chemistry Passage Sample

Styrene is used extensively in the manufacture of plastics, rubber, and resins. It is a colorless liquid with a sweet, aromatic odor at low concentrations and a sharp, penetrating, disagreeable odor at high concentrations.

Because of the reactivity of its metabolite, styrene is classified as a mutagen. Studies have not yet definitively proven that exposure leads to cancer, but a causal link is strongly suspected and the U.S. National Toxicology Program describes styrene as "reasonably accepted to be a human carcinogen."

Styrene can be synthesized in the lab either by reacting sulfuric acid with compound **A** ($C_8H_{10}O$) or using zinc metal with compound **B** ($C_8H_8Br_2$) in ethanol. Compound **B** can be made from compound **C** (C_8H_9Br) by generating Br_2 gas *in situ* from the reaction of potassium bromate and hydrobromic acid and irradiation with a lamp. Compound **A** is characterized by its mild hyacinth odor and the ester, **D** ($C_{10}H_{12}O_2$), formed by the reaction of **A** with acetic acid and sulfuric acid, has a fruity smell.

What outside science knowledge will most likely be required to answer questions based on this passage?

What information in this sample would be *likely* material for MCAT-style questions?

What information in this sample would be *unlikely* material for MCAT-style questions?

KAPLAN TIP

Don't let yourself get stressed about "non-science" material in science passages. In fact, you should see it as good news: more non-science information in the passage means less space for question-worthy material, making your job easier!

LESSON 5.1, LEARNING GOAL 3:

- Create efficient and useful passage outlines

Organic Chemistry Passage

Styrene is used extensively in the manufacture of plastics, rubber, and resins. It is a colorless liquid with a sweet, aromatic odor at low concentrations, but with a sharp, penetrating, disagreeable odor at high concentrations.

In humans, the liver metabolizes styrene into styrene oxide via the cytochrome P450 system. Both enantiomers are toxic, although (R)-styrene oxide has more pronounced health effects in mice. Long-term human exposure to styrene via inhalation, ingestion, or skin contact can lead to lethargy, memory loss, and headaches. Because of the reactivity of its metabolite, styrene is classified as a mutagen. Studies have not yet definitively proven that exposure leads to cancer, but a causal link is strongly suspected and the U.S. National Toxicology Program describes styrene as "reasonably accepted to be a human carcinogen."

Styrene can be synthesized in the lab by either reacting sulfuric acid with compound **A** ($C_8H_{10}O$) or using zinc metal with compound **B** ($C_8H_8Br_2$) in ethanol. Compound **B** can be made from compound **C** (C_8H_9Br) by generating Br_2 gas *in situ* from the reaction of potassium bromate and hydrobromic acid and irradiation with a lamp. Compound **A** is characterized by its mild hyacinth odor, and the ester, compound **D** ($C_{10}H_{12}O_2$), formed by the reaction of **A** with acetic acid and sulfuric acid, has a fruity smell.

Compound **A** will undergo oxidation to **E** (C_8H_8O) in the presence of bleach and acetic acid. Compound **E**, which is characterized by its floral aroma, has a boiling point of 202°C and a refractive index of 1.5372. The semicarbazone derivative of **E** has a melting point of 198°C.

For styrene production on an industrial scale, the preferred method of synthesis involves taking compound **F** (C_8H_{10}) through a dehydrogenation reaction catalyzed by an amalgam of iron(III) oxide and potassium carbonate.

KAPLAN TIP

Passage outlining, which you'll be doing a lot of between now and Test Day, is writing down what you notice about a passage as you read so you can store the important information more efficiently and return to it more easily when you need it for the questions.

K

Figure 1 shows selected synthesis and derivatives of styrene.

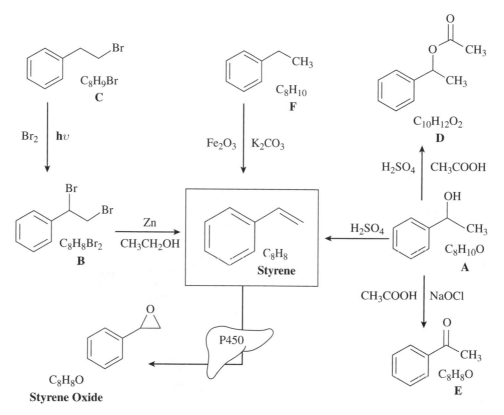

Figure 1. Selected synthesis and derivatives of styrene.

Write Your Passage Outline Here:

P1.

P2.

P3.

P4.

P5.

Fig. 1.

Sample Passage Outlines for Organic Chemistry Passage

Example 1

P1. Styrene uses and properties

P2. Styrene metabolism & risks

P3. Styrene synthesis from different compounds

P4. Compounds related to styrene (A and E)

P5. Industrial production of styrene

Fig. 1. Reactions leading to styrene

Example 2

P1. Styrene background

P2. Health risks

P3. Styrene; A, B, C, D

P4. A to E

P5. Industrial production; F

Fig. 1. Styrene synthesis

Example 3

P1. Background information, properties and uses of styrene

P2. Metabolism of styrene leads to toxic byproducts, health risks

P3. Synthesis of styrene from compounds A, B, and C. Synthesis of D from A.

P4. Compound A to compound E, and properties of E.

P5. Styrene production on industrial scale using compound F

Fig. 1. Multiple mechanisms of synthesizing styrene and related compounds

LESSON 5.1 REVIEW

MCAT Strategy—Science Passages

SCAN FOR STRUCTURE
Determine your "gut feeling" about the passage with a quick preview

READ STRATEGICALLY
Read the passage, focusing your attention on more test-worthy details

LABEL EACH COMPONENT
Write down a short label or summary for each passage as you read

REFLECT ON YOUR OUTLINE
Make a full passage summary to yourself before moving to the questions

Science Questions: Assess and Plan

In this lesson, you'll learn to:

- Assess a question and its answer choices for difficulty, science topic, and common patterns
- Plan an efficient way to answer a given question

Science Topics:

- Amino Acids, Peptides, and Proteins
- Enzyme Structure, Function, and Regulation
- Nucleic Acid Structure and Function
- Transcription
- Translation

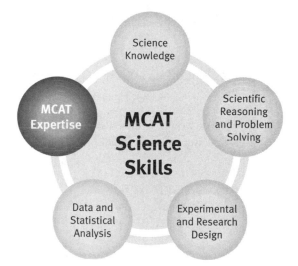

MCAT STRATEGY—SCIENCE QUESTIONS

ASSESS THE QUESTION
Read a question and its answer choices; decide whether to skip it.

PLAN YOUR ATTACK
Decide how best to approach the question, based on your experience with similar questions.

EXECUTE THE PLAN*

ANSWER BY MATCHING, ELIMINATING, OR GUESSING*

*The EXECUTE and ANSWER steps are covered in depth in Lesson 5.3.

LESSON 5.2, LEARNING GOAL 1:

- Assess a question and its answer choices for difficulty, science topic, and common patterns

Common Patterns in Questions and Answers

1. Which of the following is true about DNA synthesis?

    A. It occurs in all cells continuously.
    B. In prokaryotes, it occurs in the nucleus.
    C. It is a semiconservative process.
    D. Mitosis is a step of DNA synthesis.

What pattern or patterns are present here?

2. A segment of a DNA strand has the base sequence:

    5′—GTTCATTG—3′

    What would be the base sequence of the RNA strand transcribed from this DNA?

    A. 5′—CAATGAAC—3′
    B. 5′—GTTCATTG—3′
    C. 5′—CAAUGAAC—3′
    D. 5′—CAAGUAAC—3′

What pattern or patterns are present here?

3. A scientist has an unknown sample of an amino acid that has been determined to have an amino group, a carboxyl group, optical activity, and multiple nitrogen groups on its side chain. Of the following values, its most likely isoelectric point is:

    A. 2.65
    B. 4.77
    C. 7.10
    D. 11.15

What pattern or patterns are present here?

Common Patterns in Questions and Answers

What pattern or patterns are present here?

4. Which of the following processes is demonstrated in the regulation of enzyme A, as described in the passage?

   A. Competitive inhibition
   B. Allosteric inhibition
   C. Noncompetitive inhibition
   D. Positive feedback mechanisms

5. Which of the following is true of sample C?

   A. The amino acids are likely to have aromatic rings and appear on the inside of folded proteins.
   B. The amino acids are likely to have charged side chains and appear on the inside of folded proteins.
   C. The amino acids are likely to have aromatic rings and appear on the outside of folded proteins.
   D. The amino acids are likely to have charged side chains and appear on the outside of folded proteins.

6. Which of the following is the most likely reason for the production of faulty prelamin A in individuals with progeria?

   A. The mutation causes a termination sequence in the DNA to appear earlier than is normal.
   B. The point mutation causes a stop codon to appear earlier in protein sequencing than is normal.
   C. The DNA splices and reforms at the lamin A gene, removing part of the protein's template strand.
   D. The protein that is sequenced from prelamin A is less stable as a result of the mutation, and it denatures.

7. Is the mutation seen in paragraph 4 likely to be fatal if present in a gamete during fertilization?

   A. Yes, because proteins essential to development will not be sequenced.
   B. Yes, because the zygote will not be able to efficiently produce ATP.
   C. No, because the zygote will have access to proteins by other means.
   D. No, because proteins will be sequenced as normal with the mutation present.

KAPLAN TIP

The patterns on this page, as well as those in the rest of this lesson, will appear again and again on Test Day. Patterns indicate which strategies will be best to use and how difficult a question will be, so start noticing them now!

How to Assess a Question

Look in these places:

- The question stem
- The answer choices

For these patterns:

- Science "buzzwords"
- Passage references (e.g., "paragraph 3," "Experiment 2")
- Length and complexity of question stem
- Length, complexity, and structure of answer choices
- "Yes/No" patterns in the answer choices
- Numbers or formulas
- Figures, tables, or other graphics
- Anything else that has made questions easy, hard, or otherwise distinctive for you in the past

So you can make these judgments:

- The science being tested
- How hard the question will be for you
- How long the question will take you
- Whether you should skip the question for now

Assessing Discrete Questions

What do you notice in the ...

8. If a point mutation occurs that changes one nucleotide in an mRNA molecule, the final protein product is LEAST likely to be affected if the altered nucleotide is in the

Question stem?

   A. original start codon.
   B. original stop codon.
   C. first letter of a codon.
   D. third letter of a codon.

Answer choices?

9. Which set of graphs best depicts the optimal temperature and pH range for pepsin activity?

Question stem?

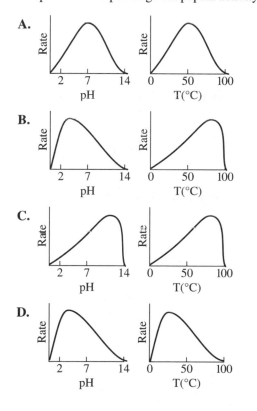

Answer choices?

KAPLAN TIP

These question and answer patterns should be relatively easy to recognize. To increase your MCAT score, try to incorporate pattern-recognition skills as you triage and attack questions on Test Day.

LESSON 5.2, LEARNING GOAL 2:

- Plan an efficient way to answer a given question

The Question

2. A segment of a DNA strand has the base sequence:

$$5'\text{—GTTCATTG—}3'$$

What would be the base sequence of the RNA strand transcribed from this DNA?

A. 5'—CAATGAAC—3'
B. 5'—GTTCATTG—3'
C. 5'—CAAUGAAC—3'
D. 5'—CAAGUAAC—3'

Plans to Answer (of varying effectiveness)

"Let me go back to the passage to see where it talks about matching DNA to RNA strands in transcription."

"This is a question where I'll have to figure out the exact answer before I go through the choices. I'd better get to work on my scratch paper!"

"Okay, DNA-to-RNA matching is A-U and C-G, and antiparallel strands mean that the 3's and 5's will be swapped...let's hit those answer choices."

The Question

3. A scientist has an unknown sample of an amino acid that has been determined to have an amino group, a carboxyl group, optical activity, and multiple nitrogen groups on its side chain. Of the following values, its most likely isoelectric point is:

    A. 2.65
    B. 4.77
    C. 7.10
    D. 11.15

Plans to Answer

"The isoelectric point of an amino acid is its pK_a, and the question says right away that this has an amino group, so I'll pick a basic answer choice."

"I know the test will sometimes expect me to know my amino acids, and I know my amino acids pretty well. Let me figure out which one this is, and then match it with the right isoelectric point in the choices."

"I know that some parts of this long question stem must be more important than others. Let me go through those molecular traits to see what makes this amino acid special, then see if that alone will point me to the right answer."

Why is the third plan the best?

KAPLAN TIP

A good way to summarize this Plan step is by asking yourself the question, *"Where have I seen this before?"* This step is about using your experience— in your science classes, your prep classes, your practice tests, and beyond— and transferring that previous knowledge to the question at hand.

LESSON 5.2 REVIEW

The Kaplan Method for Science Questions, Steps 1 and 2

ASSESS MEANS ...

Look for key details in the question stem and answer choices as you read them:

- Science "Buzzwords"
- Passage References
- Length
- Numbers or Formulas
- Common Question and Answer Patterns

Try to determine:

- Science Topic
- Difficulty
- Time Needed to Answer
- Triage (Should you skip it?)

PLAN MEANS ...

Use your judgments from the Assess step to plan your approach to the question.

Use your experience with similar questions to avoid mistakes.

Don't be afraid to change the plan if:

- You find or remember new information
- The question is harder or easier than you first thought
- The question is taking you too long

Science Questions: Execute and Answer

In this lesson, you'll learn to:

- Judge when predicting an answer is a useful strategy
- Make strong and accurate predictions for answers before reading through answer choices
- Recognize when an answer matches a prediction

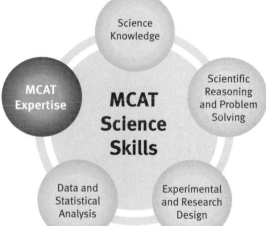

Science Topics:

- Amino Acids, Peptides, and Proteins
- Enzyme Structure, Function, and Regulation
- Nucleic Acid Structure and Function
- Transcription
- Translation

MCAT STRATEGY—SCIENCE QUESTIONS

ASSESS THE QUESTION*

PLAN YOUR ATTACK*

EXECUTE THE PLAN
Make a prediction based on your plan or decide to use elimination.

ANSWER BY MATCHING, ELIMINATING, OR GUESSING
Find your prediction within the answer choices.

The ASSESS and PLAN steps are covered in depth in Lesson 5.2.

LESSON 5.3, LEARNING GOAL 1:

- Judge when predicting an answer is a useful strategy

Consider these questions:

1. You have two fragments of DNA: fragment A melts (comes apart) at 97°C and fragment B melts at 65°C. What can you conclude about the two fragments with respect to their nucleotide composition?

What kind of prediction can you make for this question?

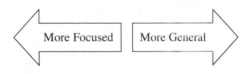

What is the prediction?

2. Which of the following is true about transcription?

What kind of prediction can you make for this question?

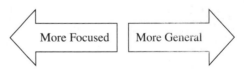

What is the prediction?

Prediction Practice

Indicate the best type of prediction:

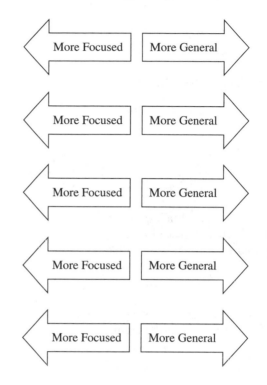

3. Researchers measure the mRNA found in a set of cells for a particular gene, and find it to be elevated. What must be occurring in the cell?

More Focused | More General

4. Which of the following statements about DNA methylation is the most accurate?

More Focused | More General

5. Polymerase chain reaction amplifies DNA by first unwinding it using heat rather than DNA helicase. What bonds must be broken in order for this reaction with heat to proceed?

More Focused | More General

6. A segment of a DNA strand has the base sequence: 5'—GTTCATTG—3'. What would be the base sequence of the RNA strand transcribed from this DNA?

More Focused | More General

7. The different antigenic blood types (A, B, and O) are inherited through allelic genes. The actual molecular difference between two blood types is in the carbohydrate that is attached to a common molecular backbone. The best explanation for how genes determine blood type, therefore, is that each gene:

More Focused | More General

8. A person has a mutation in the promoter site of the gene for the lactase enzyme, rendering the promoter site nonfunctional. What symptom(s) will occur?

More Focused | More General

   I. Less digestion of lactose by the person

  II. More digestion of lactose by the person's symbiotic gut bacteria

 III. Malnutrition due to glucose deficiency

   A. I only
   B. II only
   C. I and II only
   D. I and III only

KAPLAN TIP

You can also make a strategic guess on a question if you're not able to come up with a prediction at all. Eliminate answers for the best reasons you can think of.

LESSON 5.3, LEARNING GOAL 2:

• Make strong and accurate predictions for answers before reading through answer choices

The PLAN and EXECUTE Steps with a Passage

Practice Passage (Questions 9–13)

Hutchinson-Gilford progeria syndrome (HGPS) is a rare genetic disease that affects one in eight million live births. Individuals with progeria exhibit symptoms of aging at an early age and generally only live until their teenage years or, occasionally, their early 20s. Affected individuals experience stunted growth, musculoskeletal degeneration, loss of hair, and have a characteristic appearance.

A point mutation in position 1824 of the *LMNA* gene coding for lamin A is the typical cause of progeria. A cytosine is replaced with thymine; as a result, a shortened mRNA transcript is generated, which codes for a faulty version of unprocessed prelamin A. During post-translational processing, prelamin A is incapable of losing its farnesyl group (a 15-carbon isoprenoid), preventing the conversion of prelamin A to mature lamin A. Figure 1 shows the post-translational processing that results in mutant prelamin A, which is also called progerin. The farnesyl group locks progerin to the nuclear rim. While bound to the nuclear rim, progerin cannot offer the necessary structural support to the nuclear envelope. As a consequence, the nuclear envelope is misshapen. The structure of the nuclear envelope is essential for the proper manipulation of chromatin during mitosis.

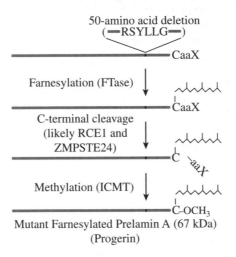

Figure 1. Mutant prelamin A post-translational processing.

Normal prelamin A post-translational modification consists of four steps. The processing begins with the farnesylation of the cysteine of the CaaX box (cysteine and three aliphatic amino acids located at the carboxyl terminus of prelamin A) by farnesyltransferase (FTase). Shortly thereafter, the –aaX portion of the CaaX box is removed. Next, the product is methylated. Finally, the carboxyl terminal as well as the modified farnesyl group is sliced off by the peptidase ZMPSTE24. Figure 2 illustrates normal prelamin A post-translational processing. FTase inhibitors have been tested with animal models and shown to reverse the malformation of the nuclear envelope caused by progerin.

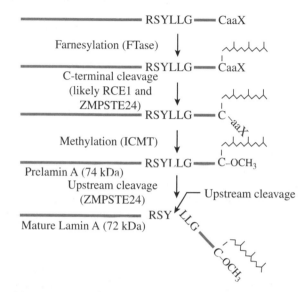

Figure 2. Normal prelamin A post-translational processing.

Passage Outline

P1.

P2.

Fig. 1.

P3.

Fig. 2.

The PLAN and EXECUTE Steps with Passage Questions

9. Why is the malformation of the nuclear envelope reversed in animal models when FTase inhibitors are used?

    A. FTase inhibitors catalyze the upstream cleavage of the modified farnesyl group.
    B. No progerin is made in the presence of FTase inhibitors.
    C. Normal prelamin A is created when FTase inhibitors are present.
    D. FTase inhibitors physically prevent progerin from locking to the nuclear rim.

    Prediction:

10. One of the three amino acids found at the carboxyl terminus of prelamin A could be:

    A. tyrosine.
    B. tryptophan.
    C. phenylalanine.
    D. alanine.

    Prediction:

11. Which of the following is the most likely reason for the production of faulty prelamin A in individuals with progeria?

    A. The mutation introduces a new splice site, resulting in a loss of RNA from one of the exons of prelamin A.
    B. The point mutation causes a stop codon to appear earlier in protein sequencing than is normal.
    C. The DNA splices and reforms at the lamin A gene, removing part of the protein's template strand.
    D. The protein that is sequenced from prelamin A is less stable as a result of the mutation, and it denatures.

    Prediction:

12. Which of the following is most likely to result in stunted growth and musculoskeletal degeneration?

    A. Structurally supported nuclear envelopes
    B. Loss of the farnesyl group by prelamin A
    C. Methylation of prelamin A during post-translational processing
    D. The improper manipulation of chromatin during mitosis

    Prediction:

13. What changes occur in the DNA when a point mutation changes a cytosine to a thymine?

    A. One fewer hydrogen bond is formed between base pairs.
    B. A pyrimidine is changed into a purine.
    C. An –OH group is added to deoxyribose.
    D. The phosphate backbone is deformed due to base-pair mismatch.

    Prediction:

LESSON 5.3, LEARNING GOAL 3:

- Recognize when an answer matches a prediction

The ANSWER Step with Passage Questions

9. Why is the malformation of the nuclear envelope reversed in animal models when FTase inhibitors are used?

   A. FTase inhibitors catalyze the upstream cleavage of the modified farnesyl group.
   B. No progerin is made in the presence of FTase inhibitors.
   C. Normal prelamin A is created when FTase inhibitors are present.
   D. FTase inhibitors physically prevent progerin from locking to the nuclear rim.

10. One of the three amino acids found at the carboxyl terminus of prelamin A could be:

    A. tyrosine.
    B. tryptophan.
    C. phenylalanine.
    D. alanine.

11. Which of the following is the most likely reason for the production of faulty prelamin A in individuals with progeria?

    A. The mutation introduces a new splice site, resulting in loss of RNA from one of the exons of prelamin A.
    B. The point mutation causes a stop codon to appear earlier in protein sequencing than is normal.
    C. The DNA splices and reforms at the lamin A gene, removing part of the protein's template strand.
    D. The protein that is sequenced from prelamin A is less stable as a result of the mutation, and it denatures.

12. Which of the following is most likely to result in stunted growth and musculoskeletal degeneration?

    A. Structurally supported nuclear envelopes
    B. Loss of the farnesyl group by prelamin A
    C. Methylation of prelamin A during post-translational processing
    D. The improper manipulation of chromatin during mitosis

13. What changes occur in the DNA when a point mutation changes a cytosine to a thymine?

    A. One fewer hydrogen bond is formed between base pairs.
    B. A pyrimidine is changed into a purine.
    C. An –OH group is added to deoxyribose.
    D. The phosphate backbone is deformed due to base pair mismatch

---

KAPLAN TIP

Don't forget your prediction when you're looking through the answers. Make sure you match your prediction carefully in the Answer step.

LESSON 5.3 REVIEW

The Kaplan Method for Science Questions: Steps 3 and 4

EXECUTE MEANS ...

Using the steps you came up with during the PLAN step, solve the problem.

Use that solution, whether general or focused, to make a prediction of the correct answer.

ANSWER MEANS ...

Find the correct answer within the given choices by either:

Choosing the answer that closely matches your focused prediction, or

Eliminating answer choices that don't fit with your general prediction until only one choice remains.

Triage in the Science Sections

In this lesson, you'll learn to:

- Utilize the triaging strategy within a science section of the MCAT
- Use question stems and answer choices to preview and triage MCAT questions
- Determine when a question is a "pseudo-discrete" question

Science Topics:

- The Nervous System
- The Endocrine System

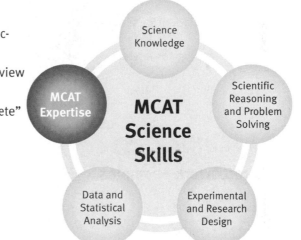

LESSON 5.4, LEARNING GOAL 1:

- Utilize the triaging strategy within a science section of the MCAT

Section Triage Strategy

- Triage Order:

    1. Discrete questions

    2. Easiest passages

    3. Passages with ambiguous difficulty

    4. Hardest passages

- Flagging for Review

- Navigation Panel

Scratchwork Examples

P1	P2	P3	P4	P5	P6	P7	P8	P9	P10
☺	☹		☺				☹		☺

1~   2✓ D 3✓   4✗   5~   D 6✓   7~   8✗ D 9~   10~

E:	M:	H:
1	13	34
5	17	52
48	21	
	29	
	39	

KAPLAN TIP

There is no single best triaging technique. Every great test-taker has their own unique method, so experiment with different techniques until you find what works for you. Just remember that the ultimate goal is to find a way to do the easiest questions first, and make sure you perfect your method before Test Day!

Sample Passage 1

Appropriate function of the nervous system, especially in regard to locomotion, relies on the ability of motor nerves to communicate with muscle tissue. Pathological conditions that inhibit the ability of neurons to communicate with muscles result in various types of muscular dysfunction. For example, myasthenia gravis (MG) is a disease in which autoantibodies target receptors located at the neuromuscular junction, resulting in the inability of the neuron to communicate with the muscle. Interestingly, many patients with MG also have an abnormal thymus. Treatment often involves pharmaceutical therapy, which generally offers only symptomatic relief. However, definitive treatment can often be achieved with removal of the thymus.

Another disease that causes a decrease in the ability of nerves to communicate with muscles is known as Lambert–Eaton myasthenic syndrome. In this condition, autoantibodies attack the presynaptic calcium channels, diminishing the signal transmitted to the postsynaptic cells. This condition is often associated with small-cell lung cancer.

Myasthenia gravis and Lambert–Eaton syndrome are often characterized by muscle weakness. However, in the absence of additional information, it can be difficult to make a differential diagnosis. One of the ways these two conditions can be distinguished is by the administration of a medication that inhibits acetylcholinesterase. Patients with MG will notice substantial improvement with administration of such a medication, while Lambert–Eaton patients will not. Another way to distinguish the two is by the use of repetitive nerve stimulation (RNS). RNS is performed by electrically stimulating a nerve and measuring the response of the muscle. Figure 1 shows the appearance of RNS muscle response. Each peak indicates a single stimulation event.

Repetitive nerve stimulation

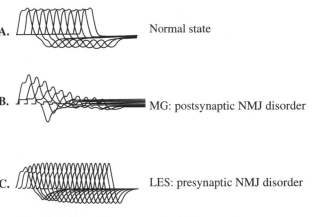

Figure 1. Repetitive nerve stimulation muscle response.

1. Why does the administration of a medication that inhibits acetylcholinesterase improve the symptoms of myasthenia gravis?

   A. It inactivates the antibodies against the receptors at the neuromuscular junction preventing the autoantibodies from attacking.
   B. It increases the concentration of acetylcholine at the synapse allowing for greater stimulation of unaffected receptors.
   C. It decreases the quantity of acetylcholine at the synapse to prevent aberrant signaling.
   D. It allows for more efficient opening of calcium channels at the neuromuscular junction.

What is your triage decision?

Sample Passage 2

Pituitary adenomas are tumors that form in the pituitary gland. The most common pituitary adenomas are known as lactotroph adenomas. They affect the cells of the anterior pituitary that produce prolactin, a hormone that encourages lactation. The incidence of lactotroph adenomas is estimated at 2.2 cases per 100,000, while the prevalence is approximately 100 cases per 1 million.

As prolactin is the primary hormone produced by a lactotroph adenoma, these adenomas are also known as prolactinomas. One of the major symptoms of these tumors is inappropriate lactation, known as galactorrhea. However, there may be other symptoms resulting simply from the size of the tumor and how it affects the surrounding tissues. When a tumor causes additional symptoms due to its size, it is known as mass effect. As the tumor grows, surrounding cells may become compressed, which results in cessation of physiological function. For example, pituitary tumors often present with changes in vision due to compression of the chiasma.

For many pituitary adenomas, transphenoidal surgery is the recommended treatment. This involves penetration of the sella turcica via the nasal and sinus passages. However, for prolactinomas, medical treatment is available in the form of medications that mimic the actions of pituitary-inhibiting factor. Generally, the application of these medications results in shrinking the tumor, but not its complete disappearance. Treatment of prolactinomas using medications is usually safer and less expensive than surgery. Surgical intervention is reserved for cases in which the tumor has become too large to be controlled by medications.

2. A researcher seeks to identify how a prolactinoma affects the production of other hormones, but can only take samples from an IV placed in the wrist. Which of the following is unlikely to be measured?

A. Thyroid-stimulating hormone
B. Cortisol-releasing hormone
C. Adrenocorticotropic hormone
D. Follicle-stimulating hormone

What is your triage decision?

Sample Passage 3

The simple nervous system of the sea snail *Aplysia* has been used as a model system to explore the processes of short-term memory. When the mollusk's siphon is touched, sensory neurons stimulate motor neurons, causing the animal's gill to withdraw. However, with repeated touching of the siphon, the animal becomes habituated to stimulus and no longer withdraws its gill in response. Electric shock resensitizes the snail and following a shock, it will once again withdraw its gill in response to a touch on the siphon. This resensitization can last for days and is a simple form of short-term memory.

The cause of habituation has been traced to a reduction in the amount of neurotransmitter released by the sensory neurons in response to repeated touching of the siphon. This leads to a decrease in the post-synaptic potential and a consequent decrease in contraction of the gill muscles.

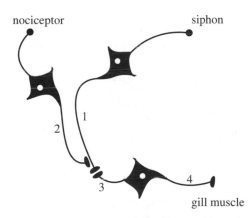

Figure 1. The nerve system of the sea snail *Aplysia*.

3. A researcher gently brushes the *Aplysia* siphon and monitors action potentials in the mollusk's nervous system. The researcher then presses the siphon more forcefully, leading to:

   A. larger action potentials at point 1.
   B. depolarization at point 2.
   C. more frequent action potentials at point 1.
   D. fewer action potentials at point 4.

What is your triage decision?

LESSON 5.4, LEARNING GOAL 2:

• Use question stems and answer choices to preview and triage MCAT questions

Practice Passage (Questions 1–7)

The simple nervous system of the sea snail *Aplysia* has been used as a model system to explore the processes of short-term memory. When the mollusk's siphon is touched, sensory neurons stimulate motor neurons, causing the animal's gill to withdraw. However, with repeated touching of the siphon, the animal becomes habituated to stimulus and no longer withdraws its gill in response. Electric shock resensitizes the snail and following a shock, it will once again withdraw its gill in response to a touch on the siphon. This resensitization can last for days and is a simple form of short-term memory.

The cause of habituation has been traced to a reduction in the amount of neurotransmitter released by the sensory neurons in response to repeated touching of the siphon. This leads to a decrease in the post-synaptic potential and a consequent decrease in contraction of the gill muscles.

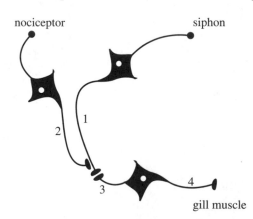

Figure 1. The nerve system of the sea snail *Aplysia*.

In sensitization, an electric shock stimulates nociceptors, which respond to pain stimuli. These neurons synapse on the presynaptic axon terminal of the siphon-touch sense neurons, as shown in Figure 1. The nociceptor terminals release serotonin, which binds to cell-surface receptors on the sensory presynaptic terminal and leads to the production of cAMP within the cell. cAMP activates a protein kinase, which phosphorylates voltage-gated K^+ channels on the membrane and causes them to remain shut. When action potentials arrive at the axon terminal, K^+ channels do not open and K^+ cannot flow out of the cell. Voltage-gated Ca^{++} channels remain open longer, allowing more Ca^{++} to flow into the cell. This leads to a larger release of neurotransmitter and a larger excited post-synaptic potential in the siphon motor neurons.

KAPLAN TIP

Remember, *you're taking the MCAT*. Don't let the test take you! You have to make strategic decisions about the questions to be efficient with your time and get the most points possible.

1. According to the information presented in the passage, which of the following is true regarding the membrane potential of the siphon axon terminal following sensitization?

   A. The axon terminal is hyperpolarized.
   B. The axon terminal is depolarized.
   C. The axon terminal remains polarized longer following action potential.
   D. The axon terminal remains depolarized longer following action potential.

   How would you triage this question?

2. A researcher gently brushes the *Aplysia* siphon and monitors action potentials in the mollusk's nervous system. The researcher then presses the siphon more forcefully, leading to:

   A. larger action potentials in the muscle neuron.
   B. depolarization at all points along the neuron.
   C. more frequent action potentials in the muscle neuron.
   D. fewer action potentials in the muscle neuron.

   How would you triage this question?

3. Which of the following effects of repeated stimulation of the siphon provides the most likely explanation for the habituation mechanism?

   A. Repeated stimulation leads to closure of calcium channels in the terminal membrane.
   B. Repeated stimulation leads to a decrease in the number of serotonin receptors in the terminal membrane.
   C. Repeated stimulation leads to a decrease in concentration of neurotransmitter-degrading enzymes in the siphon/gill muscle–nerve synapse.
   D. Repeated stimulation causes neurotransmitter vesicles to fuse with the terminal membrane in response to lower excitatory potentials.

   How would you triage this question?

4. Which of the following points indicated in Figure 1 are neuron axons?

   A. 1 and 2 only
   B. 1 and 3 only
   C. 2, 3, and 4 only
   D. 1, 2, and 4 only

   How would you triage this question?

KAPLAN TIP

The easier questions can help you understand the passage better, making you better prepared to answer the harder questions later.

LESSON 5.4, LEARNING GOAL 3:

• Determine when a question is a "pseudo-discrete" question

Practice Passage (Questions 1–7)

The simple nervous system of the sea snail *Aplysia* has been used as a model system to explore the processes of short-term memory. When the mollusk's siphon is touched, sensory neurons stimulate motor neurons, causing the animal's gill to withdraw. However, with repeated touching of the siphon, the animal becomes habituated to stimulus and no longer withdraws its gill in response. Electric shock resensitizes the snail and following a shock, it will once again withdraw its gill in response to a touch on the siphon. This resensitization can last for days and is a simple form of short-term memory.

The cause of habituation has been traced to a reduction in the amount of neurotransmitter released by the sensory neurons in response to repeated touching of the siphon. This leads to a decrease in the post-synaptic potential and a consequent decrease in contraction of the gill muscles.

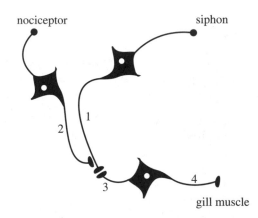

Figure 1. The nerve system of the sea snail *Aplysia.*

In sensitization, an electric shock stimulates nociceptors, which respond to pain stimuli. These neurons synapse on the presynaptic axon terminal of the siphon-touch sense neurons, as shown in Figure 1. The nociceptor terminals release serotonin, which binds to cell-surface receptors on the sensory presynaptic terminal and leads to the production of cAMP within the cell. cAMP activates a protein kinase, which phosphorylates voltage-gated K^+ channels on the membrane and causes them to remain shut. When action potentials arrive at the axon terminal, K^+ channels do not open and K^+ cannot flow out of the cell. Voltage-gated Ca^{++} channels remain open longer, allowing more Ca^{++} to flow into the cell. This leads to a larger release of neurotransmitter and a larger excited post-synaptic potential in the siphon motor neurons.

5. Ca^{++} channels in the sensory presynaptic terminal are likely to stay open longest at what voltage, due to K^+ ions being unable to leave the cell after sensitization?

   A. Less than −70 mV
   B. −70 mV
   C. 0 mV
   D. +35 mV

How would you triage this question?

What information is needed from the passage to answer this question?

6. A researcher determines the volume of serotonin released by a set of nociceptors to be 0.223 μL over 20 seconds. If this rate continues, how much serotonin could these same nociceptors produce in one hour?

   A. 2.007×10^{-3} mL/hr
   B. 4.014×10^{-2} mL/hr
   C. 8.028×10^{-1} mL/hr
   D. 4.014×10^{1} mL/hr

How would you triage this question?

What information is needed from the passage to answer this question?

7. Some anesthetics work by blocking voltage-gated Na^+ channels. These drugs work particularly well on sensory neurons, and therefore block the transmission of pain. If an anesthetic like this was applied to the habituated gill of an *Aplysia* followed by electric shock, what would the likely response be and why?

   A. The gill muscle would not become resensitized due to no serotonin being released by the nociceptor.
   B. The gill muscle would become resensitized due to serotonin being released by the nociceptor.
   C. The gill muscle would become habituated due to K^+ channels being open for longer.
   D. The gill muscle would become resensitized due to K^+ channels getting phosphorylated.

How would you triage this question?

What information is needed from the passage to answer this question?

KAPLAN TIP
Don't waste time doing questions with long calculations first. Save these questions for the end of the section.

LESSON 5.4 REVIEW

Triaging the Section:

1. Discrete questions

2. Ask yourself for each passage:

   How difficult do you find this topic?
   How difficult is the sentence structure and vocabulary?
   Are there figures, tables, graphs, or equations?
   How long is the passage?

   And then do:

   Easiest passages
   Passages with ambiguous difficulty
   Hardest passages

Triaging the Questions:

Characteristics of Easier Questions	Characteristics of Harder Questions
Shorter question stems and answer choices	Longer question stems and answer choices
Little to no passage research required	Heavy passage research required
The way to answer the question is clear	The way to answer the question is not clear and must be figured out
The question requires no calculations	The question requires calculations
The question is testing Skill 1	The question is testing Skill 2

Wrong Answer Types (Sciences)

In this lesson, you'll learn to:

- Eliminate wrong answers quickly using the repetitive structure of answers
- Recognize common wrong answer pathologies for science questions

Science Topics:

- Oxidative Phosphorylation
- Mitosis, Meiosis, and Other Factors Affecting Genetic Variability
- Endocrine System

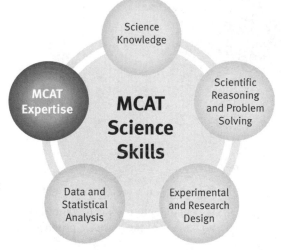

LESSON 5.5, LEARNING GOAL 1:

• Eliminate wrong answers quickly using the repetitive structure of answers

Answer Choices with Little Repetition:

1. Which is the last enzyme in the electron transport chain?

   A. Hexokinase
   B. Pyruvate decarboxylase
   C. Alcohol dehydrogenase
   D. Cytochrome c oxidase

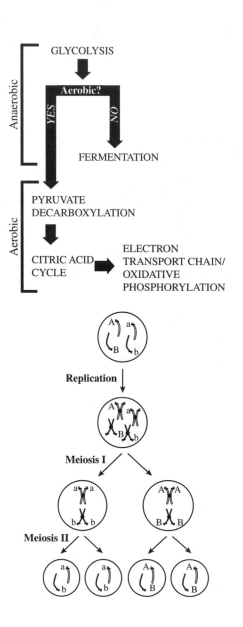

2. A mutation has occurred in one chromosome of a spermatogonium. This mutation will show up in how many of the gametes produced from this cell?

   A. None
   B. One-fourth
   C. Half
   D. All

Answer Choices with Repetition:

3. Testosterone is converted to estradiol via aromatase, a member of the CYP450 family of enzymes. Estradiol receptors fall into two classes: ER (further divided into ERα and ERβ) and G protein-coupled receptors (GPR30). Where are these receptors most likely to be located?

    A. ERα and ERβ are likely to be embedded in the cell membrane, and GPR30 is likely to be dissolved in the cytosol.
    B. ERα and ERβ are likely to be dissolved in the cytosol, and GPR30 is likely to be found embedded in the cell membrane.
    C. ERα, ERβ, and GPR30 are all likely to be found dissolved in the cytosol.
    D. ERα, ERβ, and GPR30 are all likely to be found embedded in the cell membrane.

4. During the generation of the proton-motive force:

    A. the pH of the mitochondrial matrix decreases and the pH of the intermembrane space increases.
    B. the pH of the mitochondrial matrix decreases and the pH of the intermembrane space decreases.
    C. the pH of the mitochondrial matrix increases and the pH of the intermembrane space increases.
    D. the pH of the mitochondrial matrix increases and the pH of the intermembrane space decreases.

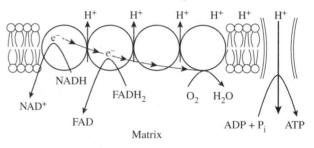

5. Crossing over, a contributor to genetic variation, most commonly occurs between:

    A. homologous chromosomes during prophase I of mitosis.
    B. homologous chromosomes during prophase I of meiosis.
    C. nonhomologous chromosomes during prophase I of mitosis.
    D. nonhomologous chromosomes during prophase I of meiosis.

KAPLAN TIP

Use the Assess Step to gain a "repetitive" advantage!

K

LESSON 5.5, LEARNING GOAL 2:

- Recognize common wrong answer pathologies for science questions

Common Wrong Answer Pathologies:

1. Which of the following would be expected to be observed in an adult with a functioning male reproductive system?

Wrong Answer Choice	FUD	OPP	OS	DIST/EXT
ADH, released in response to high plasma osmolarity, is synthesized in the hypothalamus and transported to the posterior pituitary for storage by the body's only portal system.				
GnRH stimulates the anterior pituitary to release FSH and LH, which act primarily on the Leydig and Sertoli cells, respectively.				
The presence of testosterone and its derivatives induce the development of the Wolffian duct, a key component in male sexual differentiation.				
Prolactin and oxytocin, whose secretion is increased during pregnancy, act to stimulate milk production and let down.				
During times of inadequate iodine intake, TSH levels are reduced, because iodine is necessary to produce the thyroid hormones.				
After a meal, insulin is secreted by beta cells in the pancreas, thereby maintaining elevated plasma glucose levels.				

FUD = faulty use of detail; OPP = opposite; OS= out of scope; DIST/EXT = distortion or extreme

Miscalculations:

6. Given the reduction potentials below and $\Delta G^{\circ\prime} = -nF\Delta E_0'$ (n = moles of e^- transferred and $F = 96.48$ kJ mol^{-1} V^{-1}), approximately how much energy is released by the system as a molecule of NADH is oxidized?

$$\frac{1}{2} O_2 + 2 H^+ + 2 e^- \rightarrow H_2O \qquad E_0' = +0.82\,V$$

$$NAD^+ + H^+ + 2 e^- \rightarrow NADH \qquad E_0' = -0.32\,V$$

A. 1.6×10^{-19} J
B. 1.8×10^{-19} J
C. 3.6×10^{-19} J
D. 3.6×10^{-22} J

The correct calculations:

$$\frac{1}{2} O_2 + NADH + H^+ \rightarrow H_2O + NAD^+$$

$$\Delta E_0' = E_0'\,(\textbf{cathode}) - E_0'\,(\textbf{anode})$$

$$\Delta E_0' = +0.82 - (-0.32)$$

$$\Delta E_0' = +1.14\,V$$

$$\Delta G^{\circ\prime} = -(2)\left(96.48\text{ kJ mol}^{-1}\,V^{-1}\right)\left(1.14\ V\right)$$

$$\Delta G^{\circ\prime} = -220\text{ kJ mol}^{-1}$$

$$\frac{220\text{ kJ}}{\text{mol NADH}} \times \frac{1\,\text{mol NADH}}{6.02 \times 10^{23}\text{ molecules NADH}}$$

$$= \frac{220\text{ kJ}}{6.02 \times 10^{23}\text{ molecules NADH}}$$

$$= 36 \times 10^{-23}\ \frac{\textbf{kJ}}{\textbf{molecule}}$$

$$3.6 \times 10^{-22}\ \frac{\text{kJ}}{\text{molecule}} \times \frac{1000\ \text{J}}{1\,\text{kJ}}$$

$$= 3.6 \times 10^{-19}\ \frac{\text{J}}{\text{molecule}}$$

Common miscalculations:

(A) is derived by confusing sign convention.

$$\Delta E_0' = +0.82 + (-0.32)$$

$$\Delta E_0' = +\textbf{0.50}\ V$$

(B) may be obtained by incorrectly substituting 1 for n.

(D) results from a failure to convert units.

KAPLAN TIP

The answer choices, and the relationships between them, can reveal key steps in the solution to a calculation problem.

Practice Passage (Questions 7–10)

Many genetically inherited disorders result from chromosomal abnormalities involving autosomes, sex chromosomes, or both. The abnormalities can be classified as either structural or numerical.

Structural abnormalities result from chromosome breakage and subsequent reconstitution in an abnormal combination. This often results in a translocation—the rearrangement of genetic material from one chromosome to another. The most common outcome of a translocation is a balanced rearrangement resulting in chromosome sets with the normal complement of genetic information arranged in different positions. An unbalanced rearrangement results in chromosome sets that contain additional or missing genetic information. Figure 1 shows a specific type of balanced translocation, a Robertsonian translocation.

Numerical abnormalities result when an individual is either missing a chromosome from a pair (monosomy) or has more than two chromosomes (trisomy denotes three representatives of a particular chromosome). Partial trisomy refers to trisomy for only a portion of a chromosome. The causes of these abnormalities are not entirely understood. It is supposed that most cases result from meiotic nondisjunction—the failure of a pair of chromosomes to separate normally during one of the two meiotic divisions, most often during meiosis I.

Trisomy or monosomy for a whole chromosome rarely results in a viable phenotype. Trisomy 21 (Down syndrome), trisomy 18, and trisomy 13 are the only well-defined instances of autosomal trisomy that are observed in postnatal infants, and each of these results in an abnormal phenotype. Monosomy for an entire chromosome in a live birth is only observed for the X chromosome, a condition known as Turner's syndrome. It is interesting to note that although the great majority of Down syndrome cases have 47 chromosomes, approximately 5% of Down syndrome cases have the normal chromosome number with the third copy of chromosome 21 translocated onto and fused with another chromosome.

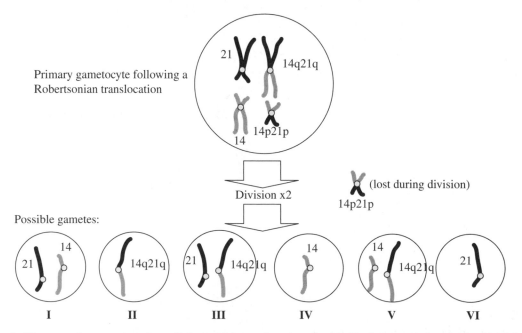

Figure 1. Diagram of segregation after a Robertsonian translocation; the 14p21p fragment is lost during division with no phenotypic effect (the genes on this fragment are also found on other chromosomes).

7. In Figure 1, which of the gametes (I, II, III, IV, V, VI) will most likely produce a viable, normal phenotype?

    A. I and II only
    B. I and III only
    C. I, II, and III only
    D. I, II, and IV only

What do you notice in the answer choices?

8. Which of the following events would most likely lead to partial trisomy?

    A. A base substitution in the DNA of a pluripotent cell
    B. An unbalanced rearrangement in germ line tissue
    C. An inversion of a single segment of an autosome
    D. The deletion of a portion of a sex chromosome

What do you notice in the answer choices?

9. Which of the following hypotheses might explain the disproportionate number of babies with Down syndrome born to mothers over 35 years of age?

    A. Older eggs require fertilization by multiple sperm.
    B. Older eggs contain a higher percentage of mutated chromosomes.
    C. Older eggs are more likely to disjoin incorrectly.
    D. Older eggs are not susceptible to translocations.

What do you notice in the answer choices?

10. Robertsonian translocation carriers contain all essential DNA and are phenotypically normal, even though they inherited two chromosomes fused together because of the Robertsonian translocation. Are zygotes fertilized by a Robertsonian translocation carrier at greater than average risk for trisomy?

    A. Yes, because the carrier's chromosomal mutation will be transmitted to all of their offspring.
    B. Yes, because of increased odds that the carrier will pass on two copies of the same genetic material.
    C. Yes, because in addition to the risk of meiotic nondisjunction, the zygote has a 5% chance of developing trisomy from a Robertsonian translocation.
    D. No, because the carrier has the normal complement of DNA and is phenotypically normal.

What do you notice in the answer choices?

KAPLAN TIP

When wrong answer pathologies show up in the science sections of the MCAT, noticing them will help your process of elimination.

LESSON 5.5 REVIEW

Wrong Answer Types (Sciences)

Miscalculation

- Is wrong because
  - It has values or units inconsistent with the correct answer
  - Often follows from common mathematical errors

Faulty Use of Detail (FUD)

- Is wrong because
  - It misrepresents information in the passage or question stem
  - Does not answer the question that was asked

Opposite (OPP)

- Is wrong because
  - It is the exact opposite concept/idea from the correct answer
  - May confuse a relationship (i.e. increase *vs.* decrease)

Out of Scope (OS)

- Is wrong because
  - It presents information irrelevant to the question

Distortion or Extreme (DIST/EXT)

- Is wrong because
  - It manipulates factual information, altering its validity

Strategic Guessing

In this lesson, you'll learn to:

- Choose the answer most likely to be correct when guessing the answer to a question

Science Topics:

- Alcohols
- Aldehydes and Ketones
- Carboxylic Acids
- Acid Derivatives
- Molecular Structure and Absorption Spectra

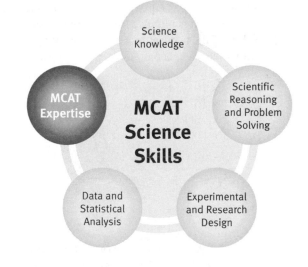

LESSON 5.6, LEARNING GOAL 1:

- Choose the answer most likely to be correct when guessing the answer to a question

Math Estimation

1. Simvastatin's concentration is measured and calculated by the following equation:

$$A = \varepsilon \times l \times c$$

   The cuvette length, l, is 0.5 cm; ε is 18,000; and absorbance, A, is equal to $2 - \log(\%T)$, where $\%T$ is the transmittance found in the experiment $\times$ 100. If the transmittance is 0.1, what is simvastatin's concentration, c?

   A. 5.7×10^{-4} M
   B. 1.1×10^{-4} M
   C. 8.2×10^{-5} M
   D. 2.5×10^{-5} M

   How can you eliminate wrong answers in this question?

2. Specific rotation, $[\alpha]$ (units of $° \cdot dm^{-1} \cdot mL \cdot g^{-1}$), for D-glucose is +52.5, and observed rotation, α, for D-glucose in an experiment is 7.80°. Using the equation:

$$[\alpha] = \frac{\alpha}{l \times c}$$

   where l is the sample tube length (1 dm in this case), what is the concentration, c, of D-glucose?

   A. 1.49×10^{-1} g/mL
   B. 1.52×10^{-2} g/mL
   C. 3.78×10^{-2} g/mL
   D. 2.56×10^{-3} g/mL

   How can you eliminate wrong answers in this question?

Answer Implications

3. The following is the chemical composition of ricinine:

    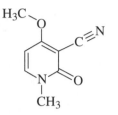

    The following IR spectrum was obtained from an unknown compound:

    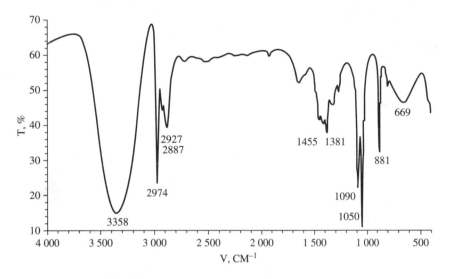

    Is this the IR spectrum for the alkaloid ricinine?

    A. Yes, as confirmed by the presence of the peak at 3300 cm^{-1}.
    B. Yes, as confirmed by the absence of the peak at 1750 cm^{-1}.
    C. No, as confirmed by the absence of the peak at 1750 cm^{-1}.
    D. Not enough information is given.

How can you eliminate wrong answers in this question?

Equivalent or Extreme Answers

4. The rate of the first step in the cross-linking reaction will be increased by acidic conditions. This is because acidic conditions:

   A. cause lysine's amino group to protonate, making it more nucleophilic.
   B. garner nucleophilic quality by attaching a hydrogen ion to the amino group of lysine.
   C. decrease the rate at which imine intermediate is formed.
   D. make the formation of an oxocarbenium intermediate more likely.

How can you eliminate wrong answers in this question?

5. The mechanism of 4-aminobutanoic acid lactam synthesis proceeds through each of the following steps EXCEPT:

   A. nucleophilic addition to form a by-product.
   B. condensation reaction involving an amine group.
   C. loss of water from the product.
   D. nucleophilic attack on the carbonyl carbon.

How can you eliminate wrong answers in this question?

Maximum and Minimum Questions

6. The figure below shows plots of the vapor pressure of several compounds as a function of temperature. Which of them has the lowest boiling point if the ambient pressure is 0.5 atm?

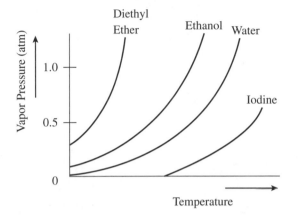

A. Diethyl ether
B. Ethanol
C. Water
D. Iodine

How can you eliminate wrong answers in this question?

7. In ozonolysis, ozone cleaves unsaturated carbon–carbon bonds and replaces those bonds with carbonyls. How many ketone groups are found in the product of the following reaction?

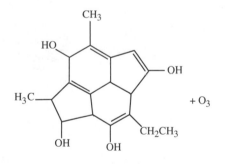

A. 0
B. 5
C. 8
D. 15

How can you eliminate wrong answers in this question?

Roman Numeral Questions

8. Which of the following is/are true of compound A, the product of the student's first experiment?

   I. It has a conjugated pi system.

   II. It has adjacent carbon atoms with unhybridized p-orbitals.

   III. It is more stable than compound B.

   A. I only
   B. I and II only
   C. II and III only
   D. I, II, and III

How can you eliminate wrong answers in this question?

KAPLAN TIP

Roman numeral questions, while rare on the MCAT, are particularly ripe for strategic guessing because there are two rounds of elimination possible: first eliminating the Roman numerals and then eliminating answer choices containing those Roman numerals.

Questions in the CARS Section

Passage Excerpt:

Since nontherapeutic experimentation confers no benefit on the subject, it has been more controversial. While the need for nontherapeutic experimentation is now generally accepted, there is still controversy over how best to select or encourage volunteers. Finally, although those conducting both therapeutic and nontherapeutic experiments have attempted to take precautions by conducting their research on animals first, there remains an inevitable risk for human volunteers. To minimize possible hazards, certain traditional safeguards have been utilized.

Tone

9. In which of the following ways do therapeutic experimentation and nontherapeutic experimentation differ?

   A. Therapeutic experimentation offers volunteers improved health as an incentive.
   B. Nontherapeutic experimentation is a relic of a bygone era in medical science.
   C. Therapeutic experimentation is performed on healthy volunteers.
   D. Nontherapeutic experimentation is not consistent with conventional medical ethics.

How can you eliminate wrong answers in this question?

Vague Language

10. On the subject of nontherapeutic experimentation, the scientific community has been:

   A. divided over the necessity of obtaining an informed consent from subjects' physicians.
   B. somewhat more receptive of therapeutic research than of nontherapeutic research.
   C. completely opposed to the sentiments expressed by other members of society on this issue.
   D. appalled by the government's delayed acceptance of nontherapeutic testing.

How can you eliminate wrong answers in this question?

KAPLAN TIP

There's no such thing as a "best" Blind Guessing strategy, but the strategies from this lesson are a good way to approximate the answer if you're stuck.

LESSON 5.6 REVIEW

Strategic Guessing—Question and Answer Characteristics

Questions have...

> Math that will take too much time or is easy to estimate
>
> Aspects about tone in a CARS passage

Answers have...

> Obvious patterns
>
> Logic dictating some choices must be wrong
>
> Extreme choices
>
> Roman numerals

Test-Specific Situations for Strategic Guessing

> When running out of time
>
> When you don't know the answer
>
> Anytime guessing is much easier or faster than answering a different way

MCAT Science Strategies in Action

In this lesson, you'll learn to:

- Use the Kaplan Triage Strategy for MCAT science passages
- Use the Kaplan Passage Strategy for MCAT science passages
- Use the Kaplan Question Strategy for MCAT science questions
- Use Kaplan methods on answer choices within MCAT science questions

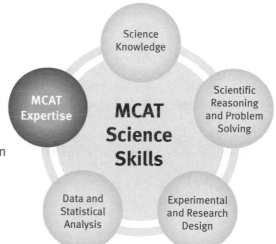

MCAT SCIENCE STRATEGY

Passage Strategy

SCAN FOR STRUCTURE

READ STRATEGICALLY

LABEL EACH COMPONENT

REFLECT ON YOUR OUTLINE

Question Strategy

ASSESS THE QUESTION

PLAN YOUR ATTACK

EXECUTE THE PLAN

ANSWER BY MATCHING, ELIMINATING, OR GUESSING

LESSON 5.7, LEARNING GOALS 1–4:

- Use the Kaplan Triage Strategy for MCAT science passages
- Use the Kaplan Passage Strategy for MCAT science passages
- Use the Kaplan Question Strategy for MCAT science questions
- Use Kaplan methods on answer choices within MCAT science questions

Practice Passage 1 (Questions 1–3)

The human kidney can concentrate the fluid it filters out of the blood up to ~1200 mOsm/L. The flow rate of this filtrate is in part what determines the amount of water resorbed by the body due to pressure change with rate of flow. The countercurrent multiplier is the method by which the kidney accomplishes this task. The steps within this countercurrent multiplier are outlined below and in Figure 1. These steps are repeated over and over so that, over time, solutes are trapped in the medulla up until a concentration of ~1200 mOsm/L is reached.

Step 1: Assume the loop of Henle is filled with fluid with a concentration of 300 mOsm/L.

Step 2: The active pump of the thick ascending limb is turned on, reducing the concentration inside the tubule and increasing the concentration of the interstitial fluid (maximum difference = 200 mOsm/L).

Step 3: Tubular fluid in the descending limb quickly reaches osmotic equilibrium with interstitial fluid because the descending limb is permeable to water.

Step 4: Additional flow of fluid into the loop of Henle from the proximal convoluted tubule causes the hyperosmotic fluid previously formed in the descending limb to flow into the ascending limb.

Step 5: Once this fluid is in the ascending limb, additional ions are pumped into the interstitium until a 200 mOsm/L gradient is established. Now the interstitial fluid osmolarity rises to 500 mOsm/L.

Step 6: The fluid in the descending limb reaches equilibrium with the hyperosmotic medullary interstitial fluid.

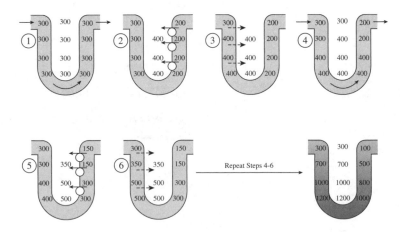

Figure 1. The countercurrent multiplier in the loop of Henle

Passage Outline

What can you learn from this passage?

P1.

List.

F1.

Questions

1. Countercurrent heat exchange is a process used by organisms to minimize heat loss through the skin's surface. The basic mechanism is outlined below.

   What can you learn from this question?

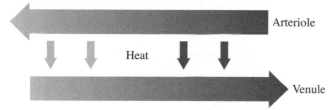

   Which of the following concepts in the kidney's countercurrent multiplier is most analogous to heat in the countercurrent heat exchange system?

   A. Filtration of blood
   B. Concentration of solutes in interstitium
   C. Active transport of ions
   D. Anti-parallel flow of fluid

2. If flow rate of filtrate through the loop of Henle increases, would membrane transport mechanisms need to act in order to prevent deviations from homeostasis?

   What can you learn from this question?

   A. Yes, to prevent a decrease in osmolarity in the filtrate in the descending limb of the loop of Henle
   B. Yes, to prevent an increase in osmolarity in the filtrate in the descending limb of the loop of Henle
   C. No, because this would cause no osmolarity change in the filtrate
   D. No, but this would cause a cessation of urine production

3. Which of the following is an accurate way of describing the thick ascending limb of the loop of Henle?

   What can you learn from this question?

   A. Site of glucose reabsorption from filtrate to body
   B. First step in filtering the blood to form urine
   C. Concentrating segment of the nephron
   D. Diluting segment of the nephron

Practice Passage 2 (Questions 4–6)

The citric acid cycle is the metabolic process by which the energy stored in pyruvate is transferred to electron carrier molecules. See Figure 1 for the steps in this cycle.

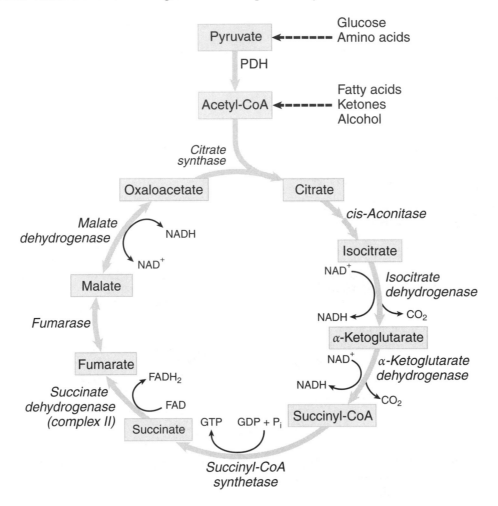

Figure 1. The citric acid cycle.

There are several metabolic disorders that originate with malfunctions of citric acid cycle enzymes; these disorders most commonly arise from deleterious mutations in the genes coding for these citric acid cycle enzymes. However, often the expression of the mutations is not uniform throughout the body. Most often, if the disorder is not uniformly expressed, the localized effects are found in the neuromuscular system.

Passage Outline

P1.

   F1.

P2.

Questions

4. Suppose a genetic defect renders the enzyme fumarase nonfunctional in some tissues of an organism. Due to this defect, it is most likely that:

   A. the citric acid cycle would cease to function in tissues where the genetic defect is not expressed.

   B. the organism would not be able to function.

   C. less NADH would be synthesized from the citric acid cycle in the mitochondria of these tissues.

   D. less succinate would be synthesized in all tissues of this organism.

5. Following a large meal, cells accumulate an excess of acetyl-CoA in mitochondria. What effect does this have on cells?

   A. Acetyl-CoA is used to form succinyl-CoA, which moves to the cytoplasm for beta oxidation.

   B. Acetyl-CoA is used to form citrate, which moves to the cytoplasm for fatty acid synthesis.

   C. Acetyl-CoA moves directly to the cytoplasm, where it is combined with oxaloacetate to form citrate.

   D. Acetyl-CoA is used to form α-ketoglutarate, which moves to the cytoplasm for ketogenesis.

6. Which of the following is NOT a potential explanation for why a genetic defect in the citric acid cycle would be observed in some tissues and not others within a single, healthy organism?

   A. Variations in regulation of gene transcription across tissues

   B. Variations in regulation of gene translation across tissues

   C. Variations in tissue capability to adapt to citric acid cycle malfunction

   D. Variations in the presence of the gene locus in cell nuclei in somatic cells

What can you learn from this passage?

What can you learn from this question?

What can you learn from this question?

What can you learn from this question?

LESSON 5.7 REVIEW

Chapter 5 Learning Goals

5.1 Science Passage Strategy

- Preview a science passage at a glance, determining likely topics and difficulty
- Identify the most question-relevant information in a science passage
- Create efficient and useful passage outlines

5.2 Science Questions: Assess and Plan

- Assess a question and its answer choices for difficulty, science topic, and common patterns
- Plan an efficient way to answer a given question

5.3 Science Questions: Execute and Answer

- Judge when predicting an answer is a useful strategy
- Make strong and accurate predictions for answers before reading through answer choices
- Recognize when an answer matches a prediction

5.4 Triage in the Science Sections

- Utilize the triaging strategy within a science section of the MCAT
- Use question stems and answer choices to preview and triage MCAT questions
- Determine when a question is a "pseudo-discrete" question

5.5 Wrong Answer Types (Sciences)

- Eliminate wrong answers quickly using the repetitive structure of answers
- Recognize common wrong answer pathologies for science questions

5.6 Strategic Guessing

- Choose the answer most likely to be correct when guessing the answer to a question

CHAPTER

6

CARS Skills

CARS Passage Structure and Strategy

In this lesson, you'll learn to:

- Utilize the Kaplan Passage Strategy, given a CARS passage

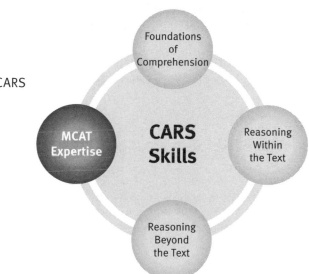

LESSON 6.1, LEARNING GOAL

- Utilize the Kaplan Passage Strategy, given a CARS passage

The Kaplan Method for CARS Passages

SCAN FOR STRUCTURE
Decide whether to read the passage now or later

READ STRATEGICALLY
Quickly read the passage, looking for keywords and connections

LABEL EACH COMPONENT
Write a brief description of each paragraph

REFLECT ON YOUR OUTLINE
Include the goal of the passage in your outline

The SCAN Step: Passage Types

HUMANITIES	SOCIAL SCIENCES
Architecture	Anthropology
Art	Archaeology
Dance	Cultural Studies
Ethics	Economics
Literature	Education
Music	Geography
Philosophy	History
Popular Culture	Linguistics
Religion	Political Science
Theater	Population Health
	Psychology
	Sociology

The SCAN Step: Triage

Read this passage excerpt:

W.H. Auden's reputation, already declining by the 1950s, reached its nadir with the publication of his posthumous collection *Thank You, Fog* (1974). Critics almost unanimously found his last work trite and garrulous. Indeed, the assessment has served as a retrospective judgment on the poet's final three decades.

What is the passage type?

Would you read this passage now or later?

Now try this one:

The simple notion that the president proposes and Congress disposes is greatly complicated by the fragmentation of power within each branch. Moreover, efforts to make fiscal policy more coherent have added new power centers without consolidating old ones. Presidents have tried various coordination mechanisms including "troika" arrangements and an almost infinite variety of committees...

What is the passage type?

Would you read this passage now or later?

Now try this one:

The notion of realism in literature is based largely on the implicit belief that writers can accurately transform common objects or ideas from life into words on a page while maintaining an accurate representation of the object or idea. If an author writes a novel which seems believable, meaning that a reader can imagine events in the novel actually happening, then that book is often considered a "realistic" work of literature.

What is the passage type?

Would you read this passage now or later?

KAPLAN TIP

Don't forget to triage on Test Day! This will increase your efficiency while taking the test.

The READ Step: Keywords

After the outbreak of World War II and his emigration to the United States, Auden, while not entirely rejecting the theme of political insecurity, manifested decidedly different concerns. Although he maintained his interest in technique by experimenting with meter and form, he increasingly felt that the lyricism that came so naturally to him gave rise to dishonest sentiment and didacticism.

Gradually, Auden developed a middle manner which was less grand and more discursive. This manner could also accommodate his new thematic interests.

Often called dry and prosaic, Auden's mature style was as an appropriate vehicle for his later concerns.

Critics should view Auden's later style as the best way to support his shift in interests.

Thematically, some say the shift might be viewed as one from society to the self.

Relation Keywords

Difference

Similarity

Author Keywords

Positive *vs.* Negative

Extreme

Moderating

The READ Step: Keywords

Because they were unwilling to come to terms with the change in Auden's intellectual concerns, and since they were misinterpreting his rejection of lyric excitement, critics therefore wrongly dismissed the later works as productions of a worn-out talent.

Much of the criticism of his tampering calls into question this wrong-headed idea that an artist must not disappoint an audience prepared to accept one point of view by evolving as a thinker.

Logic Keywords

Evidence and Conclusion

Refutation

KAPLAN TIP
Keywords are one way the testmaker says, "We'll be asking you about this later, in the questions."

The LABEL and REFLECT Steps

Those who consider the Devil to be a partisan of Evil and angels to be warriors for Good accept the demagogy of the angels. Things are clearly more complicated. Angels are partisans not of Good, but of Divine creation. The Devil, on the other hand, denies all rational meaning to God's world.

World domination, as everyone knows, is divided between demons and angels. But the good of the world does not require the latter to gain precedence over the former (as I thought when I was young); all it needs is a certain equilibrium of power. If there is too much uncontested meaning on Earth (the reign of the angels), man collapses under the burden; if the world loses all its meaning (the reign of the demons), life is every bit as impossible.

Things deprived suddenly of their putative meaning, the place assigned to them in the ostensible order of things, make us laugh. Initially, therefore, laughter is the province of the Devil, who knows what it means to be abruptly stripped of rank—he could not help but guffaw after being cast from the Heavens and plunging into the bowels of the Earth. This laughter has a certain malice to it (things have turned out differently from the way they tried to seem), but a certain beneficent relief as well (things are looser than they seemed, we have greater latitude in living with them, their gravity does not oppress us).

The first time an angel heard the Devil's laughter he was horrified. It was in the middle of a feast with a lot of people around, and one after the other they joined the Devil's laughter. It was terribly contagious. The angel was all too aware that the laughter was aimed against God and the wonder of His works. He knew he had to act fast, but felt weak and defenseless. Unable to fabricate anything of his own, he simply turned his enemy's tactics against him. He opened his mouth and let out a wobbly, breathy sound in the upper reaches of his vocal register and endowed it with the opposite meaning. Whereas the Devil's laughter pointed at the meaninglessness of things, the angel's shout rejoiced in how rationally organized, well-conceived, beautiful, good, and sensible everything on Earth was.

There they stood, Devil and angel, face to face, mouths open, both making more or less the same sound, but each expressing himself in a unique timbre—absolute opposites. And seeing the laughing angel, the Devil laughed all the harder, all the louder, and all the more openly, because the laughing angel was infinitely laughable.

Laughable laughter is cataclysmic. And even so, the angels have gained something by it. They have tricked us all with their semantic hoax. Their imitation laughter and its original (the Devil's) have the same name. People nowadays do not even realize that one and the same external phenomenon embraces two completely contradictory internal attitudes. We lack the words to distinguish these two types of laughter.

Framework for Passage Outline

P1. (A summary or label of paragraph 1)

P2. (A summary or label of paragraph 2)

P3. (A summary or label of paragraph 3)

P4. (A summary or label of paragraph 4)

P5. (A summary or label of paragraph 5)

P6. (A summary or label of paragraph 6)

Goal: (The main point and purpose of the passage)

Create your own Outline

P1.

P2.

P3.

P4.

P5.

P6.

Goal:

Example Passage Outlines

Sample Outline 1

P1. Angels aren't good; they represent creation; the Devil is anti-rational.

P2. The world needs balance between angels and demons.

P3. Devil's laughter (the initial kind) is caused by loss of meaning and has some benefit.

P4. Angel fought Devil's laughter with his own, celebrating rational order.

P5. Angels and the Devil compete.

P6. Two laughs treated alike due to ambiguity of language.

Goal: To argue that the meaning of the word "laughter" is ambiguous.

Sample Outline 2

P1. Ang not good, creat; Dev anti-rat

P2. need balance ang/dev

P3. Dev laugh 1st = loss of meaning

P4. Ang laugh, celeb order

P5. Ang/Dev compete

P6. 2 laughs = ambiguity

Goal: Argue word "laughter" ambiguous

Sample Outline 3

P1. Difference between Devil and Angels complicated

P2. Equilibrium of power necessary

P3. Laughter = loss of meaning = Devil

P4. Story of Angel's competing laugh

P5. "Laugh off"

P6. Angel wins by laughter semantics

Goal: Assert the word "laughter" is vague in meaning

LESSON 6.1 REVIEW

The Kaplan Method for CARS Passages

SCAN FOR STRUCTURE
Decide whether to read the passage now or later

- Look for passage type (humanities or social science)
- Determine the difficulty of the passage

READ STRATEGICALLY
Quickly read the passage, looking for keywords and connections

- Remember your keywords
- Find each paragraph's relation to the passage as a whole

LABEL EACH COMPONENT
Write a brief description of each paragraph

REFLECT ON YOUR OUTLINE
Include the goal of the passage in your outline

CARS Questions: Foundations of Comprehension

In this lesson, you'll learn to:

- Answer Main Idea questions
  - Identify the main idea of an MCAT CARS passage
- Answer Detail questions
  - Find the correct answer to a Detail question in a passage, and match it with an answer choice
- Answer Function questions
  - Determine the role of a portion of text as it relates to the passage as a whole
- Answer Definition-in-Context questions
  - Identify the meaning of a word or phrase in the context of where it appears in the passage

Founda-tions of Compre-hension

CARS Skills

MCAT Expertise

Reasoning Within the Text

Reasoning Beyond the Text

MCAT STRATEGY—CARS QUESTIONS

ASSESS THE QUESTION
Read the question (NOT the answers), looking for clues to the difficulty.

PLAN YOUR ATTACK
Think about question type, your outline, and researching the passage.

EXECUTE THE PLAN
Predict what you can about the answer.

ANSWER BY MATCHING, ELIMINATING, OR GUESSING
Find the right answer in the answer choices.

LESSON 6.2, LEARNING GOALS 1–4:

- Answer Main Idea questions
  - Identify the main idea of an MCAT CARS passage
- Answer Detail questions
  - Find the correct answer to a Detail question in a passage, and match it with an answer choice
- Answer Function questions
  - Determine the role of a portion of text as it relates to the passage as a whole
- Answer Definition-in-Context questions
  - Identify the meaning of a word or phrase in the context of where it appears in the passage

KAPLAN TIP

These question types may require less reasoning than others in the CARS section, but it's still important to move through them as quickly as possible to save time for other questions in the section.

CARS Question Types Map

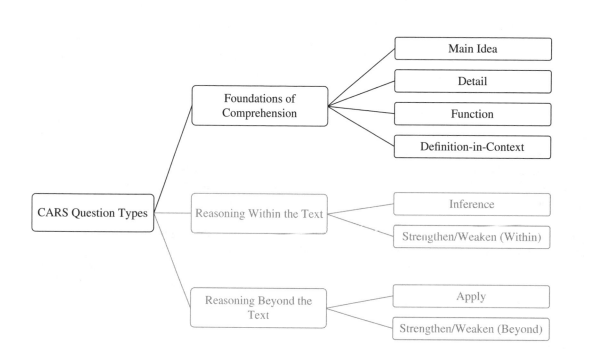

Foundations of Comprehension Introduction (Questions 1–4)

Visual art—drawing, painting, sculpture, and the like—holds a clear place and process in the mind of the general public. To clarify, I mean that the average person knows how a painting, for instance, is created, but the workings of other disciplines that craft visual experiences are less clear to the average member of their audience. The popular perception of these hard-working artists becomes the default: a hand wave of, "Oh, I'm sure it comes together somehow." This sentiment becomes progressively stronger as the creation in question becomes more collaborative, and as the final visual product is less of the audience's primary engagement with the work as a whole.

Theatrical design lies at the extreme of both the above trends: in addition to theater's status as one of the definitive collaborative art forms, the strictly visual aspects of a performance—scenic, costume, and lighting design—are not generally "why [one] goes to the theater." Because of the latter point in particular, these design aspects exist as nothing more than a subordinate credit in a play's program to most theatergoers, even as expensive modern technology and enhanced production values allow them to be an ever-larger part of the experience.

Needless to say, designers for the performing arts (which include dance and opera as well as theater) can bring a strong and definitive artistic voice to a work; and that voice is often nuanced and masterful. My own scenic design professor, who is now a Tony Award winner for his craft, was six-foot-four, with a build that would be placed by popular stereotype as more football player than dollhouse maker. But his giant hands would spend countless hours building miniature, astonishingly lifelike sets and stages out of cardstock and gesso.

Passage Outline

P1.

P2.

P3.

Goal (of P1–P3):

Main Idea Question

1. The central idea of the passage is:

   A. that the author's professor worked at the top of his field.
   B. that most visual art is misunderstood by the public.
   C. that theater is an art form equal to more popular forms.
   D. that some art requires more effort and skill than most people assume.

Detail Question

2. Which of the following is stated by the author regarding an audience's typical attitude toward theatrical productions?

   A. The audience does not notice visual design during a production.
   B. A Tony Award increases the appeal of a production.
   C. Scenic design is more noticeable than costume design.
   D. Visual design is not the primary motivation to attend a production.

Function Question

3. Drawing, painting, and sculpture are used by the author as examples of what?

   A. Reasons why theatergoers attend a production
   B. Arts whose creation process is well understood
   C. Collaborative visual art forms
   D. Crafts in which the author is trained

Definition-in-Context Question

4. In the context of the passage, "the default" (paragraph 1) most precisely means which of the following?

   A. A mistake made when attention is not paid
   B. An opinion held as a result of little thought
   C. A failure to repay a debt in a timely manner
   D. An original, natural state of a work of art

KAPLAN TIP

This passage will be continued on the next page, along with additional practice questions. For this exercise, however, you will only require the first three paragraphs (shown here).

Foundations of Comprehension Practice Passage (Questions 5–9)

Visual art—drawing, painting, sculpture, and the like—holds a clear place and process in the mind of the general public. To clarify, I mean that the average person knows how a painting, for instance, is created, but the workings of other disciplines that craft visual experiences are less clear to the average member of their audience. The popular perception of these hard-working artists becomes the default: a hand wave of, "Oh, I'm sure it comes together somehow." This sentiment becomes progressively stronger as the creation in question becomes more collaborative, and as the final visual product is less of the audience's primary engagement with the work as a whole.

Theatrical design lies at the extreme of both the above trends: in addition to theater's status as one of the definitive collaborative art forms, the strictly visual aspects of a performance—scenic, costume, and lighting design—are not generally "why [one] goes to the theater." Because of the latter point in particular, these design aspects exist as nothing more than a subordinate credit in a play's program to most theatergoers, even as expensive modern technology and enhanced production values allow them to be an ever-larger part of the experience.

Needless to say, designers for the performing arts (which include dance and opera as well as theater) can bring a strong and definitive artistic voice to a work; and that voice is often nuanced and masterful. My own scenic design professor, who is now a Tony Award winner for his craft, was six-foot-four, with a build that would be placed by popular stereotype as more football player than dollhouse maker. But his giant hands would spend countless hours building miniature, astonishingly lifelike sets and stages out of cardstock and gesso.

The models demanded absolute perfection and detail, because while the miniature is not the final product of the show itself, it is the final product of the designer. His role is to make a complete visualization of the stage and set dressings as the audience will experience it, but also to convey that vision in such a way that it can be duplicated by others who are tasked to build the full-size version out of plywood, metal, screen projections, and so on.

That flexibility given to the actual scene-builders is the heart of what makes breathtaking visual theater, and it also exposes a key tenet of collaborative art in general. The operant word is specialization: the scene is designed by a man or woman with an eye for weight, color, composition, and dramatic function; but it is then constructed by a team that knows how to build, fly, and weld. As an example, consider a designer who demands a bucking and swaying boat for the opening scene of Shakespeare's *The Tempest*. The designer will build a model with each plank on the boat just so, and that rocks back and forth to the exact angle desired of the final product. The exact mechanism of that rocking, on the other hand, whether it be hydraulic platforms, sophisticated video projections, or ultra-strong cables from the fly space above, is left to the engineers, carpenters, and technicians in the "scene shop." Compromises on the initial design may, of course, have to be made, but they are normally handled in consultation with the director and the designers, and especially in today's big-budget Broadway productions such scope adjustments are cut to an absolute minimum.

Passage Outline

P1.

P2.

P3.

P4.

P5.

Goal:

5. The passage cites the amount of money spent on a production as influencing all of the following EXCEPT:

    Question Type:

    A. the degree to which visual design can contribute to an audience's experience.
    B. the precise way in which a designer's vision is executed by the scene shop.
    C. the scope of a designer's vision as she delivers it to her colleagues.
    D. the amount by which a designer's vision is reduced during production.

6. The author mentions the size of the scenic design professor's hands to:

    Question Type:

    A. scoff at the mismatched traits of the professor.
    B. emphasize the professor's skill at model-building.
    C. make a contrast between expectation and reality.
    D. clarify how audience members feel watching a play.

7. "Visualization" (paragraph 4) is used in the passage to mean:

    Question Type:

    A. a physical portrayal of an idea.
    B. the mental image of a design concept.
    C. the final visual representation of an artistic work.
    D. forming a vision of future success.

KAPLAN TIP

Detail questions will likely be the most common question type you see in the Foundations of Comprehension category of CARS questions.

Foundations of Comprehension Practice Passage (Questions 5–9)

Visual art—drawing, painting, sculpture, and the like—holds a clear place and process in the mind of the general public. To clarify, I mean that the average person knows how a painting, for instance, is created, but the workings of other disciplines that craft visual experiences are less clear to the average member of their audience. The popular perception of these hard-working artists becomes the default: a hand wave of, "Oh, I'm sure it comes together somehow." This sentiment becomes progressively stronger as the creation in question becomes more collaborative, and as the final visual product is less of the audience's primary engagement with the work as a whole.

Theatrical design lies at the extreme of both the above trends: in addition to theater's status as one of the definitive collaborative art forms, the strictly visual aspects of a performance—scenic, costume, and lighting design—are not generally "why [one] goes to the theater." Because of the latter point in particular, these design aspects exist as nothing more than a subordinate credit in a play's program to most theatergoers, even as expensive modern technology and enhanced production values allow them to be an ever-larger part of the experience.

Needless to say, designers for the performing arts (which include dance and opera as well as theater) can bring a strong and definitive artistic voice to a work; and that voice is often nuanced and masterful. My own scenic design professor, who is now a Tony Award winner for his craft, was six-foot-four, with a build that would be placed by popular stereotype as more football player than dollhouse maker. But his giant hands would spend countless hours building miniature, astonishingly lifelike sets and stages out of cardstock and gesso.

The models demanded absolute perfection and detail because, while the miniature is not the final product of the show itself, it is the final product of the designer. His role is to make a complete visualization of the stage and set dressings as the audience will experience it, but also to convey that vision in such a way that it can be duplicated by others who are tasked to build the full-size version out of plywood, metal, screen projections, and so on.

That flexibility given to the actual scene-builders is the heart of what makes breathtaking visual theater, and it also exposes a key tenet of collaborative art in general. The operant word is specialization: the scene is designed by a man or woman with an eye for weight, color, composition, and dramatic function; but it is then constructed by a team that knows how to build, fly, and weld. As an example, consider a designer who demands a bucking and swaying boat for the opening scene of Shakespeare's *The Tempest*. The designer will build a model with each plank on the boat just so, and that rocks back and forth to the exact angle desired of the final product. The exact mechanism of that rocking, on the other hand, whether it be hydraulic platforms, sophisticated video projections, or ultra-strong cables from the fly space above, is left to the engineers, carpenters, and technicians in the "scene shop." Compromises on the initial design may, of course, have to be made, but they are normally handled in consultation with the director and the designers, and especially in today's big-budget Broadway productions such scope adjustments are cut to an absolute minimum.

8. The author describes a possible opening scene of *The Tempest* in the passage, along with the process by which it might be created. For which of the following concepts found elsewhere in the passage does this example serve as a counterpoint?

   A. "hand wave" (paragraph 1)
   B. "collaborative art" (paragraph 2)
   C. "complete visualization" (paragraph 4)
   D. "popular stereotype" (paragraph 3)

   Question Type:

9. Based on the passage, which of the following is a responsibility of directors in creating a theatrical production?

   A. Building models of what a play's set will look like
   B. Negotiating whether designers' visions will be simplified during production
   C. Acting as a manager to the actors who perform onstage
   D. Deciding how all elements of a production will be executed together on stage

   Question Type:

KAPLAN TIP

When passage references are given in a question stem, use them! There's no reason to overthink a question and tax your memory when the test itself is pointing you to the right place. Remember, though, to read text surrounding the quotation as well, so you see the context of the reference.

LESSON 6.2 REVIEW

CARS Skill 1: Foundations of Comprehension

Question Types

Main idea

- Answer will be the author's overall purpose
- Often will match the goal from your passage outline

Detail

- Demands a detail from the passage, sometimes paraphrased
- Passage outline and (optionally) highlighting will help

Function

- Asks *why* an author has included a detail or structure
- Answer will often match with your passage outline for the paragraph

Definition-in-Context

- Asks for meaning of a word or phrase, usually with a passage reference
- Don't fall for trap answers that are common (but incorrect) definitions

CARS Questions: Reasoning Within the Text

In this lesson, you'll learn to:

- Answer Inference questions
  - Identify the unstated parts of arguments in passages
- Answer Strengthen/Weaken (Within Passage) questions
  - Find text from the passage that produces the desired effect

MCAT STRATEGY—CARS QUESTIONS

ASSESS THE QUESTION
Read the question (NOT the answers), looking for clues to the difficulty.

PLAN YOUR ATTACK
Think about question type, your outline, and researching the passage.

EXECUTE THE PLAN
Predict what you can about the answer.

ANSWER BY MATCHING, ELIMINATING, OR GUESSING
Find the right answer in the answer choices.

Foundations of Comprehension

MCAT Expertise

CARS Skills

Reasoning Within the Text

Reasoning Beyond the Text

LESSON 6.3, LEARNING GOALS 1 AND 2:

- Answer Inference questions
  - Identify the unstated parts of arguments in passages
- Answer Strengthen/Weaken (Within Passage) questions
  - Find text from the passage that produces the desired effect

CARS Question Types Map

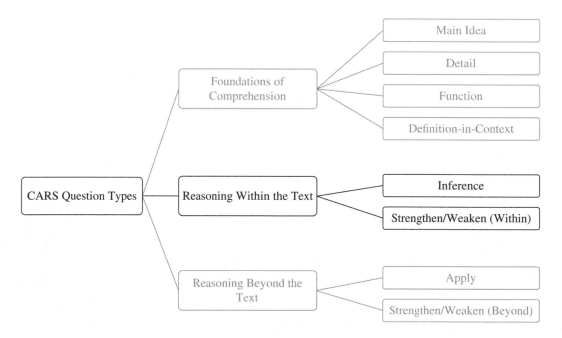

Reasoning Within the Text Introduction (Questions 1–2)

If one always ought to act so as to produce the best possible circumstances, then morality is extremely demanding. No one could plausibly claim to have met the requirements of this "simple principle." It would seem strange to punish those intending to do good by sentencing them to an impossible task. Also, if the standards of right conduct are as extreme as they seem, then they will preclude the personal projects that humans find most fulfilling.

From an analytic perspective, the potential extreme demands of morality are not a "problem." A theory of morality is no less valid simply because it asks great sacrifices. In fact, it is difficult to imagine what kind of constraints could be put on our ethical projects. Shouldn't we reflect on our base prejudices, and not allow them to provide boundaries for our moral reasoning? Thus, it is tempting to simply dismiss the objections to the simple principle. However, in *Demands of Morality*, Liam Murphy takes these objections seriously for at least two distinct reasons.

Passage Outline

P1.

P2.

Inference Question

1. The author suggests that the "simple principle":

   A. has been employed by many philosophers, including Murphy.
   B. requires humans to prioritize the personal projects they find most fulfilling.
   C. holds that decisions must be made to produce the best possible outcomes.
   D. is a theory of morality that is simple to implement.

Strengthen/Weaken (Within) Question

2. Which of the following claims provides the most support in the passage for the "simple principle"?

   A. Ethical projects should be completely without constraints.
   B. Objections to the simple principle are difficult to imagine.
   C. Moral theories are not less valid if they require great sacrifices.
   D. Nobody always acts to produce the best possible circumstances.

KAPLAN TIP

The contrapositive to a conditional ("if…then") statement is guaranteed to be a true inference. For example, the contrapositive of "if A, then B" is "if not B, then not A."

K

Reasoning Within the Text Practice Passage (Questions 3–6)

If one always ought to act so as to produce the best possible circumstances, then morality is extremely demanding. No one could plausibly claim to have met the requirements of this "simple principle." It would seem strange to punish those intending to do good by sentencing them to an impossible task. Also, if the standards of right conduct are as extreme as they seem, then they will preclude the personal projects that humans find most fulfilling.

From an analytic perspective, the potential extreme demands of morality are not a "problem." A theory of morality is no less valid simply because it asks great sacrifices. In fact, it is difficult to imagine what kind of constraints could be put on our ethical projects. Shouldn't we reflect on our base prejudices, and not allow them to provide boundaries for our moral reasoning? Thus, it is tempting to simply dismiss the objections to the simple principle. However, in *Demands of Morality*, Liam Murphy takes these objections seriously for at least two distinct reasons.

First, discussion of the simple principle provides an excellent vehicle for a discussion of morality in general. Perhaps, in a way, this is Murphy's attempt at doing philosophy "from the inside out." Second, Murphy's starting point tells us about the nature of his project. Murphy must take seriously the collisions between moral philosophy and our intuitive sense of right and wrong. He must do so because his work is best interpreted as intended to forge moral principles from our firm beliefs, and not to proscribe beliefs given a set of moral principles.

Murphy argues from our considered judgments rather than to them. For example, Murphy cites our "simple but firmly held" beliefs as supporting the potency of the over-demandingness objection, and nowhere in the work can one find a source of moral values divorced from human preferences.

Murphy does not tell us what set of "firm beliefs" we ought to have. Rather, he speaks to an audience of well-intentioned but unorganized moral realists, and tries to give them principles that represent their considered moral judgments. Murphy starts with this base sense of right and wrong, but recognizes that it needs to be supplemented by reason where our intuitions are confused or conflicting. Perhaps Murphy is looking for the best interpretation of our convictions, the same way certain legal scholars try to find the best interpretation of our Constitution.

This approach has disadvantages. Primarily, Murphy's arguments, even if successful, do not provide the kind of motivating force for which moral philosophy has traditionally searched. His work assumes and argues in terms of an inner sense of morality, and his project seeks to deepen that sense. Of course, it is quite possible that the moral viewpoints of humans will not converge, and some humans have no moral sense at all. Thus, it is very easy for the moral skeptic to point out a lack of justification and ignore the entire work.

On the other hand, Murphy's choice of a starting point avoids many of the problems of moral philosophy. Justifying the content of moral principles and granting a motivating force to those principles is an extraordinary task. It would be unrealistic to expect all discussions of moral philosophy to derive such justifications. Projects that attempt such a derivation have value, but they are hard pressed to produce logical consequences for everyday life. In the end, Murphy's strategy may have more practical effect than its first-principle counterparts, which do not seem any more likely to convince those that would reject Murphy's premises.

Passage Outline

      P1.

      P2.

      P3.

      P4.

      P5.

      P6.

      P7.

      Goal:

Questions

3. The passage implies that a moral principle derived from applying Murphy's philosophy to a particular group would be applicable to another group if:

    A. the first group recommended the principle to the second group.
    B. the moral viewpoints of the two groups do not converge.
    C. the members of the second group have no firmly held beliefs.
    D. the second group shares the same fundamental beliefs as the first group.

Question Type:

4. Murphy's position is most *weakened* in the passage by the claim that:

    A. he does not tell readers what "firm beliefs" to have.
    B. it is strange to punish those intending to do good.
    C. he is attempting philosophy "from the inside out."
    D. the moral viewpoints of humans may not converge.

Question Type:

KAPLAN TIP

Inference questions ask about the unstated parts of arguments: assumptions (implicit evidence) and implications (implicit conclusions). When all else fails with such questions, try the Denial Test: negating an inference will significantly weaken claims made in the passage.

Reasoning Within the Text Practice Passage (Questions 3–6)

If one always ought to act so as to produce the best possible circumstances, then morality is extremely demanding. No one could plausibly claim to have met the requirements of this "simple principle." It would seem strange to punish those intending to do good by sentencing them to an impossible task. Also, if the standards of right conduct are as extreme as they seem, then they will preclude the personal projects that humans find most fulfilling.

From an analytic perspective, the potential extreme demands of morality are not a "problem." A theory of morality is no less valid simply because it asks great sacrifices. In fact, it is difficult to imagine what kind of constraints could be put on our ethical projects. Shouldn't we reflect on our base prejudices, and not allow them to provide boundaries for our moral reasoning? Thus, it is tempting to simply dismiss the objections to the simple principle. However, in *Demands of Morality*, Liam Murphy takes these objections seriously for at least two distinct reasons.

First, discussion of the simple principle provides an excellent vehicle for a discussion of morality in general. Perhaps, in a way, this is Murphy's attempt at doing philosophy "from the inside out." Second, Murphy's starting point tells us about the nature of his project. Murphy must take seriously the collisions between moral philosophy and our intuitive sense of right and wrong. He must do so because his work is best interpreted as intended to forge moral principles from our firm beliefs, and not to proscribe beliefs given a set of moral principles.

Murphy argues from our considered judgments rather than to them. For example, Murphy cites our "simple but firmly held" beliefs as supporting the potency of the over-demandingness objection, and nowhere in the work can one find a source of moral values divorced from human preferences.

Murphy does not tell us what set of "firm beliefs" we ought to have. Rather, he speaks to an audience of well-intentioned but unorganized moral realists, and tries to give them principles that represent their considered moral judgments. Murphy starts with this base sense of right and wrong, but recognizes that it needs to be supplemented by reason where our intuitions are confused or conflicting. Perhaps Murphy is looking for the best interpretation of our convictions, the same way certain legal scholars try to find the best interpretation of our Constitution.

This approach has disadvantages. Primarily, Murphy's arguments, even if successful, do not provide the kind of motivating force for which moral philosophy has traditionally searched. His work assumes and argues in terms of an inner sense of morality, and his project seeks to deepen that sense. Of course, it is quite possible that the moral viewpoints of humans will not converge, and some humans have no moral sense at all. Thus, it is very easy for the moral skeptic to point out a lack of justification and ignore the entire work.

On the other hand, Murphy's choice of a starting point avoids many of the problems of moral philosophy. Justifying the content of moral principles and granting a motivating force to those principles is an extraordinary task. It would be unrealistic to expect all discussions of moral philosophy to derive such justifications. Projects that attempt such a derivation have value, but they are hard pressed to produce logical consequences for everyday life. In the end, Murphy's strategy may have more practical effect than its first-principle counterparts, which do not seem any more likely to convince those that would reject Murphy's premises.

5. The claim that not all moral philosophies have to provide readers with the motivation to be ethical is used by the author to:

    A. support the first-principle approach to ethics.
    B. bolster an assumption of the "simple principle."
    C. challenge an implication of Murphy's thesis.
    D. counter an objection to Murphy's position.

Question Type:

6. How does the author suggest that Murphy would be able to resolve the conflict between "the personal projects that humans find most fulfilling" and the demands of living ethically?

    A. By dismissing the objections to the "simple principle"
    B. By finding the best interpretation of the U.S. Constitution
    C. By starting from moral intuitions rather than principles
    D. By being more practical than his first-principle counterparts

Question Type:

KAPLAN TIP

Some Reasoning Within the Text questions do not fall neatly into the Inference or Strengthen/Weaken types. These questions, classified as "Other (Within)" questions, are relatively rare, but can require a variety of reasoning-based tasks, such as resolving apparent paradoxes, finding statements of clarification, or even appraising the quality of arguments from the passage.

LESSON 6.3 REVIEW

CARS Skill 2: Reasoning Within the Text
Question Types

Inference
- Asks for unstated claims that must be true given what is stated in the passage
- Use the Denial Test to isolate the statement most crucial to the argument

Strengthen/Weaken (Within Passage)
- Asks about logical relationships between statements and ideas in the passage
- Sometimes evidence supports an argument, other times it weakens an argument
- Find the tested claims in the passage and use your knowledge of the arguments to answer

CARS Questions: Reasoning Beyond the Text

In this lesson, you'll learn to:

- Answer Apply questions
  - Extrapolate ideas from the passage to new contexts
- Answer Strengthen/Weaken (Beyond Passage) questions
  - Determine the effect of new information on arguments from the passage

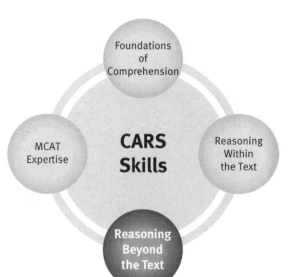

MCAT STRATEGY—CARS QUESTIONS

ASSESS THE QUESTION
Read the question (NOT the answers), looking for clues to the difficulty.

PLAN YOUR ATTACK
Think about question type, your outline, and researching the passage.

EXECUTE THE PLAN
Predict what you can about the answer.

ANSWER BY MATCHING, ELIMINATING, OR GUESSING
Find the right answer in the answer choices.

LESSON 6.4, LEARNING GOALS 1 AND 2:

- Answer Apply questions
  - Extrapolate ideas from the passage to new contexts
- Answer Strengthen/Weaken (Beyond Passage) questions
  - Determine the effect of new information on arguments from the passage

CARS Question Types Map

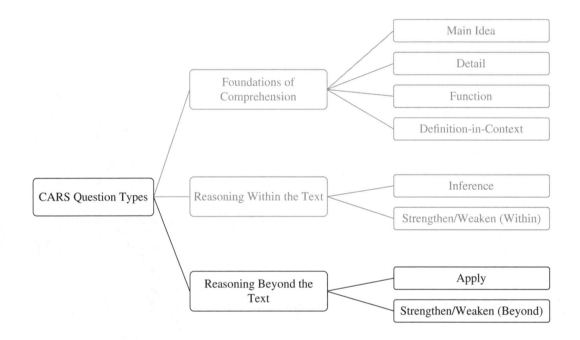

Reasoning Beyond the Text—Introduction

Does true happiness come from "within" or from "without"? Do we achieve fulfillment when external circumstances happen to satisfy our desires, as the modern Utilitarian view maintains? Or, on the contrary, is it as the ancient Stoics and Buddhists claim, and we become happy only through renouncing our desires and cultivating a proper internal attitude?

In his landmark work, *The Happiness Hypothesis*, psychologist Jonathan Haidt answers that neither is the case—or, more accurately, both. After embarking upon an ambitious project of cataloguing the world's wisdom and then looking to contemporary social science for results that verify ancient proverbs, Haidt concludes that true happiness comes from "between," requiring a mix of internal and external conditions: "Some of those conditions are within you, such as coherence among the parts and levels of your personality. Other conditions require relationships to things beyond you: Just as plants need sun, water, and good soil to thrive, people need love, work, and a connection to something larger."

Passage Outline

P1.

P2.

Apply Question

1. Which of the following is most analogous to the notion that happiness comes from "between" (paragraph 2)?

   A. Human beings are neither purely good nor entirely evil, but fall somewhere in the middle.
   B. When people get what they want, they tend to be more satisfied with their lives.
   C. True contentment is only attainable by those who can moderate their emotional reactions to events.
   D. The development of complex human traits requires a delicate balance of nature and nurture.

Strengthen/Weaken (Beyond) Question

2. Suppose an extensive cross-cultural study reveals that the happiest people tend to have few attachments to material objects and to want little besides what they already possess. What effect would this have on the passage?

   A. It would weaken the claim that happiness comes from "within."
   B. It would challenge the claim that happiness comes from "without."
   C. It would strengthen the claim that happiness comes from "without."
   D. It would support the claim that happiness comes from "between."

KAPLAN TIP

When you see a Strengthen/Weaken (Beyond) question asking for the effect of new information and the passage contains multiple views, consider the impact that the information would have on each view, and use that to make your prediction.

K

Reasoning Beyond the Text Practice Passage (Questions 3–7)

Does true happiness come from "within" or from "without"? Do we achieve fulfillment when external circumstances happen to satisfy our desires, as the modern Utilitarian view maintains? Or, on the contrary, is it as the ancient Stoics and Buddhists claim, and we become happy only through renouncing our desires and cultivating a proper internal attitude?

In his landmark work, *The Happiness Hypothesis*, psychologist Jonathan Haidt answers that neither is the case—or, more accurately, both. After embarking upon an ambitious project of cataloguing the world's wisdom and then looking to contemporary social science for results that verify ancient proverbs, Haidt concludes that true happiness comes from "between," requiring a mix of internal and external conditions: "Some of those conditions are within you, such as coherence among the parts and levels of your personality. Other conditions require relationships to things beyond you: Just as plants need sun, water, and good soil to thrive, people need love, work, and a connection to something larger."

While the above presents what Haidt calls the "final version of the happiness hypothesis," the one that stands both the test of time and empirical verification, Haidt's book as a whole is a synoptic appraisal of ten key ideas about human psychology that recur in disparate cultures and historical eras. For example, in his chapter on the "adversity hypothesis," Haidt actually evaluates two versions of the claim that suffering builds character. The weak version, "adversity *can* lead to growth," is undoubtedly supported by evidence. However, the data only support a limited version of the strong view, that it *must* cause growth: "For adversity to be maximally beneficial, it should happen at the right time (young adulthood), to the right people (those with the social and psychological resources to rise to challenges and find benefits), and to the right degree (not so severe as to cause PTSD)."

Of all the great ideas considered, perhaps the most fascinating discussion comes in Haidt's chapter on what he calls "divinity with or without God." Unpossessed of the contempt that exudes from supposed representatives of science like Richard Dawkins and Christopher Hitchens, Haidt harbors a profound—if somewhat distanced—reverence for religion. Though himself a nonbeliever, he cannot deny the power of the data on happiness, including the key finding that religious believers tend to report greater life satisfaction, especially when belonging to some kind of spiritual community. Rather than dismiss this as the product of mass delusion, Haidt instead looks for common ground, for the analogues of spiritual elevation that can be detected even by an atheist like himself.

Building on the work of his mentor, Richard Shweder, Haidt argues that social "space" can be seen to have three "dimensions," each of which corresponds roughly to a particular ethical orientation. The "ethic of autonomy," which prioritizes the prevention of harm and the removal of constraints on individual freedom, is operative in the horizontal dimension of closeness, consisting of the egalitarian bonds that humans share with their peers. With the vertical dimension of hierarchy that recognizes unequal relationships between people comes the "ethic of community," the end of which is "to protect the integrity of groups, families, companies, or nations" with an emphasis on "virtues such as obedience, loyalty, and wise leadership." Finally, there is the "ethic of divinity," which divides social space into regions that are sacred or profane, pure or polluted. This third dimension, which purports to offer "a connection to something larger," plays a crucial role in much human flourishing, which is why Haidt recognizes it as one of the key components of a happiness that comes from between.

Passage Outline

     P1.

     P2.

     P3.

     P4.

     P5.

     Goal:

3. Which of the following scenarios would most CHALLENGE the "limited version" of the strong "adversity hypothesis" that Haidt endorses?

  A. An old woman with a strong, lifelong marriage experiences significant adversity when she loses her husband, but fails to grow as a result.

  B. A middle-aged man who lives alone and has a history of depression becomes traumatized by even the slightest inconvenience.

  C. A young man with close family connections undergoes relatively minor suffering when losing his beloved cat, but is debilitated for life.

  D. A young woman with healthy coping skills loses her entire family in a tragic accident and develops post-traumatic stress disorder.

Question Type:

4. Based on the discussion in paragraph 5, a person who prioritizes an ethic of community can most reasonably be expected to:

  A. be dependent on the categories of purity and pollution for understanding the world.

  B. ignore the hierarchical dimension of human social space.

  C. demand that all human connections be viewed as relationships between equals.

  D. be willing to sacrifice the rights of individuals for the sake of the greater good of humanity.

Question Type:

KAPLAN TIP

The three most common variants of Apply questions ask for: (1) a specific example or analogy of an idea from the passage; (2) the author's response to new information; (3) the likely outcome of a novel situation, based on the logic of the passage.

Reasoning Beyond the Text Practice Passage (Questions 3–7)

Does true happiness come from "within" or from "without"? Do we achieve fulfillment when external circumstances happen to satisfy our desires, as the modern Utilitarian view maintains? Or, on the contrary, is it as the ancient Stoics and Buddhists claim, and we become happy only through renouncing our desires and cultivating a proper internal attitude?

In his landmark work, *The Happiness Hypothesis*, psychologist Jonathan Haidt answers that neither is the case—or, more accurately, both. After embarking upon an ambitious project of cataloguing the world's wisdom and then looking to contemporary social science for results that verify ancient proverbs, Haidt concludes that true happiness comes from "between," requiring a mix of internal and external conditions: "Some of those conditions are within you, such as coherence among the parts and levels of your personality. Other conditions require relationships to things beyond you: Just as plants need sun, water, and good soil to thrive, people need love, work, and a connection to something larger."

While the above presents what Haidt calls the "final version of the happiness hypothesis," the one that stands both the test of time and empirical verification, Haidt's book as a whole is a synoptic appraisal of ten key ideas about human psychology that recur in disparate cultures and historical eras. For example, in his chapter on the "adversity hypothesis," Haidt actually evaluates two versions of the claim that suffering builds character. The weak version, "adversity *can* lead to growth," is undoubtedly supported by evidence. However, the data only support a limited version of the strong view, that it *must* cause growth: "For adversity to be maximally beneficial, it should happen at the right time (young adulthood), to the right people (those with the social and psychological resources to rise to challenges and find benefits), and to the right degree (not so severe as to cause PTSD)."

Of all the great ideas considered, perhaps the most fascinating discussion comes in Haidt's chapter on what he calls "divinity with or without God." Unpossessed of the contempt that exudes from supposed representatives of science like Richard Dawkins and Christopher Hitchens, Haidt harbors a profound—if somewhat distanced—reverence for religion. Though himself a nonbeliever, he cannot deny the power of the data on happiness, including the key finding that religious believers tend to report greater life satisfaction, especially when belonging to some kind of spiritual community. Rather than dismiss this as the product of mass delusion, Haidt instead looks for common ground, for the analogues of spiritual elevation that can be detected even by an atheist like himself.

Building on the work of his mentor, Richard Shweder, Haidt argues that social "space" can be seen to have three "dimensions," each of which corresponds roughly to a particular ethical orientation. The "ethic of autonomy," which prioritizes the prevention of harm and the removal of constraints on individual freedom, is operative in the horizontal dimension of closeness, consisting of the egalitarian bonds that humans share with their peers. With the vertical dimension of hierarchy that recognizes unequal relationships between people comes the "ethic of community," the end of which is "to protect the integrity of groups, families, companies, or nations" with an emphasis on "virtues such as obedience, loyalty, and wise leadership." Finally, there is the "ethic of divinity," which divides social space into regions that are sacred or profane, pure or polluted. This third dimension, which purports to offer "a connection to something larger," plays a crucial role in much human flourishing, which is why Haidt recognizes it as one of the key components of a happiness that comes from between.

5. Which of the following would the author be most likely to characterize as an example of happiness that comes from "without"?

   Question Type:

   A. A retiree is content with life by achieving a balance between internal and external satisfaction.
   B. An addict renounces the use of drugs and turns to meditation to control his cravings.
   C. A medical student graduates and is thrilled to achieve her dream of receiving her diploma.
   D. A religious believer finds satisfaction through the inner strengths his faith has helped cultivate.

6. Which of the following statements, if true, would give the greatest support to the contention that happiness requires the recognition of something like "divinity"?

   Question Type:

   A. Writers who are contemptuous of religion tend to alienate believers more effectively than educate them.
   B. The happiest religious nonbelievers are the ones who manage to find some purpose in life greater than themselves.
   C. Religious believers are happier primarily because they succumb to the illusions of wishful thinking.
   D. Atheists report roughly equal levels of satisfaction with their lives as people who regularly attend religious services.

7. Elsewhere in *The Happiness Hypothesis*, Haidt argues that humans possess "divided selves" with conflicting parts that can make becoming happy more difficult. This argument helps to explain the claim from the passage that:

   Question Type:

   A. harmony between the different levels of one's personality is essential for happiness.
   B. adversity is most conducive to growth only under a limited set of circumstances.
   C. a connection to something larger is required for a person to achieve happiness.
   D. people who adopt the ethic of divinity divide social space into sacred and profane regions.

KAPLAN TIP

Some Reasoning Beyond the Text questions do not fall neatly into either category. For example, some questions ask for an alternative explanation to one given in the passage, while others ask for likely changes the author would make to the text in light of challenging information. These are called "Other (Beyond)" questions.

K

LESSON 6.4 REVIEW

CARS Skill 3: Reasoning Beyond the Text
Question Types

Apply
- Direction: passage → new situation
- Find the relevant ideas from the text and look for analogies

Strengthen/Weaken (Beyond Passage)
- Direction: new situation → passage
- Isolate the passage arguments and determine how new information fits in

CHAPTER

7

CARS MCAT
Expertise

Argument Structure

In this lesson, you'll learn to:

- Recognize concepts, conceptual relationships, and claims in passages
- Identify the components of an argument

Foundations of Comprehension

MCAT Expertise

CARS Skills

Reasoning Within the Text

Reasoning Beyond the Text

LESSON 7.1, LEARNING GOAL 1:

- Recognize concepts, conceptual relationships, and claims in passages

The social novel has always presupposed a substantial amount of social stability. The ideal social novel had been written by Jane Austen, a great artist who enjoyed the luxury of being able to take society for granted; it was there, and seemed steady beneath her glass, Napoleon or no Napoleon. But soon it would not be steady beneath anyone's glass, and the novelist's attention had necessarily to shift from the gradations within society to the fate of society itself. It is at this point that the political novel comes to be written—the kind in which the idea of society, as distinct from the mere unquestioned workings of society, has penetrated the consciousness of the characters in all of its profoundly problematic aspects.

The political novel—I have in mind its ideal form—is peculiarly a work of internal tensions. To be a novel at all, it must contain the usual representation of human behavior and feeling; yet it must also absorb into its stream of movement the hard and perhaps insoluble pellets of modern ideology. The conflict is inescapable: the novel tries to confront experience in its immediacy and closeness, while ideology is by its nature general and inclusive. Yet it is precisely from this conflict that the political novel gains its interest and takes on the aura of high drama: the timelessness of abstraction is confronted with the flux of life, the monolith of program with the diversity of motive, the purity of ideal with the contamination of action.

What is the defining characteristic of the author's concept of the *social novel*?

What example of the *social novel* is given?

What new concept is introduced and how does it relate to the *social novel*?

What is the defining characteristic of the author's concept of the *political novel*?

What terms are associated with the two sides of the *tension* or *conflict*?

KAPLAN TIP

Many CARS passages use parallel structures in their writing to create stark contrasts between two concepts, known as *dualisms* or *dichotomies*.

Because it exposes the impersonal claims of ideology to the pressures of private emotion, the political novel must always be in a state of internal warfare, always on the verge of becoming something other than itself. The political novelist establishes a complex system of intellectual movements, in which his own opinion is one of the most active yet not entirely dominating movers. Are we not close here to one of the secrets of the novel in general? I mean the vast respect that the great novelist is ready to offer the whole idea of opposition, the opposition he needs to allow for in his book against his own predispositions and yearnings and fantasies.

This is not to say that the political novelist's desires—both acknowledged and repressed—fail to play a pivotal role in the novel's dialectic. Indeed, the political novel turns characteristically to an apolitical temptation: in *The Possessed,* to the notion that redemption is possible only to sinners who have suffered greatly; in Conrad's *Nostromo* and *Under Western Eyes,* to the resources of private affection and gentleness; in *Man's Fate*, to the metaphysical allurements of heroism as they reveal themselves in a martyr's death; in Silone's *Bread and Wine,* to the discovery of peasant simplicity as a foil to urban corruption; and in *Darkness at Noon,* to the abandoned uses of the personal will. This, so to say, is the pastoral element that is indispensable to the political novel, indispensable for providing it with polarity and tension.

What new information is introduced in the first sentence of this paragraph?

What claim does the author make about the *political novelist's* opinion?

How could the claim in the first sentence be phrased without the double negative?

What follows the colon in the long sentence in the middle of this paragraph?

What is the author doing in the final sentence?

LESSON 7.1, LEARNING GOAL 2:

- Identify the components of an argument

Basic Arguments

A basic argument consists of:

1. Conclusion: a supported claim

2. Evidence: a supporting claim or claims

Examples

All men are mortal. Socrates is a man. Therefore, Socrates is mortal.

Conclusion:

Evidence:

That politician is lying. After all, his lips are moving.

Conclusion:

Evidence:

KAPLAN TIP   **K**
Logic keywords are a crucial tool for identifying the parts of arguments.

Inferences

Inferences are implicit parts of arguments and come in two types:

1. Assumptions: unstated evidence

2. Implications: unstated conclusions

Example

It's dangerous to drive on Main Street because Main Street is icy.

Conclusion: It's dangerous to drive on Main Street.

Evidence: Main Street is icy.

Assumption:

Implication:

Refutations

A *refutation* or *objection* is a claim that weakens an argument, making its conclusion *less likely* to be true. If backed by its own evidence, a refutation is called a *counterargument*.

Example

You can reach happiness by satisfying your desires. Thus, you should only desire what you already have.

Conclusion: You should only desire what you already have.

Evidence: You can reach happiness by satisfying your desires.

Refutation:

KAPLAN TIP

Inferences are *not* simply statements that *might* be true, but are claims that *must* be true (if not quite always, then *almost* always), given the truth of the other claims made in the argument.

Identifying Arguments in Passages

Sensing that government defined by the Articles of Confederation did not meet the needs of the newly born United States, the Congress of the Articles of Confederation authorized commissioners to "devise such further provisions as shall appear to them necessary to render the Constitution of the federal government adequate to the exigencies of the Union." These provisions were to be reported to Congress and confirmed by every state. The recommendatory acts also state that this change, to be done through alterations of the Articles of Confederation, is the most probable means of establishing a strong national government. Having given these instructions, Congress was quite surprised by the radically new terms of the Constitution submitted. In fact, some congressmen claimed that the commissioners did not have the legal authority to submit such a revolutionary document.

Why did the Articles of Confederation (AC) Congress request a new Constitution?

What conclusion did some members of the AC Congress reach about the legality of the Constitution submitted?

What reason is given for this conclusion?

In *The Federalist Papers*, James Madison defends the commissioners by returning to the terms of their mandate. Given the goals expressed in the recommendatory acts, and the principle that conflicts ought to be resolved in favor of more important goals, Madison argued that the degree to which the Constitution departs from the Articles couldn't make the Constitution illegal. Where the goal of amending the Articles conflicts with the goal of creating good government, the Articles must yield, since the goal of "good government" is an overriding consideration.

What conclusion does James Madison reach about the legality of the new Constitution?

What is Madison's reasoning?

Although Madison argued fairly convincingly that the degree of change present in the Constitution cannot be grounds for declaring it illegal, this same argument does not apply to the commissioners' decision to allow the Constitution to be ratified by only three-quarters of the states. Even though unanimous approval appears last in Madison's list of the goals of the convention, it was a fundamental aspect of national government under the Articles. Requiring non-ratifying states to be bound by the new Constitution was thus a powerful diminishment of their sovereignty.

What conclusion does the passage author seem to hold about the Constitution's legality?

What is the piece of evidence discussed here?

The new Constitution, once adopted, changed the national government from a weak union of independent states to a strong union in which the interests of the many states could outweigh the protests of the few. Although history has validated the wisdom of the change, the question of whether the change was legal is another matter. In authorizing the commissioners, the individual states requested a proposal for the alteration of the national government. They did not intend to waive their veto power. So even if Madison is correct, and the commissioners could have proposed anything they deemed likely to fulfill the goal of good government, it does not follow that their proclamations should affect the legal rights of the several states.

Does this imply that the Constitution ratified by the states has no moral authority? Not necessarily. No government ought to have the power to entrench itself against amendment, and so the fact that the government under the Articles of Confederation did not consent to the alteration of the ratification process does not establish the moral illegitimacy of the Constitution.

The ethical case for rebelling against the government under the Articles is further strengthened by the fact that the government itself admitted its unfitness for the exigencies of the Union. Indeed, the ratification process altered by the new Constitution is representative of the procedures that initially led Congress to seek reform. In addressing the relevance of opposing the government of the Articles of Confederation, we should also consider the position of the framers. They had already rebelled against England, one of the great powers of the time, and thus had demonstrated an unwillingness to tolerate bad government. Defying the government of the Articles must have seemed easy by comparison.

What is the author's counterargument against Madison's position on the Constitution's legality?

What is the author's conclusion about the moral or ethical standing of the Constitution?

What evidence does the author provide in the last two paragraphs for this conclusion?

How can you use the answers to these questions to construct a passage outline?

P1.

P2.

P3.

P4.

P5.

P6.

Goal:

LESSON 7.1 REVIEW

Know the following about **concepts**:

Concepts are characterized by their meanings or definitions.

Concepts can exist in a variety of relationships with other concepts.

Terms are words or phrases that refer to concepts.

Real-world instances of concepts are called **examples**.

Claims say things about concepts and their relations.

Recognize the different parts of an **argument**:

Conclusion: a stated supported claim

Evidence: a stated supporting claim

Assumption: an unstated supporting claim

Implication: an unstated supported claim

Refutation: a challenging claim

Wrong Answer Pathologies

In this lesson, you'll learn to:

- Recognize common wrong answer pathologies for questions in the Critical Analysis and Reasoning section

Foundations of Comprehension

MCAT Expertise

CARS Skills

Reasoning Within the Text

Reasoning Beyond the Text

LESSON 7.2, LEARNING GOAL 1:

• Recognize common wrong answer pathologies for questions in the Critical Analysis and Reasoning Section.

Identifying Wrong Answer Pathologies

Before the Voting Rights Act of 1965, some examples of the laws in place to disenfranchise minority voters were literacy tests, poll taxes, property ownership requirements, and "good character" tests. Even though these laws took away voters' rights and were a clear violation of the Fourteenth and Fifteenth Amendments, the Supreme Court usually upheld them under the protection of states' rights. In some cases, interested parties attempted to circumvent these laws with the establishment of other laws, the most common of which were grandfather clauses that preserved suffrage for otherwise (typically non-minority) disenfranchised parties.

1. According to the passage, which of the following was used to prevent the disenfranchisement of minority voters before the Voting Rights Act of 1965?

Wrong Answer Choice	FUD	OPP	OS	DIST/EXT
The passing of the Fourteenth and Fifteenth Amendments				
Abolishing grandfather clauses				
Abolishing all grandfather clause laws				
The Civil Rights Act of 1964				
Counteracting and repealing literacy tests and poll taxes				
Civil Rights advocacy geared toward non-minority voters				
Supreme Court rulings about who could and couldn't vote				

FUD = faulty use of detail; OPP = opposite; OS= out of scope; DIST/EXT = distortion or extreme

Which word/phrase makes it wrong?

2. What measures were taken to disenfranchise minority voters before the Voting Rights Act of 1965 was passed?

Literacy tests, poll taxes, property ownership requirements only

Civil Rights leaders advocating for enforcement of "good character" tests

The passing of laws that were technically legal according to the Fourteenth and Fifteenth Amendments

Racial discrimination initiatives set forth by the Supreme Court

States passing laws such as the grandfather clauses

Suppression of states' rights by the Supreme Court

KAPLAN TIP
Although it is important to identify the correct answer based on your prediction, recognizing and eliminating wrong answer choices is a skill you need to practice in order to choose the best answer on Test Day.

LESSON 7.2 REVIEW

Wrong Answer Pathologies

Faulty Use of Detail (FUD)

- Is wrong because
    - It misrepresents information in the passage
    - It does not answer the question that was asked
- Is tempting because
    - It has information that is easily recognizable from the passage
- Is recognizable by
    - Passage detail in an incorrect context

Opposite (OPP)

- Is wrong because
    - It is the exact opposite concept/idea from the correct answer
- Is tempting because
    - It will look very similar to a good prediction for the question
- Is recognizable by
    - A single word or phrase that will negate the answer (i.e., no, not, un-)

Out of Scope (OS)

- Is wrong because
    - It does not cover the same content areas as the passage
- Is tempting because
    - It will be within the overall topic of the passage
- Is recognizable by
    - The inclusion of information that is not mentioned in the passage at all

Distortion or Extreme (DIST/EXT)

- Is wrong because
    - It manipulates the author's focus or meaning in an extreme or distorted way
- Is tempting because
    - It will look very similar to the correct answer except for one word or phrase
- Is recognizable by
    - A single word or phrase that distorts the answer (i.e., always, only, must, should)

Identifying CARS Question Types

In this lesson, you'll learn to:

- Identify the question type of a given CARS question stem

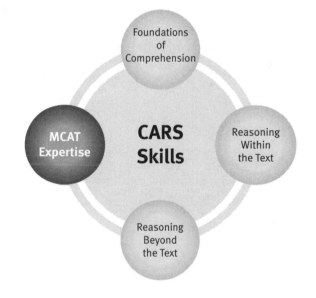

LESSON 7.3, LEARNING GOAL 1:

• Identify the question type of a given CARS question stem

CARS Question Types

Foundations of Comprehension

| Main Idea | Detail | Function | Definition-in-Context |

Reasoning Within the Text

| Inference | Strengthen/Weaken (Within the Passage) | Other |

Reasoning Beyond the Text

| Apply | Strengthen/Weaken (Beyond the Passage) | Other |

Question Stem   Question Type(s)

1. This passage primarily concerns: _____

2. Based on the passage, what theatrical concept
   was first introduced by the early musical *Pal
   Joey*?   _____ OR _____

3. The list of Luxembourg's exports is included
   in the passage because: _____

4. The phrase "offending sentiment" (paragraph 2)
   probably refers to which of the following
   remarks by Dr. Sirlin?   _____

Question Stem

Question Type(s)

5. The fact that congenital defects were more common in towns such as Beauvais casts doubt on which of the following assertions?

_____

6. Suppose that studies are conducted that determine that men with low g who regularly watch public television have higher numbers of close friends and lower divorce rates than the general population. What effect does this have on Kanazawa's opinion as it is described in the passage?

_____

7. Which of the following arguments most solidly justifies the central thesis of the passage?

_____ OR _____

8. The author of the passage would be most likely to agree with which of the following statements?

_____ OR _____

9. Based on the descriptions from the passage, which of the following situations most resembles the conflict between the ideologies of Vantas and Egbert?

_____

10. Which of the following is a statement the author makes without example, illustration, or evidence?

_____

KAPLAN TIP

Knowledge of question types, and the dependable strategies that accompany them, is one of the most important signs of expertise on the CARS section of the MCAT. Look for these patterns in question stems and answer choices, and use your previous experience to quickly answer questions on Test Day!

LESSON 7.3 REVIEW

CARS skill	Question type	What it asks you for	Common patterns or strategies
Foundations of Comprehension	Main Idea	Induce the main idea of the passage as a whole	Use the Passage Goal as a prediction
	Detail	Find one or more details in the passage	Question stems often have context clues
	Function	Explain the function of a certain part of the passage in the author's larger argument	Question stems often use "because" or "in order to"
	Definition-in-Context	Identify the meaning of a quoted word or phrase as it is used in the passage	Trap answers will often be common definitions that are incorrect in context
Reasoning Within the Text	Inference	Deduce what must be true based on the information and/or arguments in the passage	Question stems may look similar to Detail questions
	Strengthen/ Weaken (Within the Passage)	Determine how an argument in the passage is affected by another part of the passage	Answers are usually support for or contradiction to an argument's evidence
	Other	Perform other types of reasoning on the passage	Usually asks about legitimacy or flaws in passage arguments
Reasoning Beyond the Text	Apply	Apply some logic, reasoning, or process in the passage to a new situation	Often requires making one-to-one analogies to new contexts
	Strengthen/ Weaken (Beyond the Passage)	Determine how an argument in the passage is affected by newly introduced information	New information may be in question stem or answer choices
	Other	Perform other reasoning on new information from beyond the passage	Strategies from Apply questions will usually help

Triage in the CARS Section

In this lesson, you'll learn to:

- Utilize the triaging strategy within a CARS section of the MCAT
- Use question stems and answer choices to preview and triage MCAT CARS questions

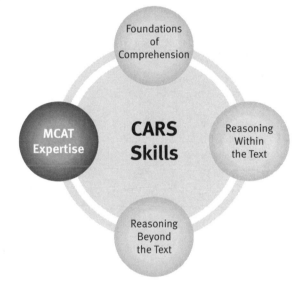

LESSON 7.4, LEARNING GOAL 1:

- Utilize the triaging strategy within a CARS section of the MCAT

Section Triage Strategy

- Triage Order:

  1. Easiest passages

  2. Passages with ambiguous difficulty

  3. Hardest passages

- Flagging for Review

- Navigation Panel

Scratchwork Examples

P1	P2	P3	P4	P5	P6	P7	P8	P9
☺	☹		☺				☹	☺

E:	M:	H:
1	19	7
13	24	36
48	30	
	42	

Later:
1 (1)
30 (5)
36 (6)

KAPLAN TIP

Remember that your ultimate triaging method should be your own style. Just make sure you practice enough to perfect that style before you take the MCAT.

Sample Passage 1

According to our traditional understanding of responsibility, we are directly responsible for our "voluntary" actions, and (at most) only indirectly responsible for the things that happen to us. It is held, for instance, that "I can't help" the surge of anger that I feel when objects in the environment present themselves to my senses in certain ways; however, I am supposed to govern my subsequent thoughts and activities regarding these objects by the force of my will. When we look inside ourselves with the goal of sorting our mental events into these two morally important categories, something peculiar happens. Events near the input and output "peripheries" fall unproblematically into place. Thus, feeling pain in my foot and seeing the desk are clearly not acts "in my control," but things that happen to me, while moving my finger or saying these words are obviously things that I do—voluntary actions.

But as we move away from those peripheries toward the presumptive center, the events we try to examine exhibit a strange flickering back and forth. It no longer seems so clear that perception is a passive matter. Do I not voluntarily contribute something to my perception, even to my recognition or "acceptance" of the desk as a desk? For after all, can I not suspend judgment in the face of any perceptual presentation, and withhold conviction? On the other side of the center, when we look more closely at action, is my voluntary act really moving my finger, or is it more properly trying to move my finger? A familiar [thought experiment] about someone willing actions while totally paralyzed attests that I am not in control of all the conditions in the world (or in my body) that are necessary for my finger actually to move.

Faced with our inability to "see" (by "introspection") where the center or source of our free actions is, and loath to abandon our conviction that we really do things (for which we are responsible), we exploit the gaps in our self-knowledge by filling it with a rather magical and mysterious entity, the unmoved mover, the active self.

1. The passage's central thesis is that:
   A. one should not be held responsible for actions over which one exerts no control.
   B. our sense that we can act voluntarily is an illusion.
   C. decisions are the instants in which we exercise our volition to the fullest.
   D. many actions cannot be classified precisely as either voluntary or involuntary.

What is your triage decision?

Sample Passage 2

The system of farming practiced in the United States today evolved during the 1950s, when the development of chemical pesticides, fertilizers, and high-yielding crop strains brought a mass shift towards specialization. Using agrochemicals, farmers found that they could grow a single crop on the same field year after year without impairing the yield or incurring pest problems. Encouraged by government programs subsidizing the production of grains such as wheat and corn, most farmers consolidated to cultivate a limited number of crops and to invest in the equipment to mechanize labor-intensive farm processes. For the last 40 years, this system has enabled American farmers to lead the world in efficiency and crop production. Today, however, rising costs and problems such as groundwater contamination, soil erosion, and declining productivity are forcing many farmers to question their dependence on agrochemicals and to investigate alternative systems.

Perhaps the most likely system to replace today's agriculture is a composite of nonconventional techniques defined as sustainable agriculture. Using a combination of organic, low-input methods that benefit the environment and preserve the integrity of the soil, many scientists believe that sustainable agriculture could reach productivity levels competitive with conventional systems. Farmers converting to sustainable systems would find themselves using the same machinery, certified seed, and feeding methods as before. But instead of enhancing productivity with purchased chemicals, sustainable farms would use, as far as possible, natural processes and local renewable resources. Returning to a system of crop rotation, where fields are used to grow a succession of different crops, would improve crop yields and bolster pest resistance. Using crop residues, manures, and other organic materials would help to restore soil quality by improving such factors as air circulation, moisture retention, and tilth, or soil structure. And systems such as integrated pest management (IPM) would combat pests by diversifying crops, regulating predators of pest species, and using pesticides intermittently when necessary.

2. Which of the following best summarizes the main idea of the passage?

   A. Sustainable agriculture should be supported for a variety of reasons.
   B. Growing only a single crop in a given tract of land can make that crop more susceptible to pests.
   C. Sustainable agriculture does not provide a viable alternative to today's farming methods.
   D. Methods of farming must be altered to prevent further damage to the environment.

What is your triage decision?

Sample Passage 3

The Modern Girl makes only a brief appearance in our histories of prewar Japan. She is a glittering, decadent, middle-class consumer who, through her clothing, smoking, and drinking, flaunts tradition in the urban playgrounds of the late 1920s. Arm in arm with her male equivalent, the Modern Boy (the *mobo*) and fleshed out in the Western flapper's garb of the roaring twenties, she engages in *ginbura* (Ginza-cruising). Yet by merely equating the Japanese Modern Girl with the flapper we do her a disservice, for the Modern Girl was not on a Western trajectory. Moreover, during the decade when this female, a creation of the mass media, excited her Japanese audience, she was not easily defined. Who was this "Modern Girl"? Why did she do what she did?

The Modern Girl is rescued from her depoliticized representation when her willful image is placed alongside the history of working, militant Japanese women. Then the depiction of the Modern Girl as apolitical (and later, as apolitical and nonworking) begins to appear as a means of displacing the very real militancy of Japanese women (just as the real labor of the American woman during the 1920s was denied by trivializing the work of the glamorized flapper). But whereas the American woman worker by the mid-1920s had allowed herself to be depoliticized by a new consumerism, the modern Japanese woman of the 1920s was truly militant. Her militancy was articulated through the adoption of new fashions, through labor in new arenas, and through political activity that consciously challenged social, economic, and political structures and relationships. The Japanese state's response encompassed attempts to revise the Civil Code, consideration of universal suffrage, organization and expansion of groups such as the Women's Alliance (*Fujin Doshikai*) and the nationwide network of *shojokai* (associations of young girls), censorship, and imprisonment of leaders. The media responded by producing the Modern Girl.

Yet the Modern Girl must have represented even more, for the determination that talk about the Modern Girl displaced serious concern about the radical nature of women's activity does not fully address her multifaceted nature.

3. According to the passage, the Modern Girl reflected tensions in all of the following issues EXCEPT:

   A. the influence of non-Japanese cultural traditions.
   B. the extent of women's participation in the workforce.
   C. whether, within Japanese families, women ought to be subordinate to men.
   D. whether the popular media should be accountable for the images they present.

What is your triage decision?

LESSON 7.4, LEARNING GOAL 2:

- Use question stems and answer choices to preview and triage MCAT CARS questions

Practice Passage 1 (Questions 1–6)

The Modern Girl makes only a brief appearance in our histories of prewar Japan. She is a glittering, decadent, middle-class consumer who, through her clothing, smoking, and drinking, flaunts tradition in the urban playgrounds of the late 1920s. Arm in arm with her male equivalent, the Modern Boy (the *mobo*) and fleshed out in the Western flapper's garb of the roaring twenties, she engages in *ginbura* (Ginza-cruising). Yet by merely equating the Japanese Modern Girl with the flapper we do her a disservice, for the Modern Girl was not on a Western trajectory. Moreover, during the decade when this female, a creation of the mass media, excited her Japanese audience, she was not easily defined. Who was this "Modern Girl"? Why did she do what she did?

The Modern Girl is rescued from her depoliticized representation when her willful image is placed alongside the history of working, militant Japanese women. Then the depiction of the Modern Girl as apolitical (and later, as apolitical and nonworking) begins to appear as a means of displacing the very real militancy of Japanese women (just as the real labor of the American woman during the 1920s was denied by trivializing the work of the glamorized flapper). But whereas the American woman worker by the mid-1920s had allowed herself to be depoliticized by a new consumerism, the modern Japanese woman of the 1920s was truly militant. Her militancy was articulated through the adoption of new fashions, through labor in new arenas, and through political activity that consciously challenged social, economic, and political structures and relationships. The Japanese state's response encompassed attempts to revise the Civil Code, consideration of universal suffrage, organization and expansion of groups such as the Women's Alliance (*Fujin Doshikai*) and the nationwide network of *shojokai* (associations of young girls), censorship, and imprisonment of leaders. The media responded by producing the Modern Girl.

Yet talk about the Modern Girl and how she displaced serious concern about the radical nature of women's activity does not fully address her multifaceted nature.

Why, in other words, was she Japanese and Western, intellectual and worker, deviant and admirable? An answer is suggested by Natalie Davis in "Women on Top," which argues that the "unruly woman" in early modern Europe served both to reinforce social structure and to incite women to militant action in public and in private. The culturally constructed figure of the Japanese Modern Girl certainly meets these two requirements. Like the disorderly woman on top, the Modern Girl as multifaceted symbol questioned relations of order and subordination.

This thesis was indeed offered by the feminist Kitamura, who claimed that "labor struggle, tenancy struggle, household struggle, struggle between man and woman" were inevitable and had recently been joined to a new battle: "a struggle over good conduct" that pitted Japanese against Western behavior and used the Modern Girl to work out the struggle.

This, then, is the significance of the Japanese Modern Girl in the broadest context of prewar Japanese history. The Modern Girl stood as the vital symbol of overwhelming "modern" or non-Japanese change instigated by both women and men during an era of economic crisis and social unrest. She stood for change at a time when state authority was attempting to reestablish authority and stability. The Modern Girl of the 1920s and early 1930s thus inverted the role of the Good Wife and Wise Mother. The ideal Meiji woman of the 1870s, 1880s, and 1890s had served as a "repository of the past," standing for tradition when men were encouraged to change their way of politics and culture in all ways.

Passage Outline

P1.

P2.

P3.

P4.

P5.

P6.

Goal:

1. According to the passage, the Modern Girl reflected tensions in all of the following issues EXCEPT:

   A. the influence of non-Japanese cultural traditions.
   B. the extent of women's participation in the workforce.
   C. whether, within Japanese families, women ought to be subordinate to men.
   D. whether the popular media should be accountable for the images they present.

How would you triage this question?

2. Which of the following, if true, would most *weaken* the author's claim about the significance of the Modern Girl?

   A. The Japanese did not associate the Modern Girl's behavior with Western influences.
   B. The Modern Girl disappeared from most popular Japanese media during World War II.
   C. Japan's social unrest in the 1920s was less than that of other countries at the time.
   D. Social change can never be solely attributed to one cultural figure.

How would you triage this question?

3. The author most likely includes the example of the "unruly woman" (paragraph 4) in order to:

   A. illustrate the extent of radical political action in 1920s Japan.
   B. suggest that gender conflicts in 1920s Japan were inevitable.
   C. help explain the complicated nature of the Modern Girl.
   D. compare the Modern Girl to her American counterpart.

How would you triage this question?

Practice Passage 1 (Questions 1–6)

The Modern Girl makes only a brief appearance in our histories of prewar Japan. She is a glittering, decadent, middle-class consumer who, through her clothing, smoking, and drinking, flaunts tradition in the urban playgrounds of the late 1920s. Arm in arm with her male equivalent, the Modern Boy (the *mobo*) and fleshed out in the Western flapper's garb of the roaring twenties, she engages in *ginbura* (Ginza-cruising). Yet by merely equating the Japanese Modern Girl with the flapper we do her a disservice, for the Modern Girl was not on a Western trajectory. Moreover, during the decade when this female, a creation of the mass media, excited her Japanese audience, she was not easily defined. Who was this "Modern Girl"? Why did she do what she did?

The Modern Girl is rescued from her depoliticized representation when her willful image is placed alongside the history of working, militant Japanese women. Then the depiction of the Modern Girl as apolitical (and later, as apolitical and nonworking) begins to appear as a means of displacing the very real militancy of Japanese women (just as the real labor of the American woman during the 1920s was denied by trivializing the work of the glamorized flapper). But whereas the American woman worker by the mid-1920s had allowed herself to be depoliticized by a new consumerism, the modern Japanese woman of the 1920s was truly militant. Her militancy was articulated through the adoption of new fashions, through labor in new arenas, and through political activity that consciously challenged social, economic, and political structures and relationships. The Japanese state's response encompassed attempts to revise the Civil Code, consideration of universal suffrage, organization and expansion of groups such as the Women's Alliance (*Fujin Doshikai*) and the nationwide network of *shojokai* (associations of young girls), censorship, and imprisonment of leaders. The media responded by producing the Modern Girl.

Yet talk about the Modern Girl and how she displaced serious concern about the radical nature of women's activity does not fully address her multifaceted nature.

Why, in other words, was she Japanese and Western, intellectual and worker, deviant and admirable? An answer is suggested by Natalie Davis in "Women on Top," which argues that the "unruly woman" in early modern Europe served both to reinforce social structure and to incite women to militant action in public and in private. The culturally constructed figure of the Japanese Modern Girl certainly meets these two requirements. Like the disorderly woman on top, the Modern Girl as multifaceted symbol questioned relations of order and subordination.

This thesis was indeed offered by the feminist Kitamura, who claimed that "labor struggle, tenancy struggle, household struggle, struggle between man and woman" were inevitable and had recently been joined to a new battle: "a struggle over good conduct" that pitted Japanese against Western behavior and used the Modern Girl to work out the struggle.

This, then, is the significance of the Japanese Modern Girl in the broadest context of prewar Japanese history. The Modern Girl stood as the vital symbol of overwhelming "modern" or non-Japanese change instigated by both women and men during an era of economic crisis and social unrest. She stood for change at a time when state authority was attempting to reestablish authority and stability. The Modern Girl of the 1920s and early 1930s thus inverted the role of the Good Wife and Wise Mother. The ideal Meiji woman of the 1870s, 1880s, and 1890s had served as a "repository of the past," standing for tradition when men were encouraged to change their way of politics and culture in all ways.

4. Which of the following is a claim made by the author that is NOT supported in the passage by evidence, explanation, or example?

    A. Japanese women in the 1920s challenged conventional notions of gender roles.
    B. Female workers in America lost their political status due to a new consumerism.
    C. The Modern Girl stood in contrast to earlier cultural exemplars.
    D. The role of the Modern Girl was not limited to strictly political issues.

How would you triage this question?

5. Implicit in the author's discussion of the Modern Girl is the assumption that:

    A. Japanese women of the 1920s viewed *ginbura* as incompatible with economic advancement.
    B. Western nations were not influenced by Japanese cultural traditions.
    C. the Modern Girl's influence contrasted with the influence of the *mobo*.
    D. political activities can be influenced by media portrayals.

How would you triage this question?

6. Which of the following pairs of entities most closely parallels the Japanese and American women workers, as described by the author?

    A. Two women who are the first and second wives, respectively, of a wealthy but dispassionate man
    B. Two picketing workers, one of whom continues pressing for better terms after a contract offer
    C. Two old friends who compete for the favor of the same employer
    D. Two sisters who work together to overcome low cultural expectations

How would you triage this question?

LESSON 7.4 REVIEW

Triaging the Section

- Read a portion (at least a sentence, plus a glance at the passage as a whole) as a rough scan to determine difficulty
- Skip the passage and return later if it looks too hard
- Use the following traits to judge a passage:
  - Subject matter
  - Complexity of writing
  - Length of paragraphs
  - Similarities to past passages you have seen
  - A rough scan of the questions
- Develop your own habits regarding checking the clock, scratchwork, and how many "passes" to make through a section

Triaging the Questions

- After reading the question stem, make a decision to skip or not
- Use the following traits to judge a question:
  - Length/complexity of question stem
  - Length/complexity of answer choices
  - Question type
  - Similarities to past questions you have seen
- Return to skipped questions before you move on to the next passage
- Consider flagging and returning to particularly hard questions at the end of a section

MCAT CARS Strategies in Action

In this lesson, you'll learn to:

- Use the Kaplan Triage Strategy for MCAT CARS passages
- Use the Kaplan Passage Strategy for MCAT CARS passages
- Use the Kaplan Question Strategy for MCAT CARS questions
- Use Kaplan methods on answer choices within MCAT CARS questions

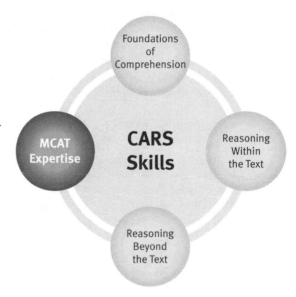

MCAT CARS STRATEGY

Passage Strategy

SCAN FOR STRUCTURE

READ STRATEGICALLY

LABEL EACH COMPONENT

REFLECT ON YOUR OUTLINE

Question Strategy

ASSESS THE QUESTION

PLAN YOUR ATTACK

EXECUTE THE PLAN

ANSWER BY MATCHING, ELIMINATING, OR GUESSING

LESSON 7.5, LEARNING GOALS 1–4:

- Use the Kaplan Triage Strategy for MCAT CARS passages
- Use the Kaplan Passage Strategy for MCAT CARS passages
- Use the Kaplan Question Strategy for MCAT CARS questions
- Use Kaplan methods on answer choices within MCAT CARS questions

Practice Passage (Questions 1–5)

Skepticism is a way of thinking or reasoning when presented with new information. Skepticism has its benefits; many mistakes can be avoided when viewing the world through the lens of a skeptic. This means looking at whether there is real and valid data to back up claims, and ensuring that data is exactly tied to the conclusions in the information. In this way, untrue information can be identified, and the pitfalls of this information can be avoided. However, skepticism has its faults as well. If skepticism is used alone, there is a risk of lack of progress. That is, just doubting all things without research or forward thinking can lead one to get mired in the muck of never moving forward. Some things must be true so that life can move on. Another disadvantage of skepticism is losing the connection with others over shared belief.

So what is the answer? When is skepticism useful? James Randi is a famous, now retired, stage magician, and is well known for his challenges to claims made by psychics, paranormal activists, and pseudoscientists. He is particularly famous for debunking Uri Geller, a world renowned, self-proclaimed psychic. In fact, each year Randi's educational foundation holds The Amazing Meeting, a conference in Las Vegas, where skeptics from all over the world come together to share in celebration of critical thinking. In this way, the connection that can potentially be lost due to not sharing beliefs with non-skeptics is gained through sharing skeptical thinking with similar-minded people. Randi also explains in his book, *Flim Flam!*, that paranormal researchers don't adhere to the scientific method as non-paranormal scientific researchers do. Randi describes this claim as a problem because people might actually make decisions based on the "results" of this paranormal research even though it's entirely possible that the paranormal data and conclusions aren't true. Randi also mentions that this sloppy following of the scientific method is less tolerated in other research fields.

There are a myriad of stories where a lack of skepticism has led people to believe false information. However, one might ask if there is any real danger in believing things like pseudoscience. For example, if someone really believes, say, that there is a ghost haunting their house, and there is, in fact, no such ghost, how does that actually hurt that person? To answer this, skeptics across the globe use online communities, books, and other media to connect and get the word out about stories of actual harm caused by belief in the unreal. Skepdic.com has archives of information about individuals experiencing everything from modern-day women being punished as witches in tribal communities to money lost in grandiose scams. Brian Dunning, host of the podcast Skeptoid, cites story after story of misinformation leading to life-ruining consequences from belief in false, supernatural claims.

So, despite the interesting prospect of a ghost in your house, a curse on your jewels, or even an unseen and benevolent protector, skepticism is a good candidate for a reasonable way to look at the world. It may not make you lots of friends or even make you happy, but skepticism does offer the prize of truth for your efforts, and this truth can be salvation from an otherwise strange and disordered world.

Passage Outline

P1.

P2.

P3.

P4.

Goal:

What can be learned from this passage?

Questions

1. Which of the following is a disadvantage of skepticism found in the first paragraph, and is also something the author fails to counter in the subsequent paragraphs?

   A. Skepticism is a method of reasoning through information
   B. Skepticism can identify untrue information
   C. The lack of progress due to skepticism
   D. The loss of connection to others through shared belief

   What can you learn from this question?

2. Suppose that Brian Dunning (paragraph 3) was recently convicted of fraud and sentenced to prison. Given this fact and the information from the passage, how should a skeptic react to the information that had been presented in Dunning's podcast?

   A. Disbelieving the information because Dunning is bad-natured
   B. Researching the information in sources other than the podcast itself
   C. Thinking the information is true because Dunning is a fellow skeptic
   D. Searching for new facts tangentially related to the podcast's information

   What can you learn from this question?

3. In regard to skepticism as a general mode of thought, the author would like to:

   A. stop readers from using skepticism so they can be happier.
   B. deter readers from skepticism if they want to make friends.
   C. increase the belief of ideas found in pseudoscience.
   D. support the use of skepticism in evaluating information.

   What can you learn from this question?

Practice Passage (Questions 1–5)

Skepticism is a way of thinking or reasoning when presented with new information. Skepticism has its benefits; many mistakes can be avoided when viewing the world through the lens of a skeptic. This means looking at whether there is real and valid data to back up claims, and ensuring that data is exactly tied to the conclusions in the information. In this way, untrue information can be identified, and the pitfalls of this information can be avoided. However, skepticism has its faults as well. If skepticism is used alone, there is a risk of lack of progress. That is, just doubting all things without research or forward thinking can lead one to get mired in the muck of never moving forward. Some things must be true so that life can move on. Another disadvantage of skepticism is losing the connection with others over shared belief.

So what is the answer? When is skepticism useful? James Randi is a famous, now retired, stage magician, and is well known for his challenges to claims made by psychics, paranormal activists, and pseudoscientists. He is particularly famous for debunking Uri Geller, a world renowned, self-proclaimed psychic. In fact, each year Randi's educational foundation holds The Amazing Meeting, a conference in Las Vegas, where skeptics from all over the world come together to share in celebration of critical thinking. In this way, the connection that can potentially be lost due to not sharing beliefs with non-skeptics is gained through sharing skeptical thinking with similar-minded people. Randi also explains in his book, *Flim Flam!*, that paranormal researchers don't adhere to the scientific method as non-paranormal scientific researchers do. Randi describes this claim as a problem because people might actually make decisions based on the "results" of this paranormal research even though it's entirely possible that the paranormal data and conclusions aren't true. Randi also mentions that this sloppy following of the scientific method is less tolerated in other research fields.

There are a myriad of stories where a lack of skepticism has led people to believe false information. However, one might ask If there is any real danger in believing things like pseudoscience. For example, if someone really believes, say, that there is a ghost haunting their house, and there is, in fact, no such ghost, how does that actually hurt that person? To answer this, skeptics across the globe use online communities, books, and other media to connect and get the word out about stories of actual harm caused by belief in the unreal. Skepdic.com has archives of information about individuals experiencing everything from modern-day women being punished as witches in tribal communities, to money lost in grandiose scams. Brian Dunning, host of the podcast Skeptoid, cites story after story of misinformation leading to life-ruining consequences from belief in false, supernatural claims.

So, despite the interesting prospect of a ghost in your house, a curse on your jewels, or even an unseen and benevolent protector, skepticism is a good candidate for a reasonable way to look at the world. It may not make you lots of friends or even make you happy, but skepticism does offer the prize of truth for your efforts, and this truth can be salvation from an otherwise strange and disordered world.

Questions

4. What is one reason the author includes the paragraph about James Randi (paragraph 2)?

   A. To counter the argument that there is no harm in belief in something unreal
   B. To show a way that skeptics can still share connections to others based on a way of thinking
   C. To demonstrate the good that can be done by pseudoscientists
   D. To highlight the harmful influence of psychics such as Uri Geller

What can you learn from this question?

5. It can reasonably be inferred that the author of this passage would react to new information in which of the following ways?

   A. The author may view the information as plausible given adequate support.
   B. The author would not believe any of the assertions in the new information.
   C. The author could consider the information valid only if other skeptics also did.
   D. The author would want to believe the information and attempt to support it.

What can you learn from this question?

LESSON 7.5 REVIEW

Chapter 6 Learning Goals

6.1 CARS Passage Structure and Strategy

- Utilize the Kaplan Passage Strategy, given a CARS passage

6.2 CARS Questions: Foundations of Comprehension

- Answer Main Idea questions
- Answer Detail questions
- Answer Function questions
- Answer Definition-in-Context questions

6.3 CARS Questions: Reasoning Within the Text

- Answer Inference questions
- Answer Strengthen/Weaken (Within Passage) questions

6.4 CARS Questions: Reasoning Beyond the Text

- Answer Apply questions
- Answer Strengthen/Weaken (Beyond Passage) questions

Chapter 7 Learning Goals

7.1 Argument Structure

- Recognize concepts, conceptual relationships, and claims in passages
- Identify the components of an argument

7.2 Wrong Answer Pathologies

- Recognize common wrong answer pathologies for questions in the Critical Analysis and Reasoning section

7.3 Identifying CARS Question Types

- Identify the question type of a given CARS question stem

7.4 Triage in the CARS Section

- Utilize the triaging strategy within a CARS section of the MCAT
- Use question stems and answer choices to preview and triage MCAT CARS questions

CHAPTER

8

Know the Test

MCAT Overview and Section Basics

In this lesson, you'll learn to:

- Describe the MCAT, its test sections, and the Kaplan MCAT course

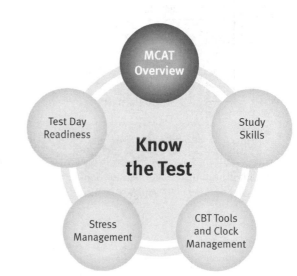

LESSON 8.1, LEARNING GOAL 1:

- Describe the MCAT, its test sections, and the Kaplan MCAT course

The Kaplan MCAT Course - Objectives and Resources

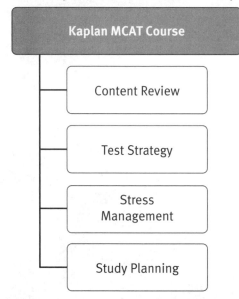

After this course, you should be able to...

Recall necessary science content when prompted by MCAT passages and questions.

Apply science knowledge and test-taking strategies to realistic MCAT questions, sections, and full-length exams.

Enact individualized clock management, stress management, and stamina-maintenance techniques on MCAT simulations and on Test Day.

Organize and follow through on the hundreds of hours of study and practice that the MCAT requires.

	Course Resource	What it's best for
Study on your own	*MCAT Review* Books (Biology, Organic Chemistry, etc.)	Science content instruction and review Integrated concept checks throughout Discrete practice questions after each chapter High-Yield Science Solutions Manual (HYSSM) for worked-out example questions
	Science Review Videos (100+ videos)	High-yield and more complex science content Interactive questions throughout
Live resources	Class Sessions (with your teacher)* Lessons On Demand (online)	Skills and test-taking strategy (always in context of specific MCAT questions) Guided practice with your class and your teacher Get your questions answered!
	The MCAT Channel (90+ unique hours)*	A little bit of everything (see schedule online) Wide range of live, expert teachers
Your practice	Full-Length Tests (including AAMC Practice)	Simulating Test Day Testing and building endurance
	Adaptive Qbank and Other Practice	Focused practice at different levels of length, structure, and difficulty
Quick hits	Flashcards App	Drills on key terms

*In Person and Live Online students only

KAPLAN TIP

In order to take full advantage of your resources, make sure to download the Kaplan Mobile Prep App! This will allow you to make use of our variety of resources even on the go, with a mobile-friendly interface.

The MCAT

Scoring on a Curve

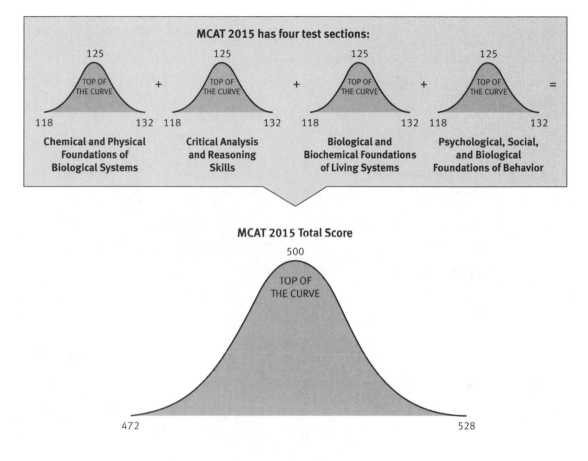

Your Goal Score

My Target Score:

The three biggest obstacles to me achieving this score are:

I can overcome these obstacles by:

How your MCAT score can help you:

An Outline of Test Day

Sections	Questions	Length, minutes
Jumpstart with Flashcard app until you check in	—	—
Examinee Agreement	—	10
Tutorial (Optional)	—	5
Chemical and Physical Foundations of Biological Systems	59	95
Optional Break	—	10
Critical Analysis and Reasoning Skills	53	90
Lunch Break	—	30
Biological and Biochemical Foundations of Living Systems	59	95
Optional Break	—	10
Psychological, Social, and Biological Foundations of Behavior	59	95
Void Question	—	5
Survey (Optional)	—	5

Total Time: 7+ hours

KAPLAN TIP

Given that the exam lasts over seven hours, you will need strategies to keep you on time and focused. The Kaplan Triaging Strategy will help you achieve this.

Science Content on the MCAT

Section	Content	Percentage*
Chemical and Physical Foundations of Biological Systems	Biochemistry	25%
	Biology	5%
	General Chem	30%
	Organic Chem	15%
	Physics	25%
Biological and Biochemical Foundations of Living Systems	Biochemistry	25%
	Biology	65%
	General Chem	5%
	Organic Chem	5%
Psychological, Social, and Biological Foundations of Behavior	Psychology	65%
	Sociology	30%
	Biology	5%

*According to the AAMC, these percentages are approximate and rounded to the nearest 5%. Exact content percentages will vary somewhat between test forms.

Section Structure Breakdown

Science Sections

Includes Chem/Phys, Bio/Biochem, and Psych/Soc Sections

44 Passage-Based questions, across 10 passages (4–6 questions per passage)

15 Discrete ("stand-alone") questions, in several sets across the section

CARS Section

53 Passage-Based questions, across 9 passages (4–7 questions per passage)

Science Skills on the MCAT

1. Knowledge of Scientific Concepts and Principles
   - Demonstrate understanding of scientific concepts and principles
   - Identify the relationships between closely related concepts

2. Scientific Reasoning and Problem Solving
   - Reason about scientific principles, theories, and models
   - Analyze and evaluate scientific explanations and predictions

3. Reasoning about the Design and Execution of Research
   - Demonstrate understanding of important components of scientific research
   - Reason about ethical issues in research

4. Data-Based and Statistical Reasoning
   - Interpret patterns in data presented in tables, figures, and graphs
   - Reason about data and draw conclusions from them

5. MCAT Expertise
   - Use strategies and thinking you need to score higher on your test

CARS Skills on the MCAT

1. Foundations of Comprehension
   - Demonstrate understanding of passage structure
   - Identify main ideas and themes in a passage

2. Reasoning Within the Text
   - Reason about arguments within a passage
   - Interpret connections between ideas and author meanings

3. Reasoning Beyond the Text
   - Apply logic from MCAT passages to novel situations
   - Determine the effect of new evidence on an author's argument

4. MCAT Expertise
   - Use strategies and thinking you need to score higher on your test

---

KAPLAN TIP

Each of the lessons in this course is organized around these Science and CARS skills. You will learn how to perform all these skills as you prepare for Test Day.

MCAT Study Skills

In this lesson, you'll learn to:

- Plan your personal course of action to raise your MCAT score

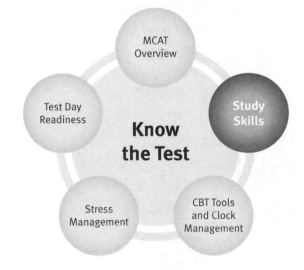

LESSON 8.2, LEARNING GOAL 1:

- Plan your personal course of action to raise your MCAT score

Register for Your MCAT

Make a Study Calendar

What to include in your calendar:

- Time for obligations
- Time for family and friends
- One day off each week
- Study time:
  - How long?
  - How often?
  - What to study?
  - Breaks

Example study day:

7 a.m.	Gym
8 a.m.	
9 a.m.	Class
10 a.m.	
11 a.m.	Lunch with Mom
12 p.m.	
1 p.m.	Volunteer at clinic
2 p.m.	
3 p.m.	Review from last MCAT class
4 p.m.	Read MCAT chapters for next class
5 p.m.	
6 p.m.	Dinner with Roommate
7 p.m.	Take a section of a practice MCAT
8 p.m.	
9 p.m.	Review MCAT practice test
10 p.m.	

KAPLAN TIP

Plan out exact details for each scheduled block of studying so you make sure to stay focused and productive during your study time.

The MCAT Lucky 7:

Study Habits for Success

1. Utilize all your resources to ensure the full study experience

2. Commit to your study and homework schedule; don't just "listen now, study later"

3. Don't just take test after test after test

4. Practice in the most test-like environment possible

5. Analyze and learn from each question you complete

6. Focus on your progress over time, not just individual scores

7. Don't let stress paralyze you—focus on success

KAPLAN TIP
Use these study habits to make the experience of studying for the MCAT
useful and productive! Make sure you make every study session count!

LESSON 8.2 REVIEW

To Do List:

Make a Study Plan

Detailed

Takes personal commitments into account

Realistic

Your Kaplan Resources

Explore your syllabus

Continue to complete your homework

CBT Tools and Clock Management

In this lesson, you'll learn to:

- Use the CBT tools provided on the MCAT effectively
- Execute a clock-monitoring strategy that promotes efficiency and prevents distractions

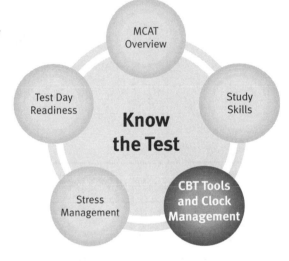

LESSON 8.3, LEARNING GOAL 1:

- Use the CBT tools provided on the MCAT effectively

What CBT tools are available, and how should you use them on Test Day?

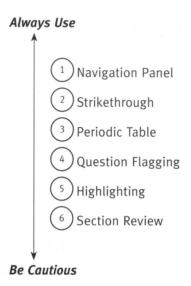

Always Use

1. Navigation Panel
2. Strikethrough
3. Periodic Table
4. Question Flagging
5. Highlighting
6. Section Review

Be Cautious

Keyboard Shortcuts (for reference):

Shortcut	Function	Shortcut (Section Review)	Function (Section Review)
Alt + N	Advance to Next; Answer No	Alt + E	End Review of Section/ Exam
Alt + P	Return to Previous	Alt + W	Return to Section Review
Alt + V	Open Navigation	Alt + A	Review All Questions
Alt + H	Highlight/Remove Highlight	Alt + I	Review Incomplete
Alt + S	Strikethrough/Remove Strikethrough	Alt + R	Review Flagged
Alt + T	Open Periodic Table	Alt + Y	Answer Yes
Alt + C	Close Navigation/Close Periodic Table	Alt + O	Answer OK
Alt + F	Flag for Review		

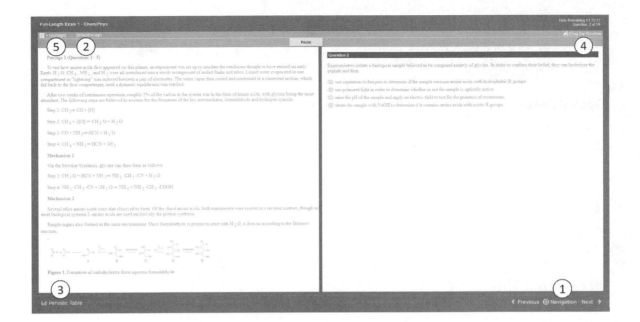

LESSON 8.3, LEARNING GOAL 2:

- Execute a clock-monitoring strategy that promotes efficiency and prevents distractions

Good Habits	Bad Habits

Facts About the Test Clock

Science Sections

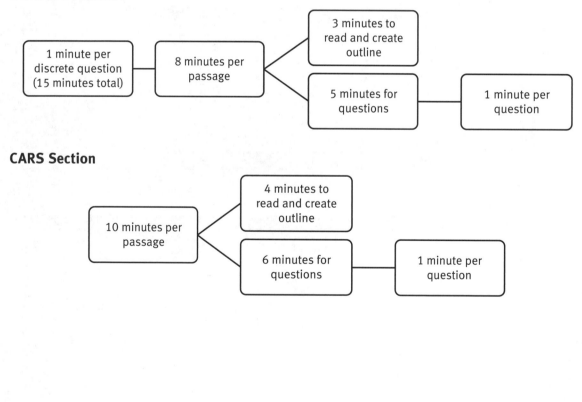

Science Sections

1 minute per discrete question (15 minutes total) → 8 minutes per passage → 3 minutes to read and create outline

5 minutes for questions → 1 minute per question

CARS Section

10 minutes per passage → 4 minutes to read and create outline

6 minutes for questions → 1 minute per question

CARS Section

KAPLAN TIP

Note that the times covered above represent an average across the entire exam. Some passages and questions may go more quickly than others. It is exactly for this reason that pacing is so important.

Section Pacing

Science Sections	Section Progress	CARS Section
95 minutes	Start	90 minutes
80 minutes	Discretes Finished	—
72 minutes	1	80 minutes
64 minutes	2	70 minutes
56 minutes	3	60 minutes
48 minutes	4	50 minutes
40 minutes	5	40 minutes
32 minutes	6	30 minutes
24 minutes	7	20 minutes
16 minutes	8	10 minutes
8 minutes	9	0 minutes
0 minutes	10	—

KAPLAN TIP

These timing benchmarks are *averages*; some passages will take longer than others on your real exam. Ideally, you also want to work slightly ahead of these numbers on Test Day, in order to keep a few minutes of buffer time to go back to difficult or flagged questions before finishing each section.

Stress Management

In this lesson, you'll learn to:

- Prevent stress from impeding your MCAT studying and Test Day performance

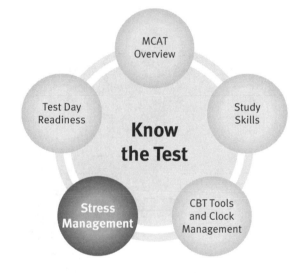

LESSON 8.4, LEARNING GOAL 1:

- Prevent stress from impeding your MCAT studying and Test Day performance

Stress Management as You Study

Positives of Your Prep

Task: Review your preparation process thus far. List all the things—large and small—that you are good at doing.

KAPLAN TIP

When there's a lot on the line, stress increases. That's normal.

Address Weaknesses as Areas of Opportunity

Task: Make a list of your test-taking weaknesses and your plans for overcoming them.

KAPLAN TIP

If you try to repair too many problems at once, you'll just get more frustrated.

KAPLAN TIP

Don't forget to exercise! This can be a good way to spend time away from the test.

Stress Management on Test Day

What will you tell yourself...

...if you fall behind in a section?

...when you can't answer a question?

...when a passage is harder than expected?

...if you start feeling overly anxious during the exam?

Task: Imagine "disaster scenarios" and visualize yourself overcoming them.

KAPLAN TIP
Thinking ahead about what problems might come up and how to tackle
them is a great way to handle these common issues.

LESSON 8.4 REVIEW

Visualize Success

Don't forget—you've been working on the psychological dimensions of test-taking since your Kaplan course began.

Task: Return to this lesson as you study and add more strengths and weaknesses as you discover them.

Task: Envision yourself successfully attacking the test.

Handling Test Anxiety

- Remember to move around or stretch during the exam
- Take the breaks given during the exam
- If your mind suddenly goes blank on a question, skip the question and come back to it later
- Take occasional deep breaths to help you relax and stay in control
- Close your eyes for a few seconds occasionally throughout the exam
- Expect some anxiety, and work toward managing it
- Remind yourself of all the great hard work you've done to get to the point of taking the MCAT

Test Day Readiness

In this lesson, you'll learn to:

- Use the time between the end of your class and Test Day efficiently

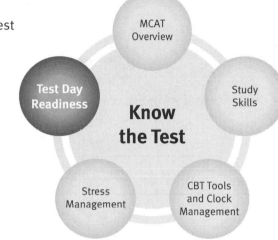

LESSON 8.5, LEARNING GOAL 1:

- Use the time between the end of your class and Test Day efficiently

Am I ready to take the MCAT?

- Have you completed relevant homework?

- Have you been *consistently* scoring in your desired range on practice tests?

- Are you experiencing understandable nervousness or actual reasons for concern?

- Make sure you talk to Kaplan before you decide to actually reschedule your exam.

Higher Score Guarantee

- You must attend all scheduled classes (and follow guidelines regarding make-up sessions).
- You must take all scheduled practice tests.
- You need to complete the "required" homework for your course *prior* to your course expiration date or exam date, whichever is earlier.
- You need to submit claim for Higher Score Guarantee within 90 days of course expiration date.

KAPLAN TIP

The decision about whether you're ready to take your MCAT is a tough one. Make sure you consider it carefully and yet still keep up your confidence!

Update Your Study Calendar

What to include in your calendar:

- Any Remaining Required Work
- Flashcards
- Full-Length Tests
- AAMC Resources
- Test Review
- Section Tests
- Adaptive QBank
- Focused Subject Review (MCAT Channel, videos, book chapters, HYPSG, etc.)
- Additional Resources

Sample Calendars: 1 Month to Test Day

Case #1: "I am not caught up with my homework from the course"

	Sunday	Monday	Tuesday	Wednesday	Thursday	Friday	Saturday
Week 4	Complete Remaining Homework from Unit 1	Complete Remaining Homework from Unit 2	Complete Remaining Homework from Unit 3	Complete Remaining Homework from Unit 3	Complete any remaining Skills Tests and Review	AAMC Section Bank, Flashcards	Day off
Week 3	Review weak content (videos), AAMC Practice, Flashcards	Review Books for weak areas, Adaptive Qbank	AAMC Practice, Flashcards	Take a practice full-length test	Review Test, Flashcards, Adaptive Qbank	Day off	AAMC Practice, Video Content Review, Flashcards
Week 2	Content Review, AAMC Practice, Adaptive Qbank, Flashcards	Take a practice full-length test	Review Test, Flashcards, Adaptive Qbank	Review Books for weak areas, Flashcards	AAMC Practice (Official Guide or similar), Flashcards	Day off	Take a practice full-length test
Last Week	Review Test, Flashcards, Adaptive Qbank	Content Review, AAMC Practice, Flashcards	AAMC Practice, Adaptive Qbank, Content Review (videos), Flashcards	Adaptive Qbank, Content Review (videos), Flashcards	Adaptive Qbank, AAMC Practice, Flashcards	Day off	**Test Day!**

> **KAPLAN TIP**
>
> Plan your study calendar in detail and stick to it to maintain great study habits all the way to Test Day.

K

Case #2: "I have a few weaker content areas but have finished all the homework"

	Sunday	Monday	Tuesday	Wednesday	Thursday	Friday	Saturday
Week 4	Review weak content areas (videos), AAMC Practice, Flashcards	Review weak content areas (books), Flashcards	AAMC Practice, Adaptive Qbank, Flashcards	Content Review (video), Flashcards	Content Review (books), Adaptive Qbank, Flashcards	Day off	Take a practice full-length test
Week 3	Review Test, Flashcards, Content Review (video)	Skills Tests + Lesson Book for Strategy, Flashcards	Content Review (books), Adaptive Qbank, Flashcards	AAMC Practice (Official Guide or similar), Flashcards	Content Review (book + video), Adaptive Qbank, Flashcards	Day off	Take a practice full-length test
Week 2	Review Test, Flashcards, Content Review (video)	Content Review (book), Adaptive Qbank, Flashcards	Content Review (video), Adaptive Qbank, Flashcards	AAMC Practice (Section Bank or similar), Flashcards	AAMC Practice (Section Bank or similar), Flashcards	Day off	Take a practice full-length test
Last Week	Review Test, Flashcards, Content Review (video)	Content Review (video), Adaptive Qbank, Flashcards	AAMC Practice, Content Review (book), Flashcards	Adaptive Qbank, Content Review (book + video), Flashcards	Short AAMC Practice/ Adaptive Qbank, Flashcards	Day off	**Test Day!**

Case #3: "I am feeling pretty confident about the test"

	Sunday	Monday	Tuesday	Wednesday	Thursday	Friday	Saturday
Week 4	Content Review (books), Adaptive Qbank, Flashcards	Content Review (video), AAMC Practice, Flashcards	AAMC Practice (Section Bank or similar), Flashcards	Take a practice full-length test	Review Test, Flashcards, Adaptive Qbank	Day off	Content Review (books + videos), Adaptive Qbank, Flashcards
Week 3	AAMC Practice (Official Guide or similar), Flashcards	Take a practice full-length test	Review Test, Flashcards, Adaptive Qbank	Content Review (video), AAMC Practice, Flashcards	Content Review (books), Adaptive Qbank, Flashcards	Day off	Take a practice full-length test
Week 2	Review Test, Flashcards, Adaptive Qbank	Content Review (video), AAMC Practice, Flashcards	Content Review (book), Adaptive Qbank, Flashcards	AAMC Practice (Section Bank or similar), Flashcards	Two practice section tests, Flashcards	Day off	Take a practice full-length test
Last Week	Review Test, Flashcards, Adaptive Qbank	Two practice section tests, Flashcards	Take a practice full-length test	Review Test, Flashcards, AAMC Practice	Short AAMC Practice or Adaptive Qbank, Flashcards	Day off	**Test Day!**

Which sample calendar most closely resembles your plans for studying up until Test Day?

Practice Tests: Problems and Solutions

What can I do if I...

...am not finishing every section in time?

...have to constantly refer back to the passage?

...keep narrowing down questions to two choices but pick the wrong answer?

...feel fatigued during the test, especially at the end?

...always end up missing questions on the same topics?

What to Do...

...until a week before the test

- Focus on weak areas.
- Read, read, read!
- Diagnose yourself with your Practice Test scores and review.
- Address any fatigue or focus issues.
- Don't get so hung up on content that you forget to evaluate things like your pacing, triaging, and endurance.
- Practice at the computer.
- Create test-friendly habits.
- Work carefully with your motivation to make sure you can stick to your study commitments.

...exactly one week before Test Day

- Get up at the same time you would on Test Day.
- Visit the test site.
- Start going to bed at an appropriate time.
- Take a practice full-length test.

...during the week of Test Day

- Eat good meals at regular times.
- Continue your sleep/wake-up schedule all week long.
- Practice in a test-like environment.
- Avoid doing anything new or unusual.

KAPLAN TIP

Thinking too much about Test Day itself can induce anxiety. Remember to focus on success and your future as a physician!

The MCAT Lucky 7 (Round Two):

Rules for the Day Before the MCAT

Rule #1: Avoid talking about the MCAT.

Rule #2: Within reason, avoid studying for the MCAT.

Rule #3: Plan your day; do something engaging that you enjoy.

Rule #4: Envision your post-MCAT activities.

Rule #5: Eat high-energy foods.

Rule #6: Get enough sleep.

Rule #7: Gather your Test Day materials.

Test Day Materials Checklist:

- Printout of your confirmation email
- Personal identification (two)
- Snacks/sports drink
- Lunch
- Tissues
- Cough drops
- Painkillers
- Antacid
- Pump-up music/good-luck token/lucky T-shirt
- Write your own list items here:

KAPLAN TIP

The day before the MCAT is the most important day of your prep in terms of getting in the right mindset for the exam. So plan it well and use it wisely to make sure the next day—Test Day—is the best that it can be.

What to do ...

... on Test Day

- Wake up on time.
- Eat your normal breakfast.
- Warm up physically and mentally.
- Wear comfortable clothing and dress in layers.
- Bring high-energy foods for snacks.
- Arrive at the test site with time to spare.
- Bring all your testing materials.

... during the MCAT

- Do the tutorial in order to get comfortable with the computer.
- Handle (the rare) test administration difficulties properly and calmly.
- Triage all passages and questions. (Remember to do the discrete questions first!)
- Answer every question.
- Reset your mind during breaks.
- Focus on what is in front of you.
- Don't discuss the test during breaks or after the exam.

KAPLAN TIP

Commonly prohibited items in the actual testing room are outerwear, hats, food, drinks, purses, briefcases, notebooks, pagers, watches, cellular telephones, recording devices, photographic equipment, and (of course) MCAT study materials.

Should I Void My Score?

No, not if you ...

- felt the test was hard.
- felt like you strategically guessed too many questions.
- didn't finish *every* passage.

Yes, if (and only if!) you ...

- left a large number of questions blank.
- got physically ill during the test.
- had extreme test administration problems.

What to Do After the Test

- Relax.
- Send Kaplan those scores when you get them!
- Continue preparing to apply to medical school.
- Secure letters of recommendation.
- Work on a personal statement.
- Keep Kaplan updated with your journey to and through medical school and your career as a physician.

KAPLAN TIP

Once you're done with the test, make sure you celebrate your hard work! In fact, looking forward to this celebration is a great way to keep yourself motivated while you are studying.

LESSON 8.5 REVIEW

What to Do Now:

- Fill in your calendar with study time and other activities.
- Stay in contact with Kaplan for questions and information.
- Focus on building stamina and endurance by completing practice tests.
- Congratulate yourself on how far you've come.
- Focus on success! Remember that you are doing all of this to become a physician!

SECTION III

Extra Practice

Chem/Phys 1: Foundations of MCAT Science

DISCRETE PRACTICE QUESTIONS (QUESTIONS 1–11)

1. Suppose that a lead ball and a plastic ball are dropped vertically from a building, and their time of flight is measured in order to calculate the gravitational constant g. Which of the following would change the measured value of g in this experiment?

   I. Increasing the mass of the Earth
   II. Using balls with different masses but the same volume
   III. Throwing the balls horizontally instead of dropping them vertically

   A. I only
   B. III only
   C. I and II only
   D. II and III only

2. Ignoring the effects of air resistance, if a ball is released from some height, the velocity of the ball just before impact with the ground does NOT depend upon:

   A. the velocity of the ball when it is released.
   B. the height from which the ball is released.
   C. the mass of the Earth.
   D. the mass of the ball.

3. A ball moving at 15 m/s decelerates uniformly at 1 m/s^2. Approximately how far does the ball travel during the first 45 ms while it decelerates?

   A. 0.121 m
   B. 0.453 m
   C. 0.674 m
   D. 0.928 m

4. A ball is thrown from a height of 10 m above the ground with a velocity of 4 m/s directed at an angle of 30° above the horizontal. What is the maximum height above the initial 10 m that the ball was released that is reached by the ball? (Note: The acceleration due to gravity is g = 9.8 m/s^2, sin 30° = 0.50, and cos 30° = 0.866.)

   A. 10.2 cm
   B. 20.4 cm
   C. 30.6 cm
   D. 61.2 cm

5. How much work is done by the force of gravity to maintain the orbit of a satellite that moves in a circular orbit if the satellite has a mass of 1×10^5 g, a velocity of 4×10^3 m/s, and a radius of orbit of 2×10^8 m from the center of the Earth?

   A. 0 J
   B. 800 J
   C. 8×10^5 J
   D. 16×10^5 J

6. In backscattering spectrometry, a beam of helium ions is directed at a sample and energy from the collision is measured. If the source aperture from which a beam of 2-MeV helium ions emerge is at a distance of 15 cm from the sample, how long does it take for one of these incident particles (each with mass 4 amu) to reach the sample? (Note: 1 amu = 1.66×10^{-27} kg; 1 eV = 1.60×10^{-19} J)

   A. 1.5×10^{-8} s
   B. 1.0×10^{-7} s
   C. 1.5×10^{-6} s
   D. 1.0×10^{-5} s

7. The most reactive functional group on the molecule 6,6-dichlorohexanal is a(n):

   A. alcohol group.
   B. carbonyl group.
   C. carboxyl group.
   D. chlorine.

8. According to the graph below, which straight-chain hydrocarbons exist in the liquid state at −50°C? (n is the number of carbons)

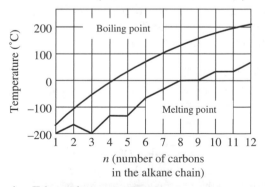

   A. Ethane, butane, pentane
   B. Pentane, hexane, octane
   C. Propane, butane, hexane
   D. Pentane, octane, urethane

9. An object in free fall first accelerates at 9.8 m/s² downwards and after a few seconds has an acceleration of 0; at no time in this span does it have a net upwards acceleration. Which of the following statements could explain these findings?

   A. The object hits the ground.
   B. Air resistance counters gravity completely at a certain speed.
   C. The object continues falling at a faster and faster rate for the whole fall.
   D. The object falls at a constant rate for the whole fall.

10. Which one of the following has the highest boiling point?

    A. Water
    B. Methane
    C. Acetic acid
    D. Acetone

11. Which of the following elements releases energy when converted to a negatively charged ion?

    I. C
    II. Na
    III. Br

    A. I only
    B. III only
    C. I and III only
    D. I, II, and III

CARS 1: Reading Passages the Kaplan Way

PASSAGE 1 (QUESTIONS 1–7)

Those who consider the Devil to be a partisan of Evil and angels to be warriors for Good accept the demagogy of the angels. Things are clearly more complicated. Angels are partisans not of Good, but of Divine creation. The Devil, on the other hand, denies all rational meaning to God's world.

World domination, as everyone knows, is divided between demons and angels. But the good of the world does not require the latter to gain precedence over the former (as I thought when I was young); all it needs is a certain equilibrium of power. If there is too much uncontested meaning on Earth (the reign of the angels), man collapses under the burden; if the world loses all its meaning (the reign of the demons), life is every bit as impossible.

Things deprived suddenly of their putative meaning, the place assigned to them in the ostensible order of things, make us laugh. Initially, therefore, laughter is the province of the Devil, who knows what it means to be abruptly stripped of rank—he could not help but guffaw after being cast from the Heavens and plunging into the bowels of the Earth. This laughter has a certain malice to it (things have turned out differently from the way they tried to seem), but a certain beneficent relief as well (things are looser than they seemed, we have greater latitude in living with them, their gravity does not oppress us).

The first time an angel heard the Devil's laughter, he was horrified. It was in the middle of a feast with a lot of people around, and one after the other they joined the Devil's laughter. It was terribly contagious. The angel was all too aware that the laughter was aimed against God and the wonder of His works. He knew he had to act fast, but felt weak and defenseless. Unable to fabricate anything of his own, he simply turned his enemy's tactics against him. He opened his mouth and let out a wobbly, breathy sound in the upper reaches of his vocal register and endowed it with the opposite meaning. Whereas the Devil's laughter pointed at the meaninglessness of things, the angel's shout rejoiced in how rationally organized, well-conceived, beautiful, good, and sensible everything on Earth was.

There they stood, Devil and angel, face to face, mouths open, both making more or less the same sound, but each expressing himself in a unique timbre—absolute opposites. And seeing the laughing angel, the Devil laughed all the harder, all the louder, and all the more openly, because the laughing angel was infinitely laughable.

Laughable laughter is cataclysmic. And even so, the angels have gained something by it. They have tricked us all with their semantic hoax. Their imitation laughter and its original (the Devil's) have the same name. People nowadays do not even realize that one and the same external phenomenon embraces two completely contradictory internal attitudes. We lack the words to distinguish these two types of laughter.

1. The primary function of the author's discussion in paragraph 3 is to:

   A. explain the character of the Devil's laughter.
   B. suggest that the Devil was justly punished for his sins.
   C. argue that the meaning of laughter is ambiguous.
   D. describe the Devil's descent from the Heavens.

2. Which of the following best characterizes the main idea of the passage?

   A. Angels learned to laugh only after observing the Devil first.
   B. Most people misunderstand the true purpose of laughter.
   C. The word "laughter" actually has at least two opposite connotations.
   D. Human laughter is an intermediate between angelic and demonic laughter.

3. In the first two paragraphs, the author is predominantly concerned with:

   A. reflecting on the errors of his youth.
   B. advocating for the superiority of the angels.
   C. finding equilibrium between two kinds of laughter.
   D. clarifying the roles of angels and demons.

4. The author's conception of laughter implies that language:

   A. is capable of concealing distinct meanings.
   B. cannot suddenly be deprived of all meaning.
   C. is always precise and unambiguous.
   D. is unnecessary for spiritual beings.

5. In the context of the passage, which of the following forms of laughter is most similar to that of the Devil?

   A. Laughing nervously in a tense situation
   B. Laughing at a joke in which the meaning of a word is twisted
   C. Laughing in satisfaction when a complicated task is completed
   D. Laughing to conceal one's true intentions

6. Based on information in the passage, with which of the following statements would the author most likely NOT agree?

   A. A balance must be struck in the world between rationality and irrationality.
   B. The Devil serves an important function for the good of the world.
   C. Laughter is the simultaneous expression of two contradictory attitudes.
   D. It is possible to laugh without having seen something deprived of meaning.

7. According to the passage, which of the following is true about the relationship between laughter and meaning?

   A. Laughter would not have come about if the meaning of everything was immutable.
   B. Without laughter, there would be no way to contest the meaning of things.
   C. The word used to denote laughter itself has no meaning.
   D. There are only two possible types of laughter that have meaning.

PASSAGE 2 (QUESTIONS 8–13)

The social novel has always presupposed a substantial amount of social stability. The ideal social novel had been written by Jane Austen, a great artist who enjoyed the luxury of being able to take society for granted; it was there, and seemed steady beneath her glass, Napoleon or no Napoleon. But soon it would not be steady beneath anyone's glass, and the novelist's attention had necessarily to shift from the gradations within society to the fate of society itself. It is at this point that the political novel comes to be written—the kind in which the idea of society, as distinct from the mere unquestioned workings of society, has penetrated the consciousness of the characters in all of its profoundly problematic aspects.

The political novel—I have in mind its ideal form—is peculiarly a work of internal tensions. To be a novel at all, it must contain the usual representation of human behavior and feeling; yet it must also absorb into its stream of movement the hard and perhaps insoluble pellets of modern ideology. The conflict is inescapable: the novel tries to confront experience in its immediacy and closeness, while ideology is by its nature general and inclusive. Yet it is precisely from this conflict that the political novel gains its interest and takes on the aura of high drama: the timelessness of abstraction is confronted with the flux of life, the monolith of program with the diversity of motive, the purity of ideal with the contamination of action.

Because it exposes the impersonal claims of ideology to the pressures of private emotion, the political novel must always be in a state of internal warfare, always on the verge of becoming something other than itself. The political novelist establishes a complex system of intellectual movements, in which his own opinion is one of the most active yet not entirely dominating movers. Are we not close here to one of the secrets of the novel in general? I mean the vast respect which the great novelist is ready to offer the whole idea of opposition, the opposition he needs to allow for in his book against his own predispositions and yearnings and fantasies.

This is not to say that the political novelist's desires—both acknowledged and repressed—fail to play a pivotal role in the novel's dialectic. Indeed, the political novel turns characteristically to an apolitical temptation: in *The Possessed*, to the notion that redemption is possible only to sinners who have suffered greatly; in Conrad's *Nostromo* and *Under Western Eyes*, to the resources of private affection and gentleness; in *Man's Fate*, to the metaphysical allurements of heroism as they reveal themselves in a martyr's death; in Silone's *Bread and Wine*, to the discovery of peasant simplicity as a foil to urban corruption; and in *Darkness at Noon*, to the abandoned uses of the personal will. This, so to say, is the pastoral element that is indispensable to the political novel, indispensable for providing it with polarity and tension.

8. The author's attitude toward literary works that focus on ideological issues can best be described as:

   A. appreciative of their ability to subordinate dramatic appeal to an exposition of serious themes.
   B. puzzled over their lack of acceptance by the general public.
   C. confident that their inherent tensions can be a source of strength.
   D. disappointed by their confusion of personal experiences with ideological arguments.

9. The author includes a discussion of Jane Austen primarily in order to:

   A. cite an example of a novelist who successfully combines elements of ideology and human experience.
   B. show the roots of the political novel in relation to earlier fiction traditions.
   C. criticize the social novel for presenting only stable social structures.
   D. argue that great novelists are not limited by their social backgrounds.

10. According to the passage, which of the following was an important factor in the emergence of the political novel?

    A. The critical success of novelists like Jane Austen
    B. The development of the "pastoral" element in novels like *Darkness at Noon*
    C. Increased awareness of the concept of societal change
    D. Agreement among critics that every great novel involves some kind of conflict

11. In paragraph 2, by "monolith of program," the author is specifically referring to:

    A. a writing method employed by political novelists.
    B. the unity inherent in a work of high drama.
    C. the conflict that characterizes political novels.
    D. the ideological aspect of a political novel.

12. Which of the following best categorizes the main content of the final paragraph?

    A. Comparing the political novel to the social novel
    B. Providing examples of certain themes in political novels
    C. Showing how all political novels are in reality apolitical
    D. Refuting the repressed desires of political novelists

13. Adopting the author's views as presented in the passage would most likely require endorsing which of the following positions?

    A. Human emotions and ideology are distinct categories that can conflict.
    B. Consciousness of societal conditions is necessary for the development of any new form of literature.
    C. The social novel owes much of its dramatic power to the conflict between rationality and human experience.
    D. Before the invention of the political novel, most novelists could not overcome their own prejudices.

PASSAGE 3 (QUESTIONS 14–18)

Sensing that government defined by the Articles of Confederation did not meet the needs of the newly born United States, the Congress of the Articles of Confederation authorized commissioners to "devise such further provisions as shall appear to them necessary to render the Constitution of the federal government adequate to the exigencies of the Union." These provisions were to be reported to Congress and confirmed by every state. The recommendatory acts also state that this change, to be done through alterations to the Articles of Confederation, is the most probable means of establishing a strong national government. Having given these instructions, Congress was quite surprised by the radically new terms of the Constitution submitted. In fact, some congressmen claimed that the commissioners did not have the legal authority to submit such a revolutionary document.

In *The Federalist Papers*, James Madison defends the commissioners by returning to the terms of their mandate. Given the goals expressed in the recommendatory acts, and the principle that conflicts ought to be resolved in favor of more important goals, Madison argued that the degree to which the Constitution departs from the Articles couldn't make the Constitution illegal. Where the goal of amending the Articles conflicts with the goal of creating good government, the Articles must yield, since the goal of "good government" is an overriding consideration.

Although Madison argued fairly convincingly that the degree of change present in the Constitution cannot be grounds for declaring it illegal, this same argument does not apply to the commissioners' decision to allow the Constitution to be ratified by only three-quarters of the states. Even though unanimous approval appears last in Madison's list of the goals of the convention, it was a fundamental aspect of national government under the Articles. Requiring non-ratifying states to be bound by the new Constitution was thus a powerful diminishment of their sovereignty.

The new Constitution, once adopted, changed the national government from a weak union of independent states to a strong union in which the interests of the many states could outweigh the protests of the few. Although history has validated the wisdom of the change, the question of whether the change was legal is another matter. In authorizing the commissioners, the individual states requested a proposal for the alteration of the national government. They did not intend to waive their veto power. So even if Madison is correct, and the commissioners could have proposed anything they deemed likely to fulfill the goal of good government, it does not follow that their proclamations should affect the legal rights of the several states.

Does this imply that the Constitution ratified by the states has no moral authority? Not necessarily. No government ought to have the power to entrench itself against amendment, and so the fact that the government under the Articles of Confederation did not consent to the alteration of the ratification process does not establish the moral illegitimacy of the Constitution.

The ethical case for rebelling against the government under the Articles is further strengthened by the fact that the government itself admitted its unfitness for the exigencies of the Union. Indeed, the ratification process altered by the new Constitution is representative of the procedures that initially led Congress to seek reform. In addressing the relevance of opposing the government of the Articles of Confederation, we should also consider the position of the framers. They had already rebelled against England, one of the great powers of the time, and thus had demonstrated an unwillingness to tolerate bad government. Defying the government of the Articles must have seemed easy by comparison.

14. According to the passage, which of the following provided justification for the revolutionary nature of the new Constitution?

    A. The current government's admission of its inadequacy in national affairs

    B. The right of any given state to refuse to ratify the new Constitution

    C. The moral right of a new government to entrench itself against amendment

    D. The recommendation that the new Constitution be created from alterations of the current Articles of Confederation

15. Which of the following assumptions can most reasonably be attributed to Madison?

    A. In the case of conflicting interests, priority should be given to the course of action that best promotes peace in the nation.

    B. Applications of conflict resolution principles can be used to determine the legality of an action.

    C. Unanimous approval is the most important objective in drafting a new constitution.

    D. The Constitution drafted by the commissioners corresponded precisely to the expectations of the Congress of the Articles of Confederation.

16. The author implies which of the following relationships between legal and moral authority?

    A. The morality of a constitution is the primary determinant of its legality.

    B. A principle lacking moral authority can still be legally binding.

    C. The morality of an action can never be determined irrespective of the legality of that action.

    D. A document lacking legal authority can still carry moral weight.

17. It can be inferred that Congress's surprise over the radical nature of the Constitution submitted by the commissioners could be attributed in part to the fact that its members did NOT foresee:

    A. the eventuality that the Constitution it requested would be adopted without the unanimous ratification of the states.

    B. the possibility that the Constitution it requested would contain provisions that jeopardized the government's moral authority.

    C. a conflict between the modification of the Articles of Confederation and the creation of a Constitution adequate to the needs of the nation.

    D. the possibility that the Constitution it requested would differ from the Articles of Confederation.

18. Which of the following, if true, would most seriously WEAKEN the argument put forth in defense of the legality of the Constitution submitted by the commissioners?

    A. Non-unanimous ratification of such a new constitution is incompatible with the goal of creating a good government.

    B. Extensive debate among statesmen is necessary in order to create a fair and legal constitution.

    C. It is nearly impossible to create an effective constitution out of the pieces of a previous constitution.

    D. No legal constitution can include provisions to safeguard the power of the ruling elite that commissioned the document.

PASSAGE 4 (QUESTIONS 19–24)

Divided power creates a built-in hurdle to making and carrying out fiscal policy. The hurdle is low when the president is articulating a policy that has broad support. It can lead to erratic shifts of policy when the president is leading in a direction in which the public and its representatives do not want to go. Deadlocks are rare, but can be serious. The failure to reduce the huge structural deficit of the mid-1980s largely reflects the fact that the president's solution—drastic reduction of the federal role in the domestic economy—did not command broad support. Prolonged government shutdowns in 1995–1996 and 2013 offer additional examples.

The simple notion that the president proposes and Congress disposes is greatly complicated by the fragmentation of power within each branch. Moreover, efforts to make fiscal policy more coherent have added new power centers without consolidating old ones. Presidents have tried various coordination mechanisms including "troika" arrangements and an almost infinite variety of committees with varying responsibilities. The system works tolerably well or exceedingly creakily, depending on the president's personal style and the personalities involved. But it encourages battling over turf as well as substance. One wonders whether it is not time to give our president the equivalent of a finance minister charged with functions now diffused to our budget director, Council of Economic Advisers, and secretary of the treasury.

The fragmentation of power and responsibility is, of course, even more extreme in the Congress. In addition to the central divide between Democrats and Republicans, a number of "parties," "caucuses," "gangs," and other voting blocs have emerged, some of which tend toward economic oversimplification and inflexible stands on the budget. The legislative branch also has a long history of attempts to make taxing and spending policy more coherent by adding new coordinating institutions—appropriations committees, budget committees, a congressional budget office—without eliminating or consolidating any old ones.

Concern that the economic policy process is not working has spawned proposals for drastic change that move in two quite different directions: one toward circumscribing the discretion of elected officials by putting economic policy on automatic pilot and the other toward making elected officials more directly responsible to voters. The automatic-pilot approach flows from the perspective that the decisions of elected officials cannot be counted on to produce economic policy in the social interest, but are likely to be biased toward excessive spending, growing deficits, special interest tax and spending programs, and easier money. A way to overcome these biases is to agree in advance on strict rules, such as a fixed monetary growth path or constitutionally required budget balance. The other direction of reform reflects the contrasting view that the diffusion of responsibility in our government makes it too difficult for the electorate to enforce its will by holding elected officials responsible for their policies. The potential for deadlock would be reduced if the country moved toward a parliamentary system, or found a way to hold political parties more strictly accountable for proposing and carrying out legislation.

19. The author's primary purpose is to:

   A. promote the automatic-pilot approach to managing fiscal policy.
   B. explain the problem that division of power poses for fiscal policy and consider solutions.
   C. describe divisions of power that occur within and between the branches of U.S. government.
   D. argue that divided power makes it impossible to execute fiscal policy effectively.

20. In paragraph 3, the author is mainly interested in:

   A. discussing how the diffusion of power in the legislative branch affects fiscal policy.
   B. advocating for the consolidation of congressional coordinating institutions.
   C. criticizing Congress for being even worse than the presidency.
   D. showing how congressional in-fighting makes solving fiscal problems hopeless.

21. Which of the following is a claim made in the passage but NOT supported by evidence, explanation, or example?

   A. Putting the economy on automatic pilot may circumvent the problems caused by elected officials.
   B. The proposals to revamp the economic policy process are based on very different assumptions.
   C. A president can have difficulty pushing through a fiscal policy when there is opposition to it.
   D. There would be less deadlock if a parliamentary system were adopted.

22. Which of the following, if true, would most strengthen the author's argument about fiscal policy-making?

   A. Countries that lack coherent and efficient procedures for determining fiscal policy also tend to have unjust electoral systems.
   B. Presidents have only been successful in making new policies when their own party controls Congress.
   C. Members of Congress whose votes do not reflect the will of the people are typically not reelected.
   D. Public opinion is often sharply divided with regard to a president's policy proposals.

23. Suppose that during the mid-1980s, Congress sought to lessen the extent of governmental influence in the domestic economy. What relevance would this have to the passage?

   A. It supports the author's claim that presidents are largely responsible for the system's inefficiency.
   B. It supports the author's claim that the system has worked tolerably well at times.
   C. It weakens the author's claim that the failure to reduce the deficit in the 1980s was the result of governmental deadlock.
   D. It weakens the author's claim that power is more fragmented in the legislative branch than in the executive branch.

24. An advocate of the "automatic-pilot approach" to fiscal reform would probably support which of the following proposals?

   A. Legislating a limit on the size of the federal budget deficit
   B. Placing all power over economic policy in the hands of an official selected by the president
   C. Publicizing the voting records of those elected officials who are involved in making fiscal policy
   D. Relying on Supreme Court rulings to determine the constitutionality of new fiscal regulations

PASSAGE 5 (QUESTIONS 25–30)

Visual art—drawing, painting, sculpture, and the like—holds a clear place and process in the mind of the general public. To clarify, I mean that the average person knows how a painting, for instance, is created, but the workings of other disciplines that craft visual experiences are less clear to the average member of their audiences. The popular perception of these hard-working artists becomes the default: a hand wave of, "Oh, I'm sure it comes together somehow." This sentiment becomes progressively stronger as the creation in question becomes more collaborative, and as the final visual product is less of the audience's primary engagement with the work as a whole.

Theatrical design lies at the extreme of both the above trends: in addition to theater's status as one of the definitive collaborative art forms, the strictly visual aspects of a performance—scenic, costume, and lighting design—are not generally "why [one] goes to the theater." Because of the latter point in particular, these design aspects exist as nothing more than a subordinate credit in a play's program to most theatergoers, even as expensive modern technology and enhanced production values allow them to be an ever-larger part of the experience.

Needless to say, designers for the performing arts (which include dance and opera, as well as theater) can bring a strong and definitive artistic voice to a work, and that voice is often nuanced and masterful. My own scenic design professor, who is now a Tony Award winner for his craft, was six-foot-four, with a build that would be placed by popular stereotypes as more football player than dollhouse maker. But his giant hands would spend countless hours building miniature, astonishingly lifelike sets and stages out of cardstock and gesso.

The models demanded absolute perfection and detail because while the miniature is not the final product of the show itself, it *is* the final product of the designer. His role is to make a complete visualization of the stage and set dressings as the audience will experience it, but also to convey that vision in such a way that it can be duplicated by others who are tasked to build the full-size version out of plywood, metal, screen projections, and so on.

That flexibility given to the actual scene-builders is the heart of what makes breathtaking visual theater, and it also exposes a key tenet of collaborative art in general. The operant word is *specialization*: the scene is designed by a man or woman with an eye for weight, color, composition, and dramatic function, but it is then constructed by a team that knows how to build, fly, and weld. As an example, consider a designer who demands a bucking and swaying boat for the opening scene of Shakespeare's *The Tempest*. The designer will build a model with each plank on the boat just so, and that rocks back and forth to the exact angle desired of the final product. The exact mechanism of that rocking, on the other hand, whether it be hydraulic platforms, sophisticated video projections, or ultra-strong cables from the fly space above, is left to the engineers, carpenters, and technicians in the "scene shop." Compromises on the initial design may, of course, have to be made to even be able to build the set, but they are normally handled in consultation with the director and the designers. Especially in today's big-budget Broadway productions, such scope adjustments are cut to an absolute minimum.

25. Which of the following is best supported by the passage?

    A. Theater is not a visual art.
    B. Scene-builders run into technical difficulties during performances.
    C. *The Tempest* is Shakespeare's best work.
    D. Some set designs are impossible to build as originally conceived.

26. Implicit in the author's discussion about the theater is the assumption that:

    A. the set design is an integral part of the theatergoer's experience.
    B. the most important aspect of the theater is the set design.
    C. collaborative art is the best visual art.
    D. most set designers do not look the part.

27. Which of the following is best supported by evidence in the passage?

    A. Engineers, carpenters, and technicians are the most important staff on a theater production.
    B. Set designers construct the objects on stage in a major theater production.
    C. Set designers are the most important staff on theater productions.
    D. The scene shop constructs the objects on stage in a major theater production.

28. Compared to earlier theater productions, a modern theater production should be:

    A. built by set designers and designed by engineers and technicians.
    B. closer to the vision of the set designer.
    C. further away from the vision of the set designer.
    D. cheaper and more cost-effective.

29. With which of the following would the author most likely agree regarding those who work on theater set design?

    A. They are usually too caught up in how something works to truly understand the art behind the design.
    B. No one appreciates their work and it goes unnoticed in the art world at large.
    C. They are underappreciated by some audiences and may receive little recognition for their contributions.
    D. Only some people appreciate their work and there are currently no avenues for them to be recognized.

30. Which of the following is implied about dance and opera?

    A. Their sets come together organically.
    B. Their set designers work less than their theater counterparts.
    C. They are both forms of collaborative art.
    D. Their sets are the main reason that people attend.

PASSAGE 6 (QUESTIONS 31–35)

Originally published in 1861, *Incidents in the Life of a Slave Girl Written by Herself* was long regarded as a powerful argument for the abolition of slavery in the United States. Recently, however, its meaning and relevance have changed. Thanks to the work of historian Jean Fagan Yellin, it has become clear that the work is not a novel, as was initially believed, but a true account by Harriet Jacobs of her own life—a primary source on the realities of an African American woman's life under slavery.

Circumstances initially led 19th-century readers to receive the book as a work of fiction in the tradition of *Uncle Tom's Cabin*, written as a thinly veiled political tract in the Abolitionist cause. *Incidents* was published anonymously. The title page provided no name other than that of its editor, Lydia Maria Child, a noted abolitionist and novelist, whose previous novels had included plotlines and themes similar to those in *Incidents*, fueling speculation that she was the author. Since the first-person narrator of the book, in consideration of others, had "concealed the names of places and given persons fictitious names," there was no way to trace the authorship of the text beyond Mrs. Child, whose denials served only to deepen the mystery surrounding the book's provenance.

But perhaps the most important reason it was insisted that *Incidents* was a novel was an inability to accept that the woman depicted in the book—who endured the brutality of slavery, hid from her owners in a garret for seven years, and then escaped to the North—could write a work so rooted in the melodramatic literary tradition popular among female readers and authors of the time. In fact, deeply ingrained racial prejudices held by most white Americans (even the abolitionists) made it difficult for them to acknowledge that an African American was capable of such a powerful and dramatic work under any circumstances.

In the 1980s, Jean Fagan Yellin, struck by the book's attempt to create a sense of sisterhood between white and black women, decided to reexamine the claims of its authenticity made by the narrator and Lydia Maria Child. While others had voiced similar arguments as early as 1947, Yellin went one step further, meticulously documenting the existence of people and events in the book. Studying the papers of Lydia Maria Child and others in her circle, Yellin found among them Jacobs's letters and other documents that led to general recognition of Jacobs as the writer.

Answering the charge that a former slave could not possibly have been familiar with the literary tradition the book reflected, Yellin demonstrated that Harriet Jacobs had access to the extensive libraries of abolitionist women. She found that Jacobs's daughter, Louisa, had been educated as a teacher and had transcribed the manuscript in preparation for its publication. Harriet Jacobs's own letters show considerable literary ability; Louisa standardized her mother's spelling and punctuation. And the author's insistence on anonymity was explained in large part by the fact that the book discussed the unique and difficult situation faced by slave women: the sexual predations of male slave owners and their powerlessness to exert on their own behalf society's standards of chaste womanhood. Such matters would be deemed inappropriate for a woman to discuss publicly in 1861, but Jacobs saw the necessity of reaching out to her female readership in this manner. *Incidents in the Life of a Slave Girl* is now recognized as a true account of the harrowing experiences of life as a slave.

31. The author probably refers to *Uncle Tom's Cabin* (paragraph 2) primarily in order to:

    A. illustrate the racial stereotyping that is also present in *Incidents*.
    B. argue that it is a poorly written novel in comparison with *Incidents*.
    C. assert that precedent existed for the type of book readers believed *Incidents* to be.
    D. provide an example of another novel that was confused with nonfiction.

32. With which of the following statements would the author of the passage most likely agree?

    A. Harriet Jacobs should not have included discussions of sexuality in her book.
    B. American standards of behavior were easy to achieve for most men who were slaves.
    C. *Incidents* was most popular among women readers when it was published.
    D. Novels can provide valuable insights into the history and politics of an era.

33. Each of the following is used by Yellin to support the idea that Harriet Jacobs wrote *Incidents in the Life of a Slave Girl* EXCEPT:

    A. her daughter was educated as a teacher.
    B. Lydia Maria Child was listed on the title page as its editor.
    C. discussions of sexuality were deemed inappropriate for a woman in 1861.
    D. the people and events cited in the book did in fact exist.

34. Which of the following ideas is most analogous to the situation described in the passage?

    A. A public figure who is identified with an important political issue writes a novel that dramatizes the issue.
    B. Thanks to the use of new technology, an oil well is discovered on land that was formerly the site of a plantation house.
    C. The value of work by a scientist who was poorly regarded during his lifetime is increasingly recognized in the years after his death.
    D. A painting that was thought to be a forgery turns out after careful analysis to be the work of a well-known artist.

35. Suppose that it was a common convention in 19th-century American literature for former slaves to dictate their memoirs to whites, who then edited the memoirs for publication. What effect would this information have had on the arguments about the authorship of *Incidents*?

    A. It would provide additional support for the idea that Lydia Maria Child wrote the book.
    B. It would lend support to the idea that the book could be a work of nonfiction.
    C. It would weaken Jean Fagan Yellin's contention that Jacobs wrote the book by herself.
    D. It would make the author's choice to remain anonymous less credible to the modern reader.

PASSAGE 7 (QUESTIONS 36–40)

The study of underwater wreckage can be a significant part of the study of human history. As early as the age of cave dwellers, mariners left the Greek mainland, taking a route across the Aegean Sea to the island of Melos in search of obsidian, a dark volcanic glass used primarily for fashioning cutting tools. Exploration of and immigration to the Americas from parts of the world lying across the Atlantic Ocean as well as from Asia to Australia and numerous islands was, until very recently, accomplished solely by some type of water transport. There have always been losses of watercraft due to storms, accidents, and wars. Underwater wrecks are, in effect, time capsules representing materials dating from the earliest historical periods to the present. At one time these sites remained largely unattended except for chance finds by fishermen, treasure hunters, or sponge divers. However, the development of the Self-Contained Underwater Breathing Apparatus (SCUBA) gear has made many more sites accessible to systematic investigation. For the value of submerged material to be realized, however, it is not sufficient for divers simply to be physically fit and skilled in aquatics. Divers, as well as everyone else involved in the recovery process, must also be educated in artifact extraction, record-keeping, and conservation techniques.

The systematic recovery and study of artifacts, as well as the development of inferences about the cultures they represent, is the particular concern of archaeology. Shipwrecks have the potential to provide almost as much archaeological data as the terrestrial sites that are more traditionally associated with this field of study. However, this potential is realized only when recovery is approached with a sensitivity to the need for both preservation of the artifacts and meticulous recording of the context in which they were found.

Artifacts in a saltwater environment are often coated with anaerobic sediment and are apparently well preserved, but nevertheless of a very friable nature. Extraction of an artifact intact requires considerable knowledge and skill. After extraction, organic materials, such as wood or textiles, can crumble in a matter of hours; iron can deteriorate over days or months; and bone, glass, and pottery can devitrify and (in extreme cases) degenerate into a pile of useless slivers. Although time-consuming and often more expensive than the original excavation, conservation must be given high priority. Otherwise, the loss will affect not only the excavator, but also archaeologists and the larger scientific community to which the results of archaeological analysis would be of interest.

To an archaeologist, human activities are far more significant than a ship or its contents. Activities are inferred not only from artifacts, but also from their context. However, the very act of recovering artifacts destroys context, which subsequently is preserved only in notes, drawings, and photographs made during recovery. Insofar as material recovered from a shipwreck is of archeological significance, documentation of its context demands attention equal to that given to its conservation. If records are neglected, the operation is not nautical archaeology, but an uncontrolled "treasure-hunting" operation.

36. The central concern of the passage is to:

   A. explain the scientific importance of exploration of and salvage from shipwrecks, and advocate adherence to appropriate methods.
   B. chronicle developments that led to the maturation of treasure-hunting into the scientific discipline of nautical archaeology.
   C. argue against adherence to standardized methods in conducting exploration of and salvage from shipwrecks.
   D. spur the discovery, exploration, and recovery of shipwrecks and their contents.

37. According to the passage, the scope of nautical archaeological discovery has been expanded by:

   A. advances in techniques for conservation of artifacts.
   B. the development of SCUBA gear.
   C. greater emphasis on systematic record-keeping.
   D. the study of underwater wreckage.

38. The passage most probably mentions the search for obsidian (paragraph 1) in order to:

   A. provide an example of one of the earlier human activities that may have resulted in underwater wreckage.
   B. indicate the type of tools that might be found in shipwrecks beneath the Aegean Sea.
   C. provide an example of a difference between the natural resources existing on the Greek mainland and the island of Melos.
   D. provide evidence for the development of an ancient trade route.

39. The passage implies that nautical archeologists are most likely to be distinguished from traditional archaeologists in that they are:

   A. more concerned with issues involved in the extraction and preservation of artifacts.
   B. more likely to be very familiar with an environment for which human beings are not naturally adapted.
   C. more concerned with meticulous recording of the context in which artifacts are found.
   D. more concerned with human activities than with physical artifacts.

40. According to the passage, a nautical archaeologist would be most interested in which of the following items discovered in a shipwreck?

   A. Pieces of a bronze statue that, when reassembled, were found to be the only surviving work of a master sculptor, suitable for museum display
   B. Well-preserved bowls, candelabras, and statuettes that could be sold at a profit, which could then be used to finance future exploration
   C. A chest of medical equipment containing implements used by the barber surgeon of the ship, including salves and bowls for draining blood
   D. Partially decayed but relatively well-preserved skeletons of rats, cats, and human beings

Bio/Biochem 1: Attacking MCAT Science Questions

PASSAGE 1 (QUESTIONS 1–5)

Proteins have several levels of structural complexity, each of which has important consequences for the protein's physical, chemical, and biological properties. A protein's primary structure is the sequence of covalent peptide bonds connecting amino acid residues, generally expressed starting with the N-terminal residue and ending with the C-terminal residue. Secondary structure deals with the presence of three-dimensional structural elements such as α-helices or β-pleated sheets. These structures are formed by short sections of the primary structural sequence and are held together by hydrogen bonds between amino acid residues. Tertiary structure expresses the complete three-dimensional arrangement of the secondary structural elements across an entire peptide chain. For example, α-helices from different sections of the primary structural sequence may be spatially close together, thus defining a portion of the peptide's tertiary structure. Quaternary structure defines the spatial relationship between two or more polypeptides in a single protein or enzyme.

The geometry of the peptide bond, which is restricted to planar conformations, is an important factor in the formation of secondary and tertiary structure. The planar restriction leads to two possible conformations, called s-*trans* and s-*cis*, shown in Figure 1.

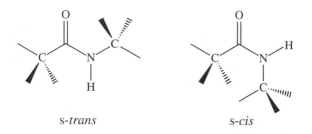

Figure 1. Peptide bonds: s-*trans* and s-*cis* conformations.

In addition to the peptide bond linking each amino acid residue, disulfide links also play important roles in determining the relationships between amino acid residues defined by secondary, tertiary, and quaternary structure. Disruption of peptide conformations or disulfide links can result in denaturation of the protein.

1. Coplanar atoms in peptide links are often shown by defining the plane that they occupy. Which of the following correctly shows the coplanar atoms in the dipeptide Gly–Ala?

   A.

   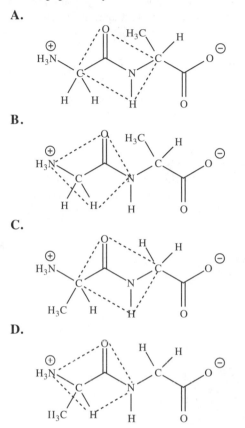

   B.

   C.

   D.

2. Disulfide links can easily be formed, as shown in the following reaction:

   $$2 \, RCH_2SH + I_2 \rightarrow RCH_2S\text{--}SCH_2R + 2 \, HI$$

   In this reaction, the two cysteine residues undergo which type of reaction?

   A. Nucleophilic substitution
   B. Reduction
   C. Nucleophilic addition
   D. Oxidation

3. The presence of s-*cis* or s-*trans* peptide links can lead to vastly different structural features in a peptide chain. However, most peptide links in a chain are of the:

   A. s-*cis* type, because of its lack of nonbonded strain.
   B. s-*cis* type, because of its excess nonbonded strain.
   C. s-*trans* type, because of its lack of nonbonded strain.
   D. s-*trans* type, because of its excess nonbonded strain.

4. A protein is subjected to conditions that cleave all disulfide links. Molecular weight determinations performed on the molecule before and after cleavage yield results that are not significantly different. Which of the following can be concluded?

   A. The protein has elements of quaternary structure.
   B. The protein does not have elements of quaternary structure.
   C. The protein has no quaternary structural elements that depend upon disulfide links.
   D. The protein has quaternary structural elements that depend upon disulfide links.

5. Because of the peptide bond restriction to planar conformations, all of the following can be concluded about the atoms in the link EXCEPT:

   A. the nitrogen lone pair has overlap with the carbonyl π-bond.
   B. there is considerable positive-charge character on the nitrogen atom.
   C. the nitrogen atom is sp^3-hybridized.
   D. there is considerable negative-charge character on the carbonyl oxygen.

PASSAGE 2 (QUESTIONS 6–10)

The immune system is a versatile and complex system that can respond to a wide variety of threats. Both nonspecific and specific mechanisms of the immune response help to protect against infection or inflammation. In fact, even the nonspecific mechanisms follow particular mechanisms.

During a successful immune response, a pathogen must first be recognized. Appropriate protein cytokines must then be produced by antigen-presenting cells. One specific class of antigen-presenting cells includes dendritic cells. Dendritic cells are some of the first targets of viruses such as HIV (human immunodeficiency virus), simian immunodeficiency virus (SIV), and feline immunodeficiency virus (FIV).

A scientist wants to determine which of the cytokines is negatively affected by FIV. In the experimental setup, dendritic cells were collected from both naïve and FIV-infected cats. The total RNA was extracted from these cells. Complementary DNA (cDNA) was made from this RNA. Finally, real-time quantitative polymerase chain reaction (PCR) was performed to quantify RNA levels of the cytokines.

Although the researcher postulated otherwise, once analyzed, the results of the experiment showed that there was no significant difference in expression of the measured cytokine levels between infected cells and cells from naïve cats, as shown in Figure 1.

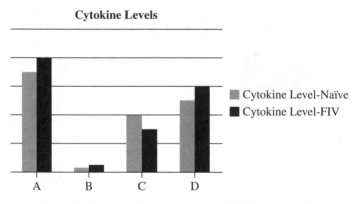

Figure 1. Cytokine levels in naïve and FIV-infected cells.

6. In the experiment, RNA was extracted from dendritic cells; however, it was then converted to cDNA. Why might this step have been included in the experimental procedure?

   A. RNA bases can make only double hydrogen bonds with one another, whereas DNA bases can make triple hydrogen bonds.
   B. DNA is more stable than RNA and can better maintain its integrity during PCR.
   C. DNA is the molecule in which genetic information is encoded, not RNA.
   D. cDNA forms more stable complexes with RNA than does genomic DNA.

7. How does the presence of RNA from the dendritic cells demonstrate cytokine levels?

   A. Cytokines are composed of RNA, so RNA levels represent cytokine levels.
   B. Cytokine DNA is translated directly into RNA molecules.
   C. Cytokine mRNA provides evidence that the cell is in the process of producing these cytokines.
   D. Total RNA shows only cytokine presence in the cell.

8. Polymerase chain reaction amplifies DNA by first unwinding it using heat rather than DNA helicase. What bonds must be broken in order for this reaction to proceed?

   A. Hydrogen bonds
   B. Phosphodiester linkages
   C. Glycosidic linkages
   D. Nucleoside–phosphate bonds

9. What modifications will be made to the nascent RNA transcript before it exits the nucleus?

   A. A poly-A tail will be added.
   B. A $3'$ guanosine cap will be added.
   C. Exons will be excised.
   D. Chaperones will assist with folding.

10. There was no significant difference between the cytokine levels found in cells from infected cats *vs.* naïve cats. What does this mean?

   A. Dendritic cells are the first step in FIV transmission.
   B. T-lymphocytes are most likely not affected by FIV infection.
   C. Dendritic cells are most likely not affected by FIV infection.
   D. These cytokines are most likely not affected by FIV infection.

DISCRETE PRACTICE QUESTIONS (QUESTIONS 11–16)

11. Amino acids are dissolved in a basic solution that is gradually titrated with HCl. Which of the following amino acids would require the most added HCl before its positively charged form predominates in solution?

   A. Lysine
   B. Aspartate
   C. Glycine
   D. Glutamine

12. Total iron binding capacity (TIBC) is a measure of how much iron can be absorbed by the binding proteins in a patient's blood. Assuming that the concentrations of these binding proteins remain constant, the TIBC in a patient with anemia due to iron deficiency would be:

   A. low, because the patient is deficient in iron.
   B. low, because the binding proteins would have a decreased affinity for iron.
   C. high, because the patient is deficient in iron.
   D. high, because the binding proteins would have a decreased affinity for iron.

13. Which of the following is a diastereomer of α-L-threose?

   I. α-D-threose
   II. β-L-threose
   III. β-D-threose

   A. I only
   B. II only
   C. I and II only
   D. II and III only

14. Why must the DNA synthesis reaction remain at a high temperature throughout the polymerase reaction in PCR?

   A. The polymerase enzyme requires a high temperature in order to proceed.
   B. The template strands would reanneal if the temperature was lowered, halting the polymerase reaction.
   C. The polymerase enzyme requires the DNA to reanneal in order to proceed with the reaction.
   D. The template strands would reanneal if the temperature was lowered, increasing the polymerase reaction.

15. A cell has lost its ability to create spliceosomes due to a mutation. What is now true of this cell?

   A. The cell can no longer do any posttranscriptional processing.
   B. The cell can no longer do any splicing as part of posttranscriptional processing.
   C. The cell can now only do some types of splicing during posttranscriptional processing.
   D. The cell will not be able to create any functional proteins.

16. RNA interference is a process by which a cell can either increase or decrease the usage of an mRNA molecule. How does RNA interference regulate gene expression in a eukaryotic cell?

   A. RNA interference regulates whether or not the mRNA is available for translation into a protein.
   B. Degradation of mRNA by RNA interference makes translation of tRNA possible.
   C. RNA interference regulates whether or not the mRNA is available for transcription into a protein.
   D. RNA interference upregulates the translation process by directly stimulating rRNA.

Extra practice for the next class session starts on the next page ▶ ▶ ▶

Psych/Soc 1: Basics of Research Design & Data

PASSAGE 1 (QUESTIONS 1–5)

Athletic skill is thought to arise from a variety of factors in an individual's genetics and environment. Having athletic skill is generally regarded as highly desirable, but determining cause-and-effect relationships associated with athletic skill level is difficult, largely due to the multitude of explanatory factors that may be involved, either alone or in combination. Because of this, the potential role of inherited factors in determining athletic ability is a robustly researched topic in the scientific community. Innate or "inborn" talent would arise from a person's genetic makeup, so researchers typically use sets of twins—comparing traits and skill among combinations of different types of twins raised in environments of varying similarity—to isolate potential causal factors.

In one such study, researchers sought to determine the extent to which genetic variation leads to differences in overall athletic ability. They compared the relative athletic skill level of identical twins raised together, identical twins raised apart, and fraternal twins raised together. Skill level was assessed through measures commonly used in exercise physiology and sports medicine research, such as maximal sprinting speed, strength of various muscle groups, and agility. Researchers then compared their data with the variability in athletic skill present in the general population. In analyzing their results, researchers discovered a negative correlation between genetic relatedness and variance in athletic skill ($p = 0.07$ and $r = -0.4$).

1. Which of the following would be the most reasonable representation of the raw data obtained on athletic skill described in the passage?

   A. A pie chart
   B. A scatterplot
   C. A bar graph
   D. A line graph

2. Based on the passage, which of the following graphs best represents the relationship between genetic variance and differences in athletic skill in the general population?

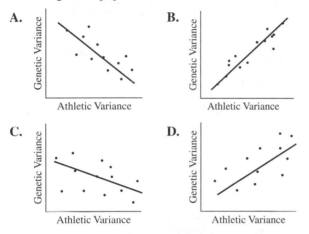

3. Which of the following statements regarding the independent variables in the study is the most accurate?

   A. They are examples of continuous variables, whereas the dependent variable is an example of a categorical variable.
   B. They allow the researchers to control for environmental factors that might contribute to variability in athletic skill.
   C. They are designed to be a reasonable, if ultimately incomplete, measure of the overall fitness of an individual.
   D. They were measured directly by examining the genome of the participants for alleles known to be associated with athletic ability.

4. Suppose that a second group of researchers repeats the study and obtains a similar result, with a p-value of 0.03. Which of the following represents the most reasonable conclusion regarding this new result?

   A. The original researchers made a mistake in their analysis of the data.
   B. Genetic variance has been confirmed to cause differences in athletic ability.
   C. The new study demonstrates a significant correlation that the original did not.
   D. The second group of researchers must have had fewer outliers in their data set.

5. In a related study, researchers determine that parental encouragement of childhood athletic activity is more highly correlated with athletic ability later in life than is genetic variability. Based on these results, which of the following groups would be expected to have the highest variance in athletic ability?

   A. Fraternal twins raised apart
   B. Fraternal twins raised together
   C. Identical twins raised apart
   D. Identical twins raised together

PASSAGE 2 (QUESTIONS 6–11)

Hormonal chemistry plays a direct role in reinforcement learning, particularly in those cases in which a reward is unexpected. The pathway for reward learning is well documented: when an individual receives a reward that is unexpected, the event is encoded in the form of a release of dopamine targeting the ventral striatum and the prefrontal cortex. It is through the resultant activity that the individual becomes better at predicting future rewards. The pathway for fear-based learning is less clear, however. Recent studies have pointed to a decay in the response of the amygdala to sequential fear-inducing stimuli as well as an increase in serotonin activity following such events as a potential explanation for prediction error conditioning in fear learning.

Researchers wishing to investigate this pathway tested two groups in a Pavlovian learning task. Prior to testing, one of the two groups followed a protein-deficient diet in order to cause tryptophan deprivation (TRP⁻), resulting in reduced serotonin activity. Researchers applied capsaicin to the forearms of members of both groups to induce increased sensitivity to temperature. Participants were presented with a stimulus consisting of a triangle shown on either the left or right side of a display; reaction times for determining on which side the triangle was shown were recorded. Eight seconds following the display of the visual stimulus, participants were sometimes subjected to a brief temperature increase to the capsaicin-treated area and sometimes were not. Skin conductance readings

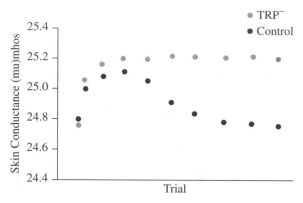

Figure 1. Skin conductance results.

were taken four seconds after the presentation of the visual stimulus as a measure of autonomic fear response, and fMRI data was acquired.

Researchers discovered no significant difference in reaction times between the two groups. fMRI data showed increased activity in the orbitofrontal cortex and the amygdala for the control group. The TRP⁻ group demonstrated no such increase. Skin conductance results are shown in Figure 1.

As a final paper for an Introduction to Psychology course, a first-year college student runs an experiment based on the results of the experiment above. He reasons that because turkey meat contains tryptophan, and the fear response is at least partly related to an increased heart rate, a large meal of turkey should have the opposite effect of the one noted in the original experiment. The student asks several of his classmates to record their resting pulse rates both before and after eating Thanksgiving dinner and other meals over the fall break. He then compares the results, which are shown in Figure 2.

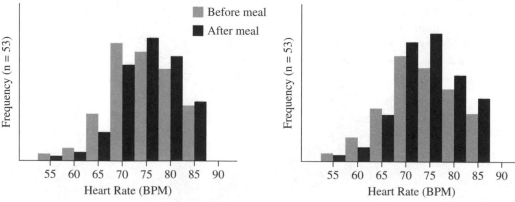

Figure 2. Pulse rates of classmates before and after eating meals.

6. Which of the following can be concluded on the basis of the researchers' study?

   A. Tryptophan deprivation may be responsible for a disruption in the ability to learn from prediction errors in anticipation of a reward.
   B. Suppression of serotonin pathways is correlated with a decrease in extinction of fear response to inconsistent stimuli.
   C. Tryptophan deprivation negatively affects the ability of an individual to develop a fear response to a novel aversive stimulus.
   D. Serotonin is largely responsible for the regulation of the physical and emotional aspects of the fear response to aversive stimuli.

7. Which of the following best describes the distribution in the student's results?

   A. It is skewed to the left.
   B. It is skewed to the right.
   C. The average and the median are the same.
   D. The standard deviation is larger on the left.

8. The student receives an "incomplete" and is asked to redo his paper and adhere more closely to the scientific method. Once the student decides on a new question to investigate, what should his next step include?

   A. Forming a hypothesis
   B. Reading previously published articles
   C. Deciding on an experimental design
   D. Applying for a research grant

9. Which of the following best describes the measurement of reaction time in the researchers' experiment?

   A. It is a dependent variable.
   B. It is an independent variable.
   C. It is used as a negative control.
   D. It is used as a positive control.

10. Which of the following best describes the use of the capsaicin-enhanced temperature increase in the first study?

    A. It is a punishment.
    B. It is a negative reinforcer.
    C. It is a conditioned stimulus.
    D. It is an unconditioned stimulus.

11. Which of the following is NOT a testable scientific hypothesis?

    A. Drug A is more effective than Drug B in reducing chemotherapy-induced nausea in cancer patients.
    B. Drug A is more effective than a placebo in reducing the number of panic attacks in patients with generalized anxiety disorder.
    C. Drug A generally reduces the intensity of auditory hallucinations in patients diagnosed with schizophrenia.
    D. Drug A is the best remedy to reduce both the severity and the intensity of a migraine headache.

PASSAGE 3 (QUESTIONS 12–17)

Color constancy is the term given to the phenomenon in which an object's perceived color remains relatively unchanged under varying conditions of illumination. As a result, an object appears to be the same color after a change in illumination, even though the absolute wavelength of the light the object reflects has changed. It has been hypothesized that the mechanism for color constancy in the brain is optimized for natural light due to its evolution under such conditions.

To test this hypothesis, a study is conducted in which participants were presented with a scene containing real objects that varied between trials. Sets of objects included various fruits and three-dimensional paper cutouts with the same surface color as the fruits. Each participant was first presented with a scene under a target illumination of a specific wavelength. Participants were then presented with the same scene under two test illuminations: one that matched the original and one that was different. Participants were asked to determine which one matched the original illumination. Illumination conditions varied along two loci. The daylight locus (*u*) corresponds roughly to changes in natural illumination throughout the day and is associated with the blue-yellow spectrum, with blue being the most common daylight illumination. A perpendicular atypical locus (*v*) corresponds to wavelengths on the red-green spectrum, typically seen only under artificial conditions, with green being the least common illumination in natural conditions.

In analyzing their results, researchers discovered that the contents of the scene had no significant effect on participants' accuracy in color matching. Results are shown in Figure 1.

Researchers then plotted a curve around the point marking a neutral illumination level in both the *u* and *v* loci. This curve marks the boundary for which participants attained a 75 percent accuracy rate in discriminating from the neutral illumination, and is presented in Figures 2 and 3.

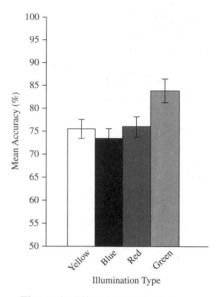

Figure 1. Effect of illumination type on color matching.

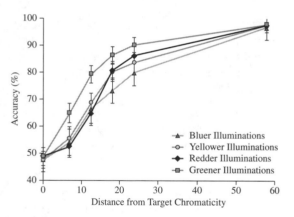

Figure 2. Distance from target chromaticity *vs.* accuracy.

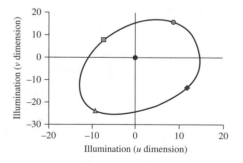

Figure 3. Illumination curve.

12. Which of the following is a potential problem with the design of the study as described?

    A. The researchers' hypothesis, as stated, cannot be feasibly investigated.
    B. The design of the experiment does not actually test the quantitative aspects of the hypothesis.
    C. The experiment has no practical benefit, and is therefore not relevant.
    D. Researchers failed to control for absolute differences in perception between participants.

13. Which of the following best summarizes a conclusion that can be made on the basis of the experiment?

    A. Evolutionary processes can be said to be responsible, at least in part, for the mechanisms responsible for color constancy.
    B. The color constancy effect is strongest under artificial lighting conditions and weakest under natural lighting conditions.
    C. The color constancy effect is strongest under natural lighting conditions and weakest under artificial lighting conditions.
    D. Color constancy has been shown to be mostly unrelated to lighting conditions as measured under both natural and artificial conditions.

14. Which of the following structures is/are most likely responsible for the phenomenon of color constancy?

    A. The primary visual cortex
    B. The cone cells of the retina
    C. The superior colliculus
    D. The lateral geniculate nucleus

15. For which of the following points on the illumination chart would participants be expected to demonstrate the highest accuracy of discrimination as compared to the neutral illumination?

    A. $u = -5, v = +10$
    B. $u = +8, v = -5$
    C. $u = +10, v = +10$
    D. $u = -15, v = -25$

16. The researchers determine that the point $u = -1$, $v = +3$ is well within the just-noticeable difference threshold for the neutral illumination. What is the expected accuracy for the discrimination task at this point?

    A. 0%
    B. 25%
    C. 50%
    D. 75%

17. Which of the following best expresses the purpose of the experiment?

    A. To determine the extent to which variations in natural and artificial light predict accuracy of color discrimination
    B. To show that the mechanisms of color constancy evolved under pressure of natural selection *in situ*
    C. To demonstrate that natural light should be preferred over artificial sources when designing interior spaces
    D. To prove that artificial light makes it more difficult to discriminate between the colors of objects

PASSAGE 4 (QUESTIONS 18–21)

In recent years, there has been a dramatic increase in the number of endurance athletes. People of varying backgrounds have become more involved in endurance sports, like obstacle racing and marathon running. More than 500,000 people complete marathons each year, an increase of more than 200,000 since 1990. Some assert that participation in these activities fulfills certain biological and psychological needs.

Extensive studies show that obesity negatively impacts the health of millions of Americans. As a result, a large segment of the population has shifted its focus toward health and wellness. Examples abound of people who have lost weight and achieved fitness through running marathons. Media attention to these stories and to the obesity epidemic is causing an infatuation with endurance sports.

Participation in these sports can have strong health benefits. Combined with proper diet, the process of training for and running a marathon can result in increasing cardiovascular strength, building muscle, and decreasing excess body fat. Yet, when asked about training for a marathon, most runners report that training is far more than developing the physical ability to complete the 26.2-mile foot race. Runners report the need to develop mental strength to continue running, even when pain and fatigue set in. Despite the pain and fatigue that these athletes experience, that same group will report a strong affinity for the sport. That people participate in and enjoy an activity that causes pain seems strange to some observers, but runners report something entirely different. Long-distance runners are more likely to say that exercise helps them to build a sense of community with other runners, to challenge themselves in new ways, and to control their own progress and success.

18. The self-determination theory would attribute the rise in the number of endurance athletes to:

   A. a response to the biological need for health.
   B. the fact that participation in endurance sports builds competence, relatedness, and autonomy, and these factors contribute to a healthy state.
   C. more people having physiological and safety needs met and therefore being able to focus on developing a sense of belonging and self-esteem.
   D. athletes being extrinsically motivated by media and our society's obsession with fitness.

19. The stressors associated with running a marathon can be numerous. Considering that runners may experience both pain and a sense of accomplishment through running, these stressors are most likely:

   A. a positive reappraisal.
   B. solely distressing for the runners.
   C. due to the repression of other emotions.
   D. eustressing and distressing in nature.

20. A woman decides to train for a marathon to lose weight. After the race, she continues to run even though she no longer needs to lose weight, but rather for the enjoyment of the sport and to win medals at races. This woman's actions:

   A. were solely extrinsically motivated.
   B. were initially extrinsically motivated, but shifted to both intrinsic and extrinsic motivation.
   C. were solely intrinsically motivated.
   D. were initially intrinsically motivated, but shifted to both intrinsic and extrinsic motivation.

21. The sense of belonging, achievement, and control satisfy which level(s) of Maslow's hierarchy of needs?

   A. Physiological needs
   B. Self-actualization and safety and security
   C. Self-esteem and love and belonging
   D. Safety and security and love and belonging

Chem/Phys 2: Scientific Reasoning on the MCAT

PASSAGE 1 (QUESTIONS 1–4)

The adult male human body is composed of approximately 60 percent water. The blood (which is largely water) is packed with various solutes that are carried to all parts of the body. Of these solutes, salt makes up a significant portion. Sparingly soluble salts are similar to the salt in the blood in that they are ionic compounds, but they only dissociate somewhat in water. Two scientists developed hypotheses to determine if one sparingly soluble salt was more or less soluble than the other.

Scientist 1
Water, a polar solvent, is better at solvating species with higher, rather than lower, polarity. The difference in the electronegativities of the ions that compose an ionic compound gives a measure of the polarity of the compound. Comparing ZnF_2 and $PbBr_2$, fluorine is more electronegative than bromine, and lead is more electronegative than zinc. The polarity of ZnF_2 is greater than the polarity of $PbBr_2$; therefore, ZnF_2 is more soluble in water than $PbBr_2$.

Element	Electronegativity
Zn	1.6
Pb	1.9
I	2.5
Br	2.8
F	4.0

Table 1. Electronegativites of commonly ionized elements.

Scientist 2
Upon dissolution, sparingly soluble salts are partially converted to ions. These ions vary in their ionic radii. Water forms hydrogen bonds with other water molecules. When ions with a smaller ionic radius are solvated, they do not significantly disrupt the hydrogen-bonding network of water. Larger ions, though, disrupt the intermolecular forces of water, and thus are less soluble. The relative sizes of the ions of the sparingly soluble salts ZnF_2 and $PbBr_2$ are: $Br^- > F^- > Pb^{2+} > Zn^{2+}$. For instance: the ions of ZnF_2 are smaller than those of $PbBr_2$; therefore, ZnF_2 is more soluble than $PbBr_2$.

1. What would Scientist 2 predict about the relative solubilities of PbF_2 and ZnF_2?

   A. PbF_2 is more soluble than ZnF_2 because the electronegativity difference of the ions that compose PbF_2 is smaller.
   B. PbF_2 is more soluble than ZnF_2 because the ions that compose PbF_2 are larger.
   C. PbF_2 is less soluble than ZnF_2 because the electronegativity difference of the ions that compose PbF_2 is smaller.
   D. PbF_2 is less soluble than ZnF_2 because the ions that compose PbF_2 are larger.

2. The solubility of ZnF_2 is 2.03 g per 100 mL at 25°C. What is the K_{sp} value for ZnF_2?

   A. 8.32×10^{-3}
   B. 3.03×10^{-2}
   C. 4.11×10^{-2}
   D. 8.21×10^{-2}

3. Which of the following is the correct order for the boiling points of the listed solutions and water? (Note: The K_b of water is $0.51°C \cdot kg/mol$.)

   I. Saturated solution of ZnF_2 in water
   II. Saturated solution of $PbBr_2$ in water
   III. Pure water

   A. III < II < I
   B. III < I < II
   C. I < II < III
   D. II < I < III

4. What would Scientist 1 predict about the relative solubilities of PbF_2 and PbI_2 in acetone?

   A. PbF_2 is more soluble than PbI_2.
   B. PbI_2 is more soluble than PbF_2.
   C. The solubilities would be roughly the same.
   D. The solubilities cannot be determined.

PASSAGE 2 (QUESTIONS 5–9)

Hydrogen peroxide is an antiseptic usually used to treat minor abrasions and scrapes. When it is applied to an open wound, the enzyme catalase in the blood converts hydrogen peroxide to water and oxygen gas. However, hydrogen peroxide will also decompose on its own when exposed to air, according to Equation 1:

$$2\ H_2O_2(aq) \longrightarrow O_2(g) + 2\ H_2O(l)$$

Equation 1

Iodide catalyzes the decomposition of hydrogen peroxide by Mechanism 1:

$$H_2O_2(aq) + I^-(aq) \longrightarrow IO^-(aq) + H_2O(l)$$

$$H_2O_2(aq) + IO^-(aq) \longrightarrow I^-(aq) + H_2O(l) + O_2(g)$$

Mechanism 1

A student decided to investigate the shelf life of hydrogen peroxide by studying the kinetics of hydrogen peroxide decomposition.

Experiment 1
The student prepares two stock solutions of 0.060 M and 0.090 M KI in water, as well as stock solutions of 0.040 M and 0.080 M H_2O_2 in water. The student stores the hydrogen peroxide solutions in the freezer until beginning the experiment. He adds 100 mL of each hydrogen peroxide solution to 100 mL of each KI solution. The student measures the rate of oxygen formation for each trial. The results are summarized in Table 1.

Trial No.	KI stock concentration (M)	H_2O_2 stock concentration (M)	Initial rate of O_2 formation (mol · L^{-1} · sec^{-1})
1	0.060	0.040	3.61×10^{-8}
2	0.060	0.080	7.25×10^{-8}
3	0.090	0.040	5.39×10^{-8}
4	0.090	0.080	1.08×10^{-7}

Table 1. Initial conditions and formation rates of product in the various trials of Experiment 1.

Experiment 2
The student repeats Experiment 1, but uses flasks that were not properly cleaned. He observes the formation of molecular iodine, but no oxygen formation.

The student suspects that acid was present in the reaction vessel. In order to test his hypothesis, the student performs a third experiment.

Experiment 3

The student repeats Experiment 1, except he adds 100 mL of nitric acid to each reaction vessel before he adds the hydrogen peroxide solutions. He measures the initial rate of I_2 formation for the various concentrations of reactants. The results are summarized in Table 2.

Trial No.	Initial KI concentration (*M*)	Initial H_2O_2 concentration (*M*)	Initial HNO_3 concentration (*M*)	Initial rate of I_2 formation $(mol \cdot L^{-1} \cdot sec^{-1})$
1	0.060	0.040	0.250	4.09×10^{-6}
2	0.060	0.080	0.250	8.23×10^{-6}
3	0.090	0.040	0.250	6.17×10^{-6}
4	0.060	0.040	0.500	8.21×10^{-6}

Table 2. Initial conditions and formation rates of product in the various trials of Experiment 3.

After analyzing the experimental results, the student determines that $k_{obs}[H^+][I^-][H_2O_2]$ is the rate expression that governs the reactions of Experiments 2 and 3. The student proposes a mechanism consistent with this rate law, as shown in Mechanism 2:

$$H_2O_2 + H^+ \rightleftharpoons H_3O_2^+ \quad \text{Step 1}$$

$$I^- + H_3O_2^+ \longrightarrow HOI + H_2O \quad \text{Step 2}$$

$$I^- + HOI \longrightarrow I_2 + OH^- \quad \text{Step 3}$$

$$H^+ + OH^- \longrightarrow H_2O \quad \text{Step 4}$$

Mechanism 2

5. What is the rate expression for the reaction in Experiment 1?

   A. rate $= k[I^-][H_2O_2]$
   B. rate $= k[H^+][I^-][H_2O_2]$
   C. rate $= k[I^-]^2[H_2O_2]$
   D. rate $= k[I^-][H_2O_2]^2$

6. What is the slowest step in the mechanism proposed for Experiments 2 and 3?

   A. Step 1
   B. Step 2
   C. Step 3
   D. Step 4

7. What type of reaction is Step 4 of Mechanism 2?

   A. Precipitation
   B. Oxidation–reduction
   C. Neutralization
   D. Displacement

8. What is the maximum mass of I_2 (*s*) that the student can obtain from Trial 2 of Experiment 3?

   A. 0.20 g
   B. 0.76 g
   C. 2.03 g
   D. 3.18 g

9. Which of the following would increase the rate of I_2 formation in Experiments 2 and 3?

   A. Adding additional H^+ to further catalyze the reaction
   B. Adding additional OH^- to drive the reaction toward the products
   C. Increasing the temperature of the reaction vessel
   D. Removing HOI to drive the reaction toward the products

PASSAGE 3 (QUESTIONS 10–15)

Magnetic therapy is a form of alternative medicine in which magnetic fields are applied to specific parts of the body. Practitioners believe this treatment has various health benefits, although there is little scientific support for this belief. It is thought that magnetic field strength must exceed 0.04 T to be effective. To determine the magnetic field strength of a magnetic therapy bracelet, a student creates a device, which is illustrated in Figure 1. The device accomplishes this task by balancing the magnetic force against a known force generated by the spring with spring constant k. The circuit consists of a DC battery supplying 100 V connected through a 2.5 Ω resistor and a metal rod. The metal rod has a near-zero resistivity, is 30 cm long, has a mass of 0.7 kg, and slides with negligible friction along the arms of the circuit. The circuit is fixed in the plane of the page, and a permanent magnetic field **B** points out of the page (the generator is not shown). A spring is connected to the metal rod on one end and to an immobile piece of nonconducting material on the other.

In the configuration shown below, the metal rod experiences a force generated by the spring and a magnetic force $F = ILB$, where I is the current through the rod, L is the length of the rod, and B is the magnitude of the external magnetic field. The spring's equilibrium length x_0 is defined as the spring length for which the rod experiences no net force. In Figure 1, the switch is open, the spring is at its relaxed length x_0, and the metal rod is at rest.

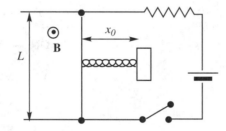

Figure 1. Student-created device for measuring magnetic strength.

10. After the switch has been closed, which of the following best describes what happens to the spring?

    A. The spring is compressed.
    B. The spring is stretched.
    C. The length of the spring does not change.
    D. The spring will either stretch or compress depending on the strength of the magnetic field.

11. If another 2.5 Ω resistor is added in series with the resistor and the battery in the circuit, what will be the approximate change in the magnetic force on the rod?

    A. It will decrease by a factor of 2.
    B. It will not change.
    C. It will increase by a factor of 2.
    D. It will increase by a factor of 4.

12. If the 2.5 Ω resistor were replaced with a 2.5 F uncharged capacitor, which of the following describes the motion of the rod when the switch is closed?

    A. It remains motionless at first.
    B. It accelerates at first.
    C. It moves with a constant velocity.
    D. It accelerates until it reaches a constant nonzero velocity.

13. If the metal rod were lengthened to 45 cm, how would the current through the circuit change?

    A. It would remain the same.
    B. It would increase.
    C. It would decrease.
    D. It would first increase, then decrease.

14. If the switch were closed, how long would it take for 16 kJ of energy to be dissipated by the 2.5 Ω resistor?

    A. 1.0 s
    B. 2.0 s
    C. 4.0 s
    D. 8.0 s

15. If a capacitor were inserted after the 2.5 Ω resistor, what is the maximum potential difference that could exist across its plates?

    A. 40 V
    B. 80 V
    C. 100 V
    D. 120 V

PASSAGE 4 (QUESTIONS 16–19)

Oxidative phosphorylation, when viewed holistically, is a combustion reaction. However, each of its constituent steps is not. It is necessarily broken up into smaller steps to prevent a rapid release of energy. The explanation for this is twofold. One, if the energy were released all at once, it would undoubtedly kill the cell. Two, it is far more efficient and manageable to harness energy that is released in smaller amounts over time. The overall energy released from NADH as a result of oxidative phosphorylation is the enthalpy of the cellular redox reaction.

All reactions result in enthalpy changes that represent the heat absorbed or lost by a system at constant pressure. The standard enthalpy of formation (ΔH_f°) is a specific case of enthalpy describing the heat lost or gained when a substance in its standard state is formed from the appropriate elements in their standard states. Enthalpy values are commonly in kJ/mol.

The enthalpy change of a reaction is often found by adding the enthalpy changes of simpler reactions that comprise the net reaction. For example, because Reaction 3 = Reaction 1 + Reaction 2 below, $\Delta H_3 = \Delta H_1 + \Delta H_2$.

$$2H_2(g) \rightarrow 4H(g)$$

Reaction 1

$$C(g) + 4H(g) \rightarrow CH_4(g)$$

Reaction 2

$$C(g) + 2H_2(g) \rightarrow CH_4(g)$$

Reaction 3

Enthalpy is important in finding the free energy of a system, which can help determine the spontaneity of the reaction. Free energy is defined by the following formula:

$$\Delta G = \Delta H - T\Delta S$$

where ΔG = the free energy change of the reaction

ΔH = the enthalpy change of the reaction

T = the absolute temperature of the reaction

ΔS = the entropy change of the reaction

The following enthalpy values were gathered to study the energies of different hydrocarbons.

Fuel	Formula	ΔH_{comb} (kJ/mol)
Hydrogen	H_2	−241.8
Ethanol	CH_3CH_2OH	−1235.4
Acetylene	C_2H_2	−1255.5
Ethane	C_2H_6	−1427.7
Propanol	C_3H_8O	−2021

Table 1. Heats of combustion of selected hydrocarbon fuels.

16. If the ΔH_f° of CO_2 (g) is -393.5 kJ/mol, and the ΔH_f° of H_2O (g) is -241.8 kJ/mol, what is the ΔH_f° of acetylene?

    A. -620.1 kJ/mol
    B. -226.7 kJ/mol
    C. 226.7 kJ/mol
    D. 620.1 kJ/mol

17. Which of the following reactions would produce the greatest increase in entropy?

    A. Combustion of hydrogen
    B. Combustion of acetylene
    C. Combustion of ethanol
    D. Combustion of propanol

18. Given that ΔS for the combustion of ethanol is 0.217 kJ/mol $\cdot$ K at 25°C, what is the value of the change in the Gibbs free energy for this reaction?

    A. -64.7 kJ/mol of ethanol
    B. -1170 kJ/mol of ethanol
    C. -1235 kJ/mol of ethanol
    D. -1300 kJ/mol of ethanol

19. Which of the following pairs of characteristics defines a reaction that is temperature dependent?

    I. Positive ΔH, positive ΔS
    II. Positive ΔH, negative ΔS
    III. Negative ΔH, positive ΔS
    IV. Negative ΔH, negative ΔS

    A. I and II only
    B. I and III only
    C. I and IV only
    D. II and III only

PASSAGE 5 (QUESTIONS 20–24)

Chronic usage of loop diuretics can induce contraction alkalosis. Contraction alkalosis is characterized by a loss of fluid in the extracellular space. Without this fluid, the concentration of bicarbonate in the blood is relatively high. The bicarbonate snatches up the H^+ in solution and increases the pH of the blood. Contraction alkalosis is identified by measuring urine $[Cl^-]$. If urine $[Cl^-]$ falls below 25 mEq/L, contraction alkalosis is indicated. $[Cl^-]$ can be determined by titrating with $AgNO_3$. It is important not to overestimate the amount of $[Cl^-]$ in order to ensure an accurate diagnosis. The Volhard method is one way to determine the exact endpoint of the titration.

The concentrations of other ions in solutions can also be determined with the Volhard method. For example, the concentration of silver ions in solution can be determined experimentally by titrating with the thiocyanate ion, SCN^-. This method uses iron(III) as an indicator because it gives a deep red color at the first excess of thiocyanate ion in solution. The solution must be kept fairly acidic to prevent $Fe(OH)_3$ formation. This titration can be utilized as a second step in determining halide concentration. After a halide solution has been titrated with silver ions to precipitate out insoluble silver halide salts, the solution can be back-titrated with thiocyanate to determine the amount of excess silver ions. This gives a more accurate reading of the halide endpoint. Relevant solubility products for the precipitates involved are given in Table 1.

A student planned to determine the concentration of chloride ion in an unknown solution. In order to obtain the best possible endpoint of silver, he filtered out the silver chloride precipitate and titrated the solution with 0.001 M sodium thiocyanate. The sodium thiocyanate was contaminated with NaOH and the red $FeSCN^{2+}$ indicator never formed.

Compound	K_{sp}
AgSCN	1.0×10^{-12}
AgCl	1.8×10^{-10}
$Fe(OH)_3$	2.6×10^{-39}

Table 1. Solubility constants of selected compounds

20. In a Volhard titration, why does AgSCN precipitate before any $FeSCN^{2+}$ forms?

    A. The anion to cation bond in silver thiocyanate has more ionic character.
    B. Silver thiocyanate is the less stable of the two compounds.
    C. Silver thiocyanate reaches equilibrium in solution at lower concentrations.
    D. Silver thiocyanate is the heavier of the two compounds.

21. Which of the following has the highest molar solubility?

    A. $BaCrO_4$ ($K_{sp} = 2.1 \times 10^{-10}$)
    B. $AgCl$ ($K_{sp} = 1.6 \times 10^{-10}$)
    C. $Al(OH)_3$ ($K_{sp} = 3.7 \times 10^{-15}$)
    D. $PbCO_3$ ($K_{sp} = 3.3 \times 10^{-14}$)

22. Why was the endpoint never indicated in the student's Volhard titration?

    A. The presence of NaOH prevented NaSCN dissociation.
    B. A hydrated AgOH complex formed, which is almost completely soluble.
    C. A hydrated $Fe(OH)_3$ complex formed, which is almost completely insoluble.
    D. The NaOH neutralized the cations in the solution.

23. When measuring $[Cl^-]$ using the Volhard method, 0.5 moles of Ag^+ were added, and it was determined that 0.1 moles of thiocyanate reacted. How many moles of Cl^- were initially present in solution?

    A. 0.3 moles
    B. 0.4 moles
    C. 0.5 moles
    D. 0.6 moles

24. What is the $[OH^-]$ contributed by $Fe(OH)_3$ in an aqueous solution of $Fe(OH)_3$ at iron (III) hydroxide's solubility equlibrium?

    A. $1 \times 10^{-11}\ M$
    B. $1 \times 10^{-10}\ M$
    C. $3 \times 10^{-10}\ M$
    D. $3 \times 10^{-9}\ M$

DISCRETE PRACTICE QUESTIONS (QUESTIONS 25–27)

25. An electron orbiting He^+ is 2×10^{-10} m from the nucleus. What is the approximate electrostatic force exerted on the electron by the nucleus? (Note: $e = 1.6 \times 10^{-19}$ C)

   A. $(6.5 \times 10^{-29})k$
   B. $(1.3 \times 10^{-28})k$
   C. $(1.3 \times 10^{-18})k$
   D. $(3.9 \times 10^{-28})k$

26. If the bond length between two phosphate groups in ATP is 9×10^{-11} m, by how much would the electrical potential energy change if the bond length were three times shorter?

   A. It would decrease by three times.
   B. It would decrease by nine times.
   C. It would increase by three times.
   D. It would increase by nine times.

27. Two charged objects, particles, or molecules will exert force on one another when juxtaposed in space. Of the following arrangements of objects A and B, the largest magnitude of force is exerted when their two charges and the distance between them are:

   A. 2 μC, 4 μC, and 4 mm, respectively.
   B. 2 μC, 3 μC, and 3 mm, respectively.
   C. 2 μC, 2 μC, and 2 mm, respectively.
   D. 1 μC, 5 μC, and 2 mm, respectively.

Extra practice for the next class session starts on the next page ▶ ▶ ▶

CARS 2: Advanced Reasoning on the CARS Section

PASSAGE 1 (QUESTIONS 1–6)

The rise of the FIRE (Finance, Insurance, and Real Estate) sector in the global economy, but especially in the "Western" democratic nations of North America and Europe, has forever altered the face of modern capitalism. While for decades Western democracies allowed for the empowerment of workers who crafted goods or provided services that led to a net increase in economic value, an orchestrated capture of the levers of power by the FIRE sector has led to the political dominance of the *rentier* class, the elite whose wealth increases solely through "rent-seeking," that is, exploitation of the monopolistic privileges associated with property rights. In short, the West has been transformed from a *productive* economy to an *extractive* one.

Evidence of this transformation can be found in the remarkable shift in behavior of companies that were once titans of manufacturing, that established their market share through efficient production of vital consumer goods, but which have now become "financialized," increasingly seeking more profit through the heavy deployment of financial instruments. For example, in 2006 both Ford and General Motors earned more income through the interest-based lending associated with purchasing their vehicles than through the actual manufacture and sale of the vehicles themselves.

Though not a distinction typically recognized by the ascendant neoclassical tradition—today's answer to medieval Scholasticism's apologetics—the difference between productive and extractive economies could not be starker. What is the true economic value of a home? The laborers who build the house and implement the architect's vision create far more real value than the landlord who purchases the property and rents it out to hapless tenants to try and turn a profit. Meanwhile, the landlord will have to deal with a host of other middlemen, all scrumming for their cut of the action, from calculating bankers seeking to capitalize on their control of the currency supply through usurious lending, to opportunistic realtors looking to "flip" properties for a quick buck. Each party takes as much as it can and gives back as little as it has to—and the consumer always picks up the tab.

Centuries of human economic enterprise have created an abundance of valuable commodities and, thus, from the standpoint of individuals who want more for themselves regardless of the cost to others, it makes more sense to exploit the wealth that already exists rather than take the risk of trying to create value anew. For the relatively small cost of campaign contributions and other forms of legalized bribery, a wealthy donor can purchase pliant politicians who will overturn unprofitable regulations and enact new laws to ensure that rent-seeking can proceed unimpeded. With democracy effectively subverted, the enforcement mechanisms of the state (ultimately grounded in violence, and the threat thereof, posed by police, military, and private security forces) ensure that monopolies are protected, so that the *rentier* class need not worry about the dangers that actual competition could pose to their profit margins.

Of course, considering the matter more broadly, humanity would do well to combat such corruption and, more generally, to avoid encouraging people to play zero-sum games. An extractive economy necessitates the immiseration of the masses who lack monopoly privileges, who must continually be servicing debts, paying fees, and selling themselves piecemeal simply to satisfy their basic needs. Hence, the *rentier* class would do well to reconsider its myopic focus on immediate profitability: history shows that the polarization of wealth rarely contributes to social stability and long-term prosperity.

1. The author of the passage most likely assumes that:

   A. There are no more productive economies in the world today.
   B. Economic value can be neither created nor destroyed.
   C. Landlords and bankers produce virtually nothing of real value.
   D. Extractive economies are no worse than productive economies.

2. What role does the claim that it is easier to exploit existing wealth than to try to create new value play in the passage's argument?

   A. It offers a potential explanation for the behavior of members of the *rentier* class.
   B. It directly strengthens the author's central thesis.
   C. It indirectly weakens the author's central thesis.
   D. It offers a potential challenge to the stance taken by members of the *rentier* class.

3. The author of the passage probably views members of the *rentier* class:

   A. as short-sighted business people only focused on a production-based economy.
   B. with contempt for their immoral exploitation of lower class production.
   C. as a powerful class who need to reassess their position to ensure future stability.
   D. with admiration for their financial success in the face of a slowing economy.

4. According to the author, which of the following would be considered to have the least real value?

   A. An investor giving money to a scientist to invent a new hair-loss drug
   B. A potter creating bowls, mugs, and plates to sell at a local farmers' market
   C. An investment banker buying bitcoins and trading them against other cryptocurrencies
   D. A musician recording music and marketing that music via the Internet

5. The author's example of Ford and General Motors is used to support his argument about:

   A. the change from a productive economy to an extractive one.
   B. the difference between a productive economy and an extractive one.
   C. the political action of the *rentier* class.
   D. the abundance of valuable commodities in today's economy.

6. According to the passage, which of the following first allowed the change from a productive economy to an extractive one?

   A. The apologetics of the proponents of Scholasticism
   B. Ford and General Motors changing to producing less and extracting more
   C. The abundance of valuable commodities
   D. The FIRE act in the United States

PASSAGE 2 (QUESTIONS 7–12)

Innovative and influential, science fiction is a large and rich literary genre that has transcended literature and become part of the larger culture. With visions of fantastical worlds and future technologies, science fiction has won the hearts of millions of people around the world. With its future-leaning viewpoints, science fiction is able to provide commentary and guidance on many different issues, such as technology, politics, the military, gender politics, and dealing with the unknown. Science fiction has pervaded modern media, and it has produced some of the most recognizable franchises and cultural artifacts in today's world.

Science fiction as a literary genre has recently been cast under the broad umbrella term of speculative fiction. Speculative fiction is a much broader category that includes science fiction, fantasy, horror fiction, supernatural fiction, and superhero fiction, as well as historical fiction and alternate history. All of these genres rely on imagining what would happen in alternate realities; the differences between genres lie in what respect the story's reality differs from the real world. Science fiction, specifically, relies on extrapolating current technology to determine the future course of human development. This includes social and political development, as well as technological and scientific advances.

Even within the genre itself, there are further divisions. The two major divisions, hard and soft science fiction, are demarcated by the scientific rigor behind the innovations discussed in the work. Hard science fiction advocates using only very precise and accurate extrapolation of scientific principles; authors make sure to research their background material extensively to maintain an internal logic and make sure to explain any apparent phenomena in terms of biology, physics, and chemistry. This mostly precludes the inclusion of any fantastical creatures, especially those based in fantasy realms such as dragons, vampires, and wyverns.

Soft science fiction, on the other hand, has a much more general definition and a looser interpretation that allows all kinds of works to be included in the genre. Soft science fiction also coincides with the "soft" sciences such as sociology, psychology, and political science. It focuses on the more human side of the future, dealing with how the future, including future technology, will affect interpersonal relationships and the culture of the human race. These futures are usually utopian, dystopian, or, even better, a utopian façade covering a dystopia such as in Huxley's *Brave New World*. Soft science fiction is also allowed more leeway in the rigor of the underlying science. Fantastical mechanisms and technology, such as FTL (faster-than-light) travel, are more widespread and accepted as the rigors of hard science fiction give way to enable the story to proceed.

In reality, hard and soft science fiction operate more on a continuum. Strict taxonomy of something as fluid as literature is merely a mental exercise for those who want the world to be black and white. With arbitrarily advanced technology, even the lines between science fiction and fantasy become blurred. Arthur C. Clarke, a famed science fiction writer, said, "any sufficiently advanced technology is indistinguishable from magic" and indeed it has recently become popular to have a scientific basis for magic in more traditional "sword-and-sorcery" fantasy novels. Clarke's quote rings true in our own world, as more technologies get so advanced that the average person might as well consider them magic, for all they know of their internal workings.

7. Which of the following viewpoints could reasonably be attributed to the author?

   A. Hard science fiction is the purest and objectively best form of science fiction.
   B. Soft science fiction is inferior because of its lack of scientific rigor.
   C. Science fiction is an influential genre that is not easily categorized.
   D. There are no clear characteristics of different kinds of science fiction.

8. How does the author regard works that comment on dystopian futures with exaggerated political climates of today?

   A. With disdain for their treatment of the hard sciences
   B. As valuable commentary that can steer society's views
   C. With admiration that they can predict the future evolution of technology
   D. As a perversion of the science that will make the future possible

9. The information in the passage best supports the author's conclusion that:

   A. some science fiction works are neither completely hard nor soft science fiction.
   B. almost all science fiction writers start out writing hard science fiction before moving to soft.
   C. the scientific rigor needed to write hard science fiction is impossible without a PhD.
   D. science fiction works based on current technology focus too much on politics.

10. What does the author assume about faster-than-light travel?

    A. It is a characteristic of hard science fiction.
    B. It is not scientifically feasible as a logical extension of current technology.
    C. It is used only in books that are purely soft science fiction.
    D. It is a main plot point in most science fiction today.

11. As used in the passage, the term "scientific rigor" (paragraph 3) most closely means:

    A. how much time it takes for one to get a degree in the natural sciences.
    B. the increasing difficulty as one progresses to higher sciences.
    C. the extent to which the science affects the story's plot.
    D. how accurate and logically the science follows today's knowledge.

12. The author includes a discussion of speculative fiction primarily in order to:

    A. describe the hierarchical quality of different forms of fiction.
    B. give context to where science fiction currently exists in literary taxonomy.
    C. show that critics have always been critical of science fiction writers.
    D. offer a conclusion about the origins of science fiction.

PASSAGE 3 (QUESTIONS 13–20)

If one always ought to act so as to produce the best possible circumstances, then morality is extremely demanding. No one could plausibly claim to have met the requirements of this "simple principle." It would seem strange to punish those intending to do good by sentencing them to an impossible task. Also, if the standards of right conduct are as extreme as they seem, then they will preclude the personal projects that humans find most fulfilling.

From an analytic perspective, the potential extreme demands of morality are not a "problem." A theory of morality is no less valid simply because it asks great sacrifices. In fact, it is difficult to imagine what kind of constraints could be put on our ethical projects. Shouldn't we reflect on our base prejudices, and not allow them to provide boundaries for our moral reasoning? Thus, it is tempting to simply dismiss the objections to the simple principle. However, in *Demands of Morality*, Liam Murphy takes these objections seriously for at least two distinct reasons.

First, discussion of the simple principle provides an excellent vehicle for a discussion of morality in general. Perhaps, in a way, this is Murphy's attempt at doing philosophy "from the inside out." Second, Murphy's starting point tells us about the nature of his project. Murphy must take seriously the collisions between moral philosophy and our intuitive sense of right and wrong. He [must do so] because his work is best interpreted as intended to forge moral principles from our firm beliefs, and not to prescribe beliefs given a set of moral principles.

Murphy argues from our considered judgments rather than to them. For example, Murphy cites our "simple but firmly held" beliefs as supporting the potency of the over-demandingness objection, and nowhere in the work can one find a source of moral values divorced from human preferences.

Murphy does not tell us what set of "firm beliefs" we ought to have. Rather, he speaks to an audience of well-intentioned but unorganized moral realists, and tries to give them principles that represent their considered moral judgments. Murphy starts with this base sense of right and wrong, but recognizes that it needs to be supplemented by reason where our intuitions are confused or conflicting. Perhaps Murphy is looking for the best interpretation of our convictions, the same way certain legal scholars try to find the best interpretation of our Constitution.

This approach has disadvantages. Primarily, Murphy's arguments, even if successful, do not provide the kind of motivating force for which moral philosophy has traditionally searched. His work assumes and argues in terms of an inner sense of morality, and his project seeks to deepen that sense. Of course, it is quite possible that the moral viewpoints of humans will not converge, and some humans have no moral sense at all. Thus, it is very easy for the moral skeptic to point out a lack of justification and ignore the entire work.

On the other hand, Murphy's choice of a starting point avoids many of the problems of moral philosophy. Justifying the content of moral principles and granting a motivating force to those principles is an extraordinary task. It would be unrealistic to expect all discussions of moral philosophy to derive such justifications. Projects that attempt such a derivation have value, but they are hard pressed to produce logical consequences for everyday life. In the end, Murphy's strategy may have more practical effect than its first-principle counterparts, which do not seem any more likely to convince those that would reject Murphy's premises.

13. According to Murphy, the application of reason is necessary for forming moral principles when:

    A. the beliefs of one group supersede the beliefs of another.
    B. people's firmly held beliefs are conflicting or confused.
    C. the belief system of a group conflicts with an overriding ethical principle.
    D. individuals have no moral sense at all.

14. In the context of the passage, the Constitution serves as the basis of:

    A. a logical proof.
    B. the author's main point.
    C. an analogy.
    D. a rebuttal.

15. According to the passage, evidence of the existence of individuals who entirely lack a moral sense would:

    A. confirm the notion that moral principles should be derived from the considered judgments of individuals.
    B. substantiate a potential disadvantage of Murphy's philosophical approach.
    C. support Murphy's belief that reason is necessary when intuitions are conflicting or confused.
    D. prove that first-principle strategies of ethical theorizing are passé.

16. Which of the following would be the most appropriate title for the passage?

    A. "The 'Simple Principle': Deceptively Complex"
    B. "The Philosophy of Right and Wrong"
    C. "Addressing Objections to *Demands of Morality*"
    D. "Murphy's Law: Everything Can Go Wrong"

17. The phrase "human preferences" (paragraph 4) refers to which of the following concepts?

    A. Intuitive beliefs people hold
    B. The popularity of Murphy's philosophy
    C. The appeal of absolute moral principles
    D. Human desire for codes of morality

18. The "analytic perspective" the author mentions (paragraph 2) is most clearly presented as:

    A. a viewpoint held by the author.
    B. a viewpoint of *Demands of Morality*.
    C. a viewpoint that Murphy opposes.
    D. a viewpoint taken by Murphy's critics.

19. Which of the following does the author NOT state regarding the "simple principle"?

    A. Its drawbacks are not necessarily problematic.
    B. It is a result of philosophy "from the inside out."
    C. No individual has ever satisfied its requirements.
    D. Studying it requires confronting our base prejudices.

20. Based on the first paragraph, which of the following statements must be true?

    A. If morality is extremely demanding, then one always ought to act so as to produce the best possible circumstances.
    B. If moral standards do not preclude the personal projects humans find most fulfilling, then they are not that extreme.
    C. Some people always act in ways that produce the best possible circumstances.
    D. Morality precludes the personal projects that humans find most fulfilling.

PASSAGE 4 (QUESTIONS 21–25)

Does true happiness come from "within" or from "without"? Do we achieve fulfillment when external circumstances happen to satisfy our desires, as the modern Utilitarian view maintains? Or, on the contrary, is it as the ancient Stoics and Buddhists claim, and we become happy only through renouncing our desires and cultivating a proper internal attitude?

In his landmark work, *The Happiness Hypothesis*, psychologist Jonathan Haidt answers that neither is the case—or, more accurately, both are. After embarking upon an ambitious project of cataloguing the world's wisdom and looking to contemporary social science for results that verify ancient proverbs, Haidt concludes that true happiness comes from "between," requiring a mix of internal and external conditions: "Some of those conditions are within you, such as coherence among the parts and levels of your personality. Other conditions require relationships to things beyond you: Just as plants need sun, water, and good soil to thrive, people need love, work, and a connection to something larger."

While the above presents what Haidt calls the "final version of the happiness hypothesis," which stands both the test of time and empirical verification, Haidt's book as a whole is a synoptic appraisal of ten key ideas about human psychology that recur in disparate cultures and historical eras. For example, in his chapter on the "adversity hypothesis," Haidt actually evaluates two versions of the claim that suffering builds character. The weak version, "adversity *can* lead to growth," is undoubtedly supported. However, the data only support a limited version of the strong view, that it *must* cause growth: "For adversity to be maximally beneficial, it should happen at the right time (young adulthood), to the right people (those with the social and psychological resources to rise to challenges and find benefits), and to the right degree (not so severe as to cause PTSD)."

Of all the great ideas considered, perhaps the most fascinating discussion comes in Haidt's chapter on what he calls "divinity with or without God." Unpossessed of the contempt that exudes from supposed representatives of science like Richard Dawkins and Christopher Hitchens, Haidt harbors a profound—if somewhat distanced—reverence for religion. Though himself a nonbeliever, he cannot deny the power of the data on happiness, including the key finding that religious believers tend to report greater life satisfaction, especially when belonging to some kind of spiritual community. Rather than dismiss this as the product of mass delusion like Dawkins and Hitchens—who essentially renounce any internal contribution to happiness—Haidt instead looks for common ground, for the analogues of spiritual elevation that can be detected by an atheist like himself.

Building on the work of his mentors, Haidt argues that social "space" has three "dimensions," each of which corresponds roughly to a particular ethical orientation. The "ethic of autonomy," which prioritizes the prevention of harm and the removal of constraints on individual freedom, is operative in the horizontal dimension of closeness, consisting of the egalitarian bonds that humans share with their peers. With the vertical dimension of hierarchy that recognizes unequal relationships between people comes the "ethic of community," the end of which is "to protect the integrity of groups, families, companies, or nations" with an emphasis on "virtues such as obedience, loyalty, and wise leadership." Finally, there is the "ethic of divinity," which divides social space into regions that are sacred or profane, pure or polluted. This third dimension, which purports to offer "a connection to something larger," plays a crucial role in much human flourishing, which is why Haidt recognizes it as one of the key components of a happiness that comes from between.

21. The primary purpose of the passage is:

    A. to extol the virtues of Jonathan Haidt's work in *The Happiness Hypothesis.*
    B. to put forth the ideas of philosophers like Dawkins, Hitchens, Shweder, and Haidt.
    C. to show how *The Happiness Hypothesis* makes the case that true happiness requires a mix of internal and external conditions.
    D. to argue against the simplistic assumption that happiness comes either from "within" or "without" and to propose a more balanced view in its place.

22. Based on the information provided in the passage, which of the following views about religion is most likely held by Richard Dawkins and Christopher Hitchens?

    A. The positive influence of religion on happiness is supported by empirical evidence.
    B. Religion can be worthy of a distant yet profound reverence, even if you aren't religious yourself.
    C. The greater life satisfaction reported by religious believers is likely a product of mass delusion.
    D. Religion can be a source of happiness as long as its believers emphasize its spiritual aspects over outdated rites and traditions.

23. The author's attitude toward Jonathan Haidt's work in *The Happiness Hypothesis* can be described as one of:

    A. reluctant agreement.
    B. restrained admiration.
    C. impartial appraisal.
    D. contemptuous dismissal.

24. As used in the passage, the phrase "a connection to something larger" could refer to:

    A. an altruistic approach to life.
    B. a spiritual connection with a higher power.
    C. a feeling of being connected and accepted within one's family and community.
    D. an alignment between one's personal mission and the mission of an organization that one belongs to.

25. Which of the following individuals is most likely to hold views similar to the modern Utilitarian view?

    A. The author of the passage
    B. Jonathan Haidt
    C. An ancient Stoic
    D. Richard Dawkins

PASSAGE 5 (QUESTIONS 26–32)

According to our traditional understanding of responsibility, we are directly responsible for our "voluntary" actions, and (at most) only indirectly responsible for the things that happen to us. It is held, for instance, that "I can't help" the surge of anger that I feel when objects in the environment present themselves to my senses in certain ways; however, I am supposed to govern my subsequent thoughts and activities regarding these objects by the force of my will. When we look inside ourselves with the goal of sorting our mental events into these two morally important categories, something peculiar happens. Events near the input and output "peripheries" fall unproblematically into place. Thus, feeling pain in my foot and seeing the desk are clearly not acts "in my control," but things that happen to me, while moving my finger or saying these words are obviously things that I do—voluntary actions.

But as we move away from those peripheries toward the presumptive center, the events we try to examine exhibit a strange flickering back and forth. It no longer seems so clear that perception is a passive matter. Do I not voluntarily contribute something to my perception, even to my recognition or "acceptance" of the desk as a desk? For after all, can I not suspend judgment in the face of any perceptual presentation, and withhold conviction? On the other side of the center, when we look more closely at action, is my voluntary act really moving my finger, or is it more properly trying to move my finger? A familiar [thought experiment] about someone willing actions while totally paralyzed attests that I am not in control of all the conditions in the world (or in my body) that are necessary for my finger actually to move.

Faced with our inability to "see" (by "introspection") where the center or source of our free actions is, and loath to abandon our conviction that we really do things (for which we are responsible), we exploit the gaps in our self-knowledge by filling it with a rather magical and mysterious entity—the unmoved mover, the active self.

This theoretical leap is nowhere more evident than in our reaction to our failures of "willpower." "I'm going to get out of bed and get to work right now!" I say to myself, and go right on lying drowsily in bed. Did I or did I not just make a decision to get up? Perhaps I just seem to myself to have made a decision. Once we recognize that our conscious access to our own decisions is problematic, we may realize how many of the important events in our lives were unaccompanied, so far as retrospective memory of conscious experience goes, by conscious decisions. "I have decided to take the job," one says. And very clearly one takes oneself to be reporting on something one had done recently, but reminiscence shows only that yesterday one was undecided, and today one is no longer undecided; at some moment in the interval the decision must have happened, without fanfare. Where did it happen? At Central Headquarters, of course.

But such a deduction reveals that we are building a psychological theory of "decision" by idealizing and extending our actual practice, by inserting decisions where theory demands them, not where we have any firsthand experience of them. I must have made a decision, one reasons, since I see that I have definitely made up my mind, and hadn't made up my mind yesterday. The mysterious inner sanctum of the central agent begins to take on a mysterious life of its own.

26. Post hoc rationalization is a term used to describe an automatic process whereby individuals try to justify decisions that were made irrationally rather than logically. The author is most likely to be of the opinion that the phenomenon of post hoc rationalization provides more evidence that:

    A. decision-making is not always a conscious process.
    B. we falsely believe we have the capacity to make decisions voluntarily.
    C. decisions are the instances in which we exercise our volition to the fullest.
    D. many actions cannot be classified precisely as either voluntary or involuntary.

27. According to the passage, if an individual has made a decision in the past, it:

    A. automatically follows that the individual must assume full responsibility.
    B. is sufficient proof that the individual possesses free will.
    C. often cannot be ascertained how the individual knows he made the decision.
    D. may not seem to the individual that there was any decision made at all.

28. Which of the following is a statement with which the author would most probably agree?

    A. People often exaggerate how much conscious thought went into their actions.
    B. A decision usually takes longer to make than one anticipates.
    C. Problems are better addressed through philosophical analysis than through science.
    D. More careful thought should go into decision-making

29. Judging from the context, the "unmoved mover" (paragraph 3) could best be described as:

    A. the divine being that many think guides one's actions.
    B. the inherent core of irrationality in human behavior.
    C. the part of the human psyche that governs decision-making.
    D. the natural tendency to pursue one's self-interest.

30. The author most probably cites "our failures of 'willpower'" (paragraph 4) in order to show that:

    A. some people have more willpower than others.
    B. one could possibly make a decision and yet not act on it.
    C. some decisions are much more difficult to make than others.
    D. the concept of willpower makes sense in theory but not in real life.

31. Aristotle characterized a voluntary act as one with a source "within the agent" and an involuntary act as one in which "the moving principle is outside." Based on the passage, the author would most likely respond to this by pointing out that:

    A. we are only responsible for our voluntary actions.
    B. many actions contain elements of both categories.
    C. there is no conscious judgment involved in an involuntary act.
    D. the external moving principle is actually our own creation.

32. Suppose that a person heats a kettle of water on a stove, takes it off the stove, and then accidentally spills some of the hot water on his skin. According to the passage, which of the following perceptions has a voluntary element?

    I. Perceiving that the hot stove caused the water to become hot
    II. Perceiving that the kettle is made of steel
    III. Perceiving the hot water as painful

    A. I only
    B. III only
    C. I and II only
    D. I, II, and III

PASSAGE 6 (QUESTIONS 33–38)

The system of farming practiced in the United States today evolved during the 1950s when the development of chemical pesticides, fertilizers, and high-yielding crop strains brought a mass shift toward specialization. Using agrochemicals, farmers found that they could grow a single crop on the same field year after year without impairing the yield or incurring pest problems. Encouraged by government programs subsidizing the production of grains such as wheat and corn, most farmers consolidated to cultivate a limited number of crops and to invest in the equipment to mechanize labor-intensive farm processes. In addition, crop strains were modified, initially using the traditional method of breeding and crossbreeding over generations, and later with genetic engineering (also known as "recombinant DNA technology"), which involves splicing a gene from one organism into another in order to confer a trait, such as resistance to insects or increase in edible portion, improved flavor, or longer shelf life. For the last 40 years, these practices have enabled American farmers to lead the world in efficiency and crop production. Today, however, rising costs and problems such as groundwater contamination, soil erosion, declining productivity, and unintended adverse health consequences of genetically modified food consumption are forcing many farmers to question their dependence on agrochemicals and genetically modified crops and to investigate alternative systems.

Perhaps the most likely system to replace today's agriculture is a composite of nonconventional techniques defined as sustainable agriculture. Using a combination of organic, low-input methods that benefit the environment and preserve the integrity of the soil, many scientists believe that sustainable agriculture could reach productivity levels competitive with conventional systems. Farmers converting to sustainable systems would find themselves using the same machinery, certified seed, and feeding methods as before. But instead of enhancing productivity with purchased chemicals, sustainable farms would use, as far as possible, natural processes and local renewable resources. Returning to a system of crop rotation, where fields are used to grow a succession of different crops, would improve crop yields and bolster pest resistance. Using crop residues, manures, and other organic materials would help to restore soil quality by improving such factors as air circulation, moisture retention, and tilth, or soil structure. And systems such as integrated pest management (IPM) would combat pests by diversifying crops, regulating predators of pest species, and using pesticides intermittently when necessary.

In order to gain acceptance, however, sustainable agriculture must also be shown to be sufficiently productive and profitable to support farmers economically. Federal farm programs currently encourage mono-cropping by providing subsidies for only a limited number of crops. Extending price supports to a wide variety of crops would promote diversification and crop rotation, and perhaps make sustainable agriculture feasible on a national scale. Comparative studies suggest that under the present conditions, sustainable farms are capable of producing greater returns than conventional farms due to lower production costs. And yet, the majority of today's farmers elect to use specialized, chemical-dependent systems on the basis of their short-term profitability. If efforts to establish an ecologically sustainable agriculture are to succeed, higher priority must not only be given to researching alternative technology. The fruits of such research must also be made available to farmers.

33. Which of the following best summarizes the main idea of the passage?

    A. Sustainable agriculture should be supported for a variety of reasons.
    B. Growing only a single crop in a given tract of land can make that crop more susceptible to pests.
    C. Sustainable agriculture does not provide a viable alternative to today's farming methods.
    D. Methods of farming must be altered to prevent further damage to the environment.

34. According to the passage, all of the following are advantages of sustainable agriculture EXCEPT:

    A. increased resistance to pests.
    B. decreased damage to the environment.
    C. more efficient feeding methods.
    D. decreased costs.

35. Suppose a farmer regularly uses locally sourced agrochemicals to grow the same three crops on his field each year. What element(s) of this practice would the author consider to be characteristic of sustainable agriculture?

    A. The locally sourced agrochemicals
    B. The growing of three crops on the same field every year
    C. The locally purchased agrochemicals and the growing of three crops on the same field every year
    D. Neither the locally sourced agrochemicals nor the growing of three crops on the same field every year

36. Which of the following, if true, would most WEAKEN the author's argument concerning the extension of price supports?

    A. Most of today's farmers consider economic issues to be more important than environmental concerns.
    B. Increasing the number of crops grown on a single farm would require expensive alterations to farming machinery.
    C. Damage caused by pests is a more pressing concern now than it was in the 1950s.
    D. The total number of functioning farms has declined steadily since the 1950s even though the total number of acres farmed has been relatively constant.

37. Which of the following does the author suggest is a barrier to more widespread use of sustainable agriculture techniques?

    I. Uncertainty among U.S. farmers concerning its effects on productivity
    II. The economic attitudes of many U.S. farmers
    III. U.S. farmers' alarm over its potential to harm the environment

    A. I only
    B. II only
    C. I and II only
    D. I, II, and III

38. According to the passage, all of the following are elements of a sustainable system EXCEPT:

    A. rotating the crops grown in a single field.
    B. organic soil preservation methods.
    C. implementing natural techniques for improving crop yields.
    D. reducing the number of crops grown on a given farm.

Bio/Biochem 2: Section-Wide Strategy & Answer Choice Analysis

PASSAGE 1 (QUESTIONS 1–5)

Pituitary adenomas are tumors that form in the pituitary gland. The most common pituitary adenomas are known as lactotroph adenomas. They affect the cells of the anterior pituitary that produce prolactin, a hormone that encourages lactation. The incidence of lactotroph adenomas is estimated at 2.2 cases per 100,000, while the prevalence is approximately 100 cases per 1 million.

As prolactin is the primary hormone produced by a lactotroph adenoma, these adenomas are also known as prolactinomas. One of the major symptoms of these tumors is inappropriate lactation, known as galactorrhea. However, there may be other symptoms resulting simply from the size of the tumor and how it affects the surrounding tissues. When a tumor causes additional symptoms due to its size, it is known as mass effect. As the tumor grows, surrounding cells may become compressed, which results in cessation of physiological function. For example, pituitary tumors often present with changes in vision due to compression of the chiasma.

For many pituitary adenomas, transsphenoidal surgery is the recommended treatment. This involves penetration of the sella turcica via the nasal and sinus passages. However, for prolactinomas, medical treatment is available in the form of medications that mimic the actions of pituitary-inhibiting factor. Generally, the application of these medications results in shrinking the tumor, but not its complete disappearance. Treatment of prolactinomas using medications is usually safer and less expensive than surgery. Surgical intervention is reserved for cases in which the tumor has become too large to be controlled by medications.

1. A researcher seeks to identify how a prolactinoma affects the production of other hormones, but can only take samples from an IV placed in the wrist. Which of the following is unlikely to be measured?

    A. Thyroid-stimulating hormone
    B. Corticotropin-releasing factor
    C. Adrenocorticotropic hormone
    D. Follicle-stimulating hormone

2. Within a certain population, the incidence of lactotroph adenomas is consistent with the general population, but the prevalence is much higher than expected, at 225 cases per million. Which of the following is likely to account for the increased prevalence in this population?

    A. Lactotroph adenomas occur more often in this population due to founder effect.
    B. This population has a decreased diagnosis of prolactinomas.
    C. This population has a longer life span and better nutrition.
    D. Transsphenoidal surgery is more common in this population.

3. A disease known as Conn's syndrome causes high concentrations of mineralocorticoids to be secreted. Which of the following is a likely indicator of this disease?

    A. High blood pressure
    B. Galactorrhea
    C. High blood glucose
    D. Low blood sodium

4. A study is designed to determine if people with a thyroid tumor are also more likely than the general population to develop a pituitary tumor. Which of the following study designs is LEAST likely to provide information to confirm or deny the correlation?

    A. A longitudinal study in which a large population is followed to identify those who develop thyroid tumors and subsequently develop a pituitary tumor
    B. A retrospective study in which 2,000 patients with known thyroid tumors are surveyed to determine how many also developed pituitary tumors
    C. A series of case studies that identifies ten cases in which patients first developed thyroid tumors and were later diagnosed with pituitary tumors
    D. A study in multiple medical centers over several years that tracks the development of thyroid tumors and pituitary tumors in a multicultural population

5. As a prolactinoma becomes larger, it begins to exhibit mass effect. Which of the following hormones is most likely to be diminished in a patient experiencing mass effect from a prolactinoma?

    A. Antidiuretic hormone
    B. Thyroid-stimulating hormone
    C. Oxytocin
    D. Serotonin

PASSAGE 2 (QUESTIONS 6–11)

Appropriate function of the nervous system, especially with regard to locomotion, relies on the ability of motor nerves to communicate with muscle tissue. Pathological conditions that inhibit the ability of neurons to communicate with muscles result in various types of muscular dysfunction. For example, myasthenia gravis (MG) is a disease in which autoantibodies target receptors located at the neuromuscular junction, resulting in the inability of the neuron to communicate with the muscle. Interestingly, many patients with MG also have an abnormal thymus. Treatment often involves pharmaceutical therapy, which generally offers only symptomatic relief. However, definitive treatment can often be achieved with removal of the thymus.

Another disease that causes a decrease in the ability of nerves to communicate with muscles is Lambert–Eaton myasthenic syndrome (LEMS). In this condition, autoantibodies attack the presynaptic calcium channels, diminishing the signal transmitted to the postsynaptic cells. This condition is often associated with small cell lung cancer.

MG and LEMS are often characterized by muscle weakness. However, in the absence of additional information, it can be difficult to differentiate between the two disorders. One of the ways these two conditions can be distinguished is by the administration of a medication that inhibits acetylcholinesterase. Patients with MG will notice substantial improvement with administration of such a medication, while LEMS patients will not. Another way to distinguish the two is by the use of repetitive nerve stimulation (RNS). RNS is performed by electrically stimulating a nerve and measuring the response of the muscle. Figure 1 shows the appearance of RNS muscle response. Each peak indicates a single stimulation event.

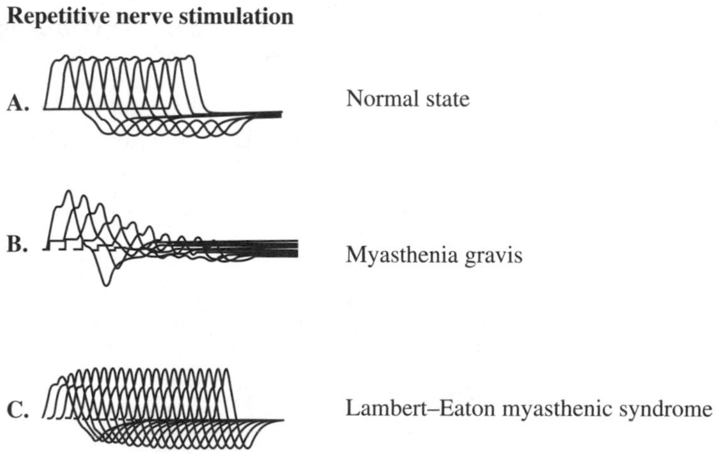

Figure 1. Repetitive nerve stimulation muscle response.

6. Why does the administration of a medication that inhibits acetylcholinesterase improve the symptoms of myasthenia gravis?

   A. It inactivates the antibodies against the receptors at the neuromuscular junction, preventing the autoantibodies from attacking.
   B. It increases the concentration of acetylcholine in the synaptic cleft, allowing for greater stimulation of unaffected receptors.
   C. It decreases the quantity of acetylcholine in the synaptic cleft to prevent aberrant signaling.
   D. It allows for more efficient opening of calcium channels at the neuromuscular junction.

7. In Lambert–Eaton myasthenic syndrome, the attack of autoantibodies on calcium channels in presynaptic cells results in muscle weakness. What causes this weakness?

   A. Action potential conduction is slowed.
   B. Acetylcholine does not bind to receptors.
   C. Neurotransmitter release is reduced.
   D. Calcium efflux is inhibited.

8. In myasthenia gravis, the speed at which an action potential travels down the axon is unchanged. Which of the following is likely to result in slower conduction of action potentials down the axon?

   A. Saltatory conduction
   B. Loss of myelin from axons
   C. Increased extracellular sodium
   D. Autoantibodies to calcium channels

9. A researcher is planning a study to determine the effect of a new medication on signal transmission at the synapse in patients with myasthenia gravis. Which of the following control groups would provide the most accurate information to help determine the efficacy of this new medication?

   A. People who do not have myasthenia gravis and have normal nerve conduction
   B. People who have Lambert–Eaton myasthenic syndrome and have not been treated
   C. People who have myasthenia gravis and are being treated with another drug
   D. People with myasthenia gravis who have not been treated with another drug

10. Which of the following is a possible interpretation of the repetitive nerve stimulation studies in Figure 1?

    A. People with Lambert–Eaton myasthenic syndrome experience increasing weakness with repetitive stimulation.
    B. People with myasthenia gravis experience increasing weakness with repetitive nerve stimulation.
    C. People with myasthenia gravis experience decreasing weakness with repetitive nerve stimulation.
    D. People with Lambert–Eaton myasthenic syndrome experience slower nerve conduction than people with myasthenia gravis.

11. A nerve conducts an action potential, but is unable to conduct a second action potential due to a highly negative membrane potential. This phenomenon is known as:

    A. depolarization.
    B. repolarization.
    C. a refractory period.
    D. threshold.

DISCRETE PRACTICE QUESTIONS (QUESTIONS 12–23)

12. In order for a zygote to have the appropriate number of genes, each gamete must be haploid. During what stage of cell division does this occur?

    A. Mitosis
    B. Meiosis I
    C. Meiosis II
    D. Cytokinesis

13. A cell is treated with a cancer drug that stabilizes microtubules, preventing degradation. Which phase of mitosis is this drug targeting?

    A. Prophase
    B. Metaphase
    C. Anaphase
    D. Telophase

14. Mitochondrial inheritance has been used to trace genetic lineage for certain groups. Which of the following relationships may be supported by similarities in mitochondrial DNA?

    A. Maternal grandmother–grandchild
    B. Maternal grandfather–grandchild
    C. Paternal grandmother–grandchild
    D. Paternal grandfather–grandchild

15. A known disease is characterized by a prolonged startle response. Which division of the nervous system is primarily responsible for returning physiology to its relaxed state after a startle response?

    A. Somatic nervous system
    B. Central nervous system
    C. Parasympathetic nervous system
    D. Peripheral nervous system

16. In order to transmit an action potential, a neuron requires stimulation from multiple presynaptic cells at the same time. Which of the following concepts best describes this phenomenon?

    A. Threshold potential
    B. Dendritic stimulation
    C. Temporal summation
    D. Spatial summation

17. Anaerobic exercise causes cessation of oxidative phosphorylation and falling pH within muscle tissue. Why does this occur?

    A. Pyruvate cannot enter the citric acid cycle and is converted to ethanol.
    B. Pyruvate cannot enter the citric acid cycle and is converted to lactic acid.
    C. The protons in the inner membrane of the mitochondria leak into the cytoplasm.
    D. ATP synthase is inhibited because electrons cannot be transferred to oxygen.

18. Apoptosis is induced in a cell and small pores are created in the mitochondrial membrane. What is the effect of this process on oxidative phosphorylation?

    A. Oxidative phosphorylation will continue because parts of the membrane are still intact.
    B. Oxidative phosphorylation will continue because ATP is required for apoptosis.
    C. Oxidative phosphorylation will cease because the electrochemical gradient required will not be present.
    D. Oxidative phosphorylation will cease because cell death causes a lack of oxygen and ATP.

19. Increased levels of ADP trigger an increase in ATP synthesis. What is the mechanism by which this occurs?

    A. Increased ADP triggers increased activity of ATP synthase.
    B. Increased ADP causes an increase in production of NADH.
    C. Decreased ATP inactivates isocitrate dehydrogenase.
    D. Decreased ATP increases available NAD^+ and FAD.

20. Which of the following is true regarding ATP synthesis?

    A. The formation of ATP is exergonic and electron transport is endergonic.
    B. The formation of ATP is endergonic and electron transport is exergonic.
    C. The formation of ATP is exothermic and electron transport is endothermic.
    D. The formation of ATP is spontaneous while electron transport is nonspontaneous.

21. Suppose an individual lacked an enzyme necessary for proper functioning of Complex II and, as a result, significant energy was lost during electron transfer to this portion of the electron transport chain. Which of the following describes the mostly likely pattern of ATP production from mitochondrial electron carriers in this individual?

    A. Mitochondrial NADH generates 1 ATP per molecule, while mitochondrial $FADH_2$ generates 1.5 ATP per molecule.
    B. Mitochondrial NADH generates 2.5 ATP per molecule, while mitochondrial $FADH_2$ generates 0.5 ATP per molecule.
    C. Mitochondrial NADH generates 1 ATP per molecule, while mitochondrial $FADH_2$ generates 0.5 ATP per molecule.
    D. Mitochondrial NADH generates 2.5 ATP per molecule while mitochondrial $FADH_2$ generates 1.5 ATP per molecule.

22. Which of the following is true regarding the extracellular environment immediately surrounding the ATP synthases of a eukaryotic cell during a high rate of oxidative phosphorylation?

    A. The area gains an increasing concentration of inorganic phosphate.
    B. The area becomes more acidic.
    C. The area becomes more basic.
    D. The area gains an increasing concentration of ADP.

23. Prokaryotes are able to produce more net ATP per molecule of glucose than eukaryotes. Why is this?

    A. Prokaryotes live longer than eukaryotes because of the additional ATP production.
    B. Prokaryotes have fewer lysosomal units than eukaryotes, so they use less ATP than eukaryotes in transferring NADH into the lysosome.
    C. Prokaryotes do not need to use ATP to transfer NADH into the mitochondrion.
    D. Prokaryotes do not lose potential energy from carriers as electrons enter the mitochondrion, whereas eukaryotes do.

Psych/Soc 2: The Psychology Behind the Test

PASSAGE 1 (QUESTIONS 1–4)

Advances in the understanding of the neuroscience of conscious thought have brought back previously marginalized psychodynamic theories of the unconscious and its role in determining behavior. One such idea that has been investigated is the use of psychoanalysis to recognize and treat repressed childhood traumas. Psychoanalysts hold that childhood trauma is often expressed through differences in behavior and explanatory style. Siblings of children who died of cancer, for example, may experience guilt associated with the wish-fulfillment of evicting a competitor, which can manifest in behavior later in life.

To test the hypothesis that childhood trauma affects explanatory style, researchers recruited two sets of participants. One set, the "patients," consisted of 14 individuals. Seven members of this set had the experience of living with a sibling who survived childhood cancer; the other seven were selected at random from a pool of volunteers. A second set of "raters" consisted of groups of three subjects each: trained psychoanalysts (PSYANs), trained cognitive behavioral therapists (CBTs), inexperienced professionals who were residents specializing in psychiatry (INXPs), experienced oncologists (ONCs), and individuals who shared the same experiences as the patients whose siblings developed cancer (SEs).

Patients were recorded giving a five-minute spontaneous speech on the way they experience their inner and outer worlds. While this topic was intentionally ambiguous, patients were asked, when applicable, not to speak about their siblings. Raters then watched the videos and received written instructions asking them to determine whether or not the patient had a sibling afflicted with childhood cancer. A score was obtained for each group by coding responses as follows: +2 when raters correctly responded yes or no, +1 when raters correctly responded probably yes or probably no, −1 when raters incorrectly responded probably yes or probably no, and −2 when raters incorrectly responded yes or no. Scores for the rater groups are tabulated in Figure 1.

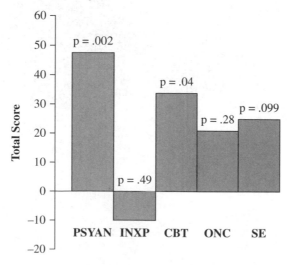

Figure 1. Scores for the rater groups.

1. Based on the passage, which of the following statements reflecting Hill's criteria for causation could be used to criticize the results of the study?

   A. The results suggest a weak correlation between the independent and dependent variables.
   B. The study violates the criterion of temporality based on its time course.
   C. The study lacks coherence with current scientific knowledge.
   D. The trauma investigated may have unique effects on behavior that other traumas do not.

2. The experimental procedure, as described in the passage, is designed to make use of which of the following defense mechanisms in the 14 patient participants?

   A. Repression
   B. Displacement
   C. Rationalization
   D. Reaction formation

3. Based on the information in the passage, a Jungian theorist might most reasonably explain the ability of the psychoanalysts to differentiate between the patient groups in which of the following ways?

   A. The psychoanalysts were able to see past the personas of the patients in order to discover their true feelings.
   B. The psychoanalysts were able to tap into the collective unconscious to sense differences between patients.
   C. The psychoanalysts perceived the patients' anima schemas and could tell who was more emotional.
   D. The psychoanalysts knew that victims of childhood trauma tend to be more introverted than the general population.

4. Based on the power of the observed effect for the inexperienced professionals being 12 percent, researchers determined that this sample did no better than chance. From this information, what is the probability that inexperienced professionals would be able to successfully sort patients into their correct groups?

   A. 0.12
   B. 0.49
   C. 0.51
   D. 0.88

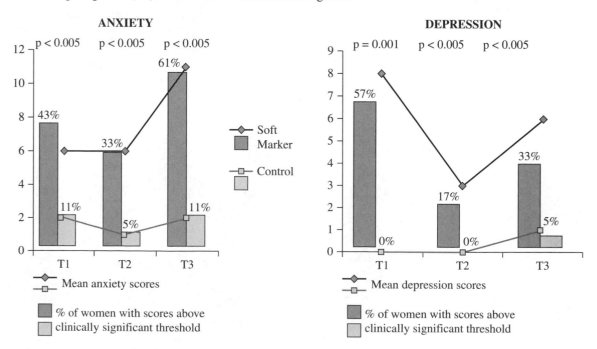

PASSAGE 2 (QUESTIONS 5–8)

Two experiments were conducted to examine the effects of false positives in prenatal testing on expectant parents.

Experiment 1
Researchers surveyed 88 mothers of newborns who had been screened for genetic abnormalities using mass spectrometry. While all of the infants in the study were born without abnormality, 49 of the infants had received a false-positive screen and 42 had received a normal screen. The screenings have a false-positive rate of 0.09 percent, with a positive predictive value (PPV) of 41 percent (PPV = number of true positive tests/number of positive tests).

Researchers found that the two groups of infants were demographically similar, although those in the false-positive group were an average of about nine days older at the time of screening and tended to be from families of lower socioeconomic status. Mothers in the false-positive group were more likely to worry about their child's future development (21 percent vs. 5 percent for the normal screen group) and were more likely to have visited a primary care physician or hospital within the first six months of the infant's life. Furthermore, 17 percent of mothers in the false-positive group received scores on a stress inventory that were indicative of the necessity for treatment. No mothers in the normal screen group scored within this range.

Experiment 2
A similar study included a false-positive group of infants ($n = 18$) who had shown soft markers for potential abnormalities on a prenatal ultrasound and required further testing. This group was compared against a normal control group in which ultrasounds revealed no such potential abnormalities ($n = 17$). Mothers in both groups were compared on scales for anxiety and depression three times during and after their pregnancy: once during the third trimester (T1), once at birth (T2), and once two months after giving birth (T3). Results are summarized in Figure 1.

Figure 1. Anxiety and depression in mothers during and after pregnancy.

5. The circumstances of the experimental groups in both studies described in the passage can be said to result most specifically from which of the following?

   A. Random error
   B. Systematic error
   C. Type I error
   D. Type II error

6. Congenital adrenal hyperplasia (CAH) has an incidence of one in 15,000 and its screening test has a PPV of 0.53%. A newborn included in the study for Experiment 1 tests positive for CAH. Which of the following describes the infant's chances of having the disease?

   A. The newborn has a one in 15,000 chance of having CAH.
   B. The newborn has a 0.53% chance of having CAH.
   C. The newborn has a 53% chance of having CAH.
   D. The newborn has a 99.47% chance of having CAH.

7. Researchers found that while most mothers in the false-positive group of Experiment 2 reported a negative experience, the 17 percent that required clinical intervention for stress felt less able to cope with their circumstances. This result can be most accounted for by differences in:

   A. primary appraisal.
   B. secondary appraisal.
   C. social readjustment.
   D. the exhaustion stage.

8. The researchers who published the results of Experiment 1 could investigate a potential confounder of their original study by attempting to find:

   A. hospital admission rates of children born with genetic abnormalities.
   B. the original ultrasound testing results of their study participants.
   C. baseline levels of postpartum stress at different income levels.
   D. the percentage of infants who receive false-negative results on genetic tests.

PASSAGE 3 (QUESTIONS 9–14)

The search for an accurate theory of moral reasoning has gone through several iterations, beginning with the work of Lawrence Kohlberg, whose stages of morality are based loosely on the ideas of Jean Piaget. Several psychologists, including Carol Gilligan, have criticized Kohlberg's stages as being androcentric and focusing too much on ideas of justice. Gilligan herself proposed an alternative scale of morality based on emotion and social interactions. This perspective is also not without its critics. Many, such as social psychologist Jonathan Haidt and cultural anthropologist Richard Shweder, cite research that supports the notion that there is very little correlation between gender and style of moral reasoning, and feel that Gilligan has gone too far in the other direction in her framework.

Furthermore, Haidt holds that morality comes most often not from well-reasoned arguments, but rather from inborn intuitions; the reasoning cited in Kohlberg's studies is no more than a post-hoc explanation of an emotional, unconscious reaction to a moral dilemma. To demonstrate this, he presented individuals with ambiguous moral situations somewhat like the Heinz dilemma that Kohlberg used in his assessment of moral reasoning, with the difference being that these were meant to elicit a more visceral reaction. It is Haidt's position that people have an intuitive "moral disgust" reaction that is an evolutionary byproduct of the disgust reaction that people have to tainted foods that protects us against pathogens. This position is the basis of Haidt's Social Intuitionist Model.

Building upon these concepts and other work by Shweder, Haidt attempted to categorize the kinds of instincts that people have when reacting to moral stimuli. According to the Moral Foundations Theory, there are six such building blocks of moral reaction, stated as opposing ideas on a scale: care vs. harm (of others); fairness vs. cheating; liberty vs. oppression; loyalty vs. betrayal; authority vs. subversion; and sanctity vs. degradation (which Haidt described as the tendency to avoid disgusting things, food, and actions). In his book *The Righteous Mind: Why Good People Are Divided by Politics and Religion*, Haidt's central thesis is the idea that differing political views often come from differences between individuals in focusing on some of these building blocks over others, and that the varied focus is closely related to the identity and socialization of the individual.

9. Suppose a person responded to Haidt's theory by saying, "People shouldn't do things that others find disgusting." Which of Kohlberg's stages of moral reasoning best describes this response?

   A. The preconventional stage
   B. The conventional stage
   C. The postconventional stage
   D. This response does not correspond with Kohlberg's stages

10. Which of the following scenarios is most closely related to Erikson's views on identity?

    A. A child develops rudimentary political views through role-playing the positions of others.
    B. A twelve-year-old is able to begin thinking about the political beliefs of others using abstract reasoning.
    C. An adolescent begins to question her political beliefs and distances herself from her parents.
    D. An adult finds that his beliefs about personal responsibility come from reactions to parental neglect in his childhood.

11. A three-year-old looks at a series of pictures depicting a boy accidentally throwing away his brother's toy while taking out the garbage. Which of the following describes the three-year-old's most likely appraisal of this story?

    A. The boy should be punished to the same degree as someone who threw away the toy on purpose.
    B. The boy should be punished because the three-year-old understands that the brother values his toys.
    C. The boy should not be punished because he was not aware he was doing anything wrong.
    D. The boy should not be punished because the three-year-old would also not like to be punished for accidental actions.

12. A child, going to school for the first time, learns that raising her hand and waiting to be called on, while not necessary at home, is an appropriate behavior in a school setting. This is an example of:

    A. primary socialization.
    B. secondary socialization.
    C. anticipatory socialization.
    D. group socialization.

13. A new law restricts the definition of free speech as it applies to corporations and draws fervent support from some but is vehemently opposed by others. According to the Moral Foundations Theory, which of the following is the most likely cause for this difference of opinion?

    A. Emotional reactions to political ideologies that are automatic and subconscious
    B. Strongly held and abstract beliefs regarding the right to express one's views freely
    C. Socialization and identification with groups that share political norms
    D. Understanding and valuation of the concepts of justice and the social contract

14. Moral beliefs arc at least in part a result of group identity and observation. Which of the following is usually the strongest source of moral guidance for an adolescent?

    A. A same-sex peer
    B. A same-sex parent
    C. An opposite-sex parent
    D. An opposite-sex celebrity

PASSAGE 4 (QUESTIONS 15–20)

In 1902, Charles Horton Cooley coined the term "looking-glass self," a social psychological concept stating that a person's self-concept is influenced by interpersonal relationships and the perceptions of others.

In 1976, sociologists Arthur Beaman, Edward Diener, and Soren Svanum performed an experiment on the effect of interpersonal relationships on the self-concepts of children by examining two distinct factors: self-awareness and individuation. The experiment was conducted on Halloween, an event during which, in America, children dress up in costumes and go door-to-door in their neighborhoods to receive candy. The researchers sent 363 children to 18 participating homes. Each time a child rang the doorbell, a woman answered the door, asked the child to pick one piece of candy, and excused herself from the room. The child would be left in the entryway, unaware of an observer hidden behind a festive backdrop. In the self-awareness condition, the entryway of the home contained a mirror placed so that the children could see themselves taking candy. Observers recorded each child's estimated age, gender, and whether or not he or she took more than one piece of candy. In the individuation condition, the woman asked the children questions about where they lived and how old they were before excusing herself. Observers in these houses recorded the same information about each child.

Of the 363 children in the study, 70 children transgressed during their time alone in the entryway. In both gender groups, fewer children transgressed when the mirror was present than when it was not (15.6 percent to 35.8 percent and 8.4 percent to 13.2 percent, respectively). It was also found that more children transgressed when they were not asked personal details. Furthermore, it was found that the rate of transgression rose with the age of the child, as can be seen in Table 1.

Age	Rate of Transgression
1–4	6.5%
5–8	9.7%
9–12	23.6%
13+	41.9%

Table 1. Ages and transgression rates.

15. The concept of the "looking-glass self" is most related to which of the following sociological paradigms?

    A. Social constructionism
    B. Symbolic interactionism
    C. Functionalism
    D. Conflict theory

16. If it were found that the observers consistently underestimated the age of children in the self-awareness group, but did not make this error with the other groups, what effect would this have on the results of the experiment?

    A. It would strengthen the hypothesis that all children are equally likely to transgress, regardless of age.
    B. It would strengthen the hypothesis that young children develop at different rates.
    C. It would weaken the hypothesis that age is related to transgression rate.
    D. It would have little effect on the overall results, though the study would need to be rerun.

17. Which of the following is true of functionalism?

    I. It is a macrosociological perspective.
    II. It focuses on the inequalities between functional societal groups.
    III. It maintains that function can be manifest or latent.

    A. III only
    B. I and II only
    C. I and III only
    D. II and III only

18. Suppose that an adult observes one of the children taking extra candy and reasons that the child transgressed because his family is less affluent and is unable to afford many snacks. This is an example of:

    A. a consistency cue.
    B. the fundamental attribution error.
    C. a dispositional attribution.
    D. a situational attribution.

19. What purpose did the act of asking the children about their ages and where they lived serve in the experiment?

    A. It encouraged the children to see themselves as real people, rather than the personae of their costumes.
    B. It was designed to be a qualitative measure of the degree of self-awareness exhibited by the children.
    C. It was an attempt to gain demographic information from the children to be used in statistical analysis.
    D. It reminded the children of their age and social background, making it more likely that they would transgress.

20. The adult participants in the study, seeing the level of transgression perpetrated by the children in the study, decide to avoid leaving candy out unattended during future Halloween celebrations. This decision is best described as:

    A. an adaptive attitude.
    B. a social interaction.
    C. a social action.
    D. a stereotype.

PASSAGE 5 (QUESTIONS 21–26)

The Elaboration Likelihood Model (ELM) is a theoretical framework for examining the strength of a persuasive message. The central route is used by an individual when she is highly invested or motivated in the subject of the argument and is capable of taking the time to think carefully about the message. Not surprisingly, individuals who process an argument centrally are more likely to make changes in their behavior and will resist the fading of new attitudes over time.

The peripheral route is used when individuals are uninterested or unable to fully engage the argument being made. This might result from distraction on the part of the listener, or it might result from what is called low "need for cognition," or a low valuation of engagement in effortful cognitive activities. People using the peripheral route tend to focus on qualities of the presenter, the sheer number of arguments presented, or their own mood when they hear the argument. People using the peripheral route also tend to be susceptible to the "mere exposure effect," a phenomenon by which an argument that is simply presented many times becomes more persuasive as a result of its familiarity. Peripherally processed arguments tend to produce a stronger persuasive effect than centrally processed arguments initially, but fade quickly and lead to little behavior change in the long term.

In 2003, the Centers for Disease Control and Prevention (CDC) implemented a program designed to take advantage of ELM principles to reduce the spread of HIV. The program's first phase focused on the population of individuals in the United States who were identified as living with an HIV-positive diagnosis. The CDC expanded voluntary counseling and testing programs for these individuals in an effort to promote lasting behavioral changes and increase the use of prophylactic prevention and antiretroviral therapy.

21. Which of the following best explains why the CDC would begin its program in the manner described in the passage?

    A. HIV-positive individuals are at a higher behavioral risk than the general population.

    B. Individuals who agree to voluntary counseling will be more likely make further changes asked of them.

    C. The CDC is counting on its credibility with the population in question to increase prevention behaviors.

    D. HIV-positive individuals find the CDC's outreach to be more personally relevant.

22. According to the Elaboration Likelihood Model, which of the following best explains the observation that patients on a course of antibiotics often stop taking the drug before the course is over, despite the doctor's instructions to continue taking the pills until they are gone?

    A. The doctors have not provided enough reasons to continue the course of the drug once symptoms cease.

    B. As patients begin to feel better their motivation to continue taking the drug decreases.

    C. Once symptoms are gone, patients reason that their doctors prescribed the wrong amount of the drug.

    D. Most patients are aware that overuse of antibiotics can cause drug resistance and be harmful to the population.

23. Suppose that individuals diagnosed with HIV go to a weekly support group. Which of the following social processes would NOT affect the likelihood of treatment compliance?

    A. Social facilitation

    B. Group polarization

    C. Peer pressure

    D. Socialization

24. Which of the following concepts is an example of a change in behavior causing a change in attitude?

    A. Cognitive dissonance

    B. Observational learning

    C. The foot-in-the-door phenomenon

    D. Stereotype threat

25. A public initiative is aimed at increasing the overall health and fitness of a population. According to the passage, which of the following messages would be useful in persuading an individual with low need for cognition to begin an exercise program?

    I. A series of lectures given by medical experts and physically fit celebrities, aired through several media outlets

    II. A newspaper article that thoroughly discusses several research findings related to the effectiveness of exercise

    III. A 30-second television ad that airs during each commercial break on major networks for three weeks

    A. II only

    B. I and II only

    C. I and III only

    D. I, II, and III

26. The CDC wishes to maximize its efforts to increase childhood vaccination. Which of the following programs would best accomplish this goal?

    A. Funding government studies providing strong evidence for the effectiveness of childhood vaccination in the prevention of harmful diseases

    B. Airing a series of television ads targeted to parents that warn of the risks of childhood illness and use fear as an emotional tool

    C. Having experts and celebrities speak at events during which vaccinations can be obtained held at pharmacies typically frequented by families

    D. Commissioning posters to be placed in doctors' offices providing statistics that show that the vast majority of young children obtain vaccinations

Chem/Phys 3: Turning Practice Into Points

PASSAGE 1 (QUESTIONS 1–6)

Antibiotics are naturally derived substances released by microorganisms for defense against pathogens in their environment. Discovered in 1928, penicillin, a product of a genus of mold called *Penicillium*, instigated the recognition that antibacterial agents can be used within the body to combat human pathogens. Penicillin itself is a member of the lactam group, a type of cyclic amide. These molecules are most commonly formed through the reaction of an amino group with a carboxylic acid group of an amino acid.

An example of a general lactam formation reaction is the reaction of 4-aminobutanoic acid. The addition of heat results in 4-aminobutanoic acid lactam. The product is named by adding the word *lactam* to the IUPAC name of the acid. See Figure 1.

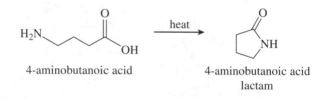

4-aminobutanoic acid   4-aminobutanoic acid
                                            lactam

Figure 1. Lactam formation reaction.

In contrast to other lactams, beta-lactams are unusually reactive. Due to considerable ring strain, the beta-lactam will acylate other nucleophiles. During the acylation reaction, opening of the ring allows the release of strain. See Figure 2.

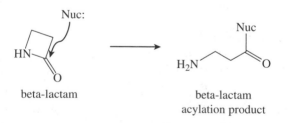

beta-lactam   beta-lactam
                                        acylation product

Figure 2. Beta-lactam acylation reaction.

The ring-opening acylation reaction provides the critical functionality of penicillin, which contains a beta-lactam ring coupled with a saturated pentane ring that contains a sulfur atom. Antibiotics such as penicillin provide therapeutic action by acylating serine residues on essential bacterial enzymes located along the pathway for cell wall synthesis. During the acylation, penicillin takes advantage of the hydroxyl group of serine to convert its amide to an ester, simultaneously freezing the conformation of the serine residue and thus inactivating the enzyme for cell wall synthesis. Without a cell wall, the bacterium cannot survive.

1. To synthesize 4-aminobutanoic acid, a primary amine must be added to butanoic acid. Butanoic acid can be produced via the oxidation of butanal. Which of the following accurately ranks the predicted boiling points of these three compounds important for 4-aminobutanoic acid lactam synthesis?

   A. Butanoic acid > butanal > 4-aminobutanoic acid

   B. 4-Aminobutanoic acid > butanal > butanoic acid

   C. 4-Aminobutanoic acid > butanoic acid > butanal

   D. Butanal > butanoic acid > 4-aminobutanoic acid

2. The mechanism of 4-aminobutanoic acid lactam synthesis involves the formation and breaking of bonds. Which of the following indicates the bonds formed, and bonds broken, respectively?

   A. N—H, O—H; N—C, O—C
   B. N—C, N—H; O—C, N—C
   C. N—O, N—H; O—C, N—C
   D. N—C, O—H; N—H, O—C

3. The mechanism of 4-aminobutanoic acid lactam synthesis proceeds through each of the following steps EXCEPT:

   A. nucleophilic addition to form a byproduct.
   B. condensation reaction involving an amine group.
   C. loss of water from the product.
   D. nucleophilic attack on the carbonyl carbon.

4. A likely intermediate in beta-lactam synthesis is:

   A. a carbanion.
   B. a carbocation.
   C. an oxygen anion.
   D. a nitrogen anion.

5. Which of the following functional groups is present in the core ring structure of penicillin?

   A. Ether
   B. Thiol
   C. Thioether
   D. Amine

6. Penicillin acts by acylating the hydroxyl group of a serine residue on a key bacterial biosynthetic enzyme. The reaction converts an amide to an ester, which is not what one would predict given the two functional groups' relative reactivities. The most plausible explanation for this reversal is that:

   A. the energetic release of ester formation is overwhelmed by the energetic cost of amide-ring breakage.
   B. the energetic cost of ester formation is overwhelmed by the energetic release of amide-ring breakage.
   C. the energetic cost of amide formation is overwhelmed by the energetic release of ester-ring breakage.
   D. the energetic release of amide formation is overwhelmed by the energetic cost of ester-ring breakage.

PASSAGE 2 (QUESTIONS 7–11)

Hydrogen gas has a variety of industrial uses. It can be used to produce refined hydrocarbon products from raw petroleum. It enhances the quality of argon-based welding applications. It also has the potential to be a fuel for alternative-fuel automobiles, if certain technical hurdles can be overcome.

Hydrogen cannot be mined or refined, however, since it is far too reactive with oxygen gas to be present in significant quantities anywhere in nature. Instead, essentially all hydrogen gas used on the planet has to be created. By far the most common method for making hydrogen gas is the electrolysis of water. A simple apparatus for the electrolysis of water is shown in Figure 1.

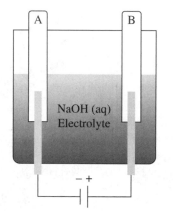

Figure 1. Apparatus for the electrolysis of water.

Two inert metal electrodes are placed in a solution of aqueous inert electrolyte, such as NaOH. The electrodes are attached to the two poles of a power source and current flows through the solution. Test tubes A and B are used to collect the gases, which are the byproducts of electrolysis.

The chemical reactions that take place at the cathode and anode, respectively, are:

Cathode: $2\,H_2O\,(l) + 2\,e^- \rightarrow H_2\,(g) + 2\,OH^-\,(aq)$ $E°_{red} = 0.0\ V$

Anode: $2\,H_2O\,(l) \rightarrow O_2\,(g) + 4\,H^+\,(aq) + 4\,e^-$ $E°_{ox} = -1.23\ V$

7. When the battery is hooked up to the electrolysis cell, which of the following best characterizes what happens?

   A. Electrons flow from cathode to anode, and oxygen gas is collected in test tube A.
   B. Electrons flow from cathode to anode, and hydrogen gas is collected in test tube A.
   C. Electrons flow from anode to cathode, and oxygen gas is collected in test tube A.
   D. Electrons flow from anode to cathode, and hydrogen gas is collected in test tube A.

8. What is the role of NaOH in the electrolysis of water?

   A. NaOH provides OH^- ions, a necessary catalyst for the cathodic reaction.
   B. NaOH dissociates into ions, which increase the conductivity of water, improving efficiency.
   C. NaOH increases the pH of the solution, preventing undesired cross-reactions.
   D. NaOH provides OH^- ions, which help limit the rate of the cathodic reaction.

9. If a 20 A current flows through a water electrolysis cell for ten minutes, what is the volume of oxygen generated at the anode if it is at STP?

   A. 45 mL
   B. 696 mL
   C. 2.69 L
   D. 20.0 L

10. Which of the following metals reacts vigorously with water to release hydrogen gas?

    A. Mg
    B. Au
    C. K
    D. Al

11. What is the oxidation state of the chromium atoms in the dichromate ion, $Cr_2O_7^{2-}$?

    A. -7
    B. 0
    C. $+4$
    D. $+6$

PASSAGE 3 (QUESTIONS 12–16)

Esters are carboxylic acid derivatives that have a variety of industrial uses. Because they have pleasant odors, they are often used in fruit drinks, soaps, and perfumes. They are also used as solvents and softeners in the polymer industry. In alcoholic beverages, especially beer, ester usage has to be carefully monitored depending on whether the taste requirements of the beverage include a fruity flavor.

Esters can be synthesized by a process known as esterification, in which a carboxylic acid and an alcohol are reacted with a catalytic amount of a mineral acid. The reaction is very slow, and the ester is produced in equilibrium concentrations. Formation of the ester can be favored by using an excess of one of the reactants, as shown in Reaction 1.

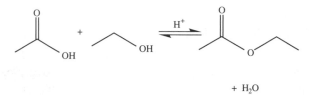

+ H_2O

Reaction 1. Formation of the ester.

One way to avoid the rate and equilibrium problems of esterification is by reacting an acyl chloride with an alcohol. Ethanoyl chloride is synthesized by the reaction of acetic acid and thionyl chloride, as shown in Reaction 2. Ethanoyl chloride is then reacted with ethanol in the presence of pyridine, as shown in Reaction 3, to produce ethyl acetate. HCl is a byproduct of this reaction.

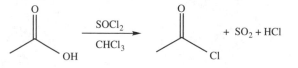

Reaction 2. Ethanoyl chloride formation.

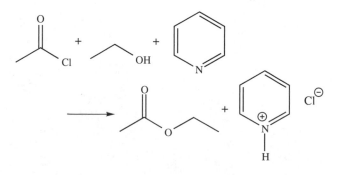

Reaction 3. Ethyl acetate formation.

12. Which of the following correctly represents the intermediate of the esterification after nucleophilic attack by the alcohol?

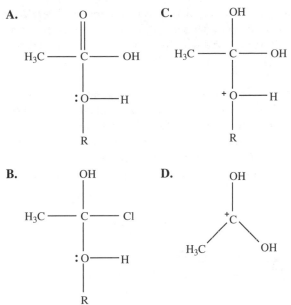

A.

H_3C — C — OH (with =O above C, and :O—H below, R below)

B.

H_3C — C — Cl (with OH above C, and :O—H below, R below)

C.

H_3C — C — OH (with OH above C, and $^+$O—H below, R below)

D.

$^+$C (with OH above, H_3C and OH below)

13. What is the role of pyridine in Reaction 3?

   A. To neutralize the inorganic acid product, preventing catalysis of ester hydrolysis upon aqueous workup
   B. To neutralize the inorganic acid product, preventing the formation of the ester product
   C. To neutralize the organic acid product, preventing catalysis of ester hydrolysis upon aqueous workup
   D. To neutralize the organic acid product, preventing catalysis of the reverse reaction

14. Why should esterification reactions not be carried out in water?

   A. Acetic acid is insoluble in water.
   B. The polar nature of water overshadows the polar nature of the carboxyl group.
   C. The extensive hydrogen bonding of water interferes with the S_N2 reaction mechanism.
   D. Water molecules would hydrolyze useful products back to the parent carboxylic acid.

15. Which of the following represents an increasing order of acidity in organic compounds?

   A. CH_3OCH_3, CH_3CHO, CH_3COOH, CH_3CH_2OH
   B. CH_3OCH_3, CH_3CH_2OH, CH_3CHO, CH_3COOH
   C. CH_3CHO, CH_3OCH_3, CH_3COOH, CH_3CH_2OH
   D. CH_3CHO, CH_3OCH_3, CH_3CH_2OH, CH_3COOH

16. What are Compounds I and II in the following reaction?

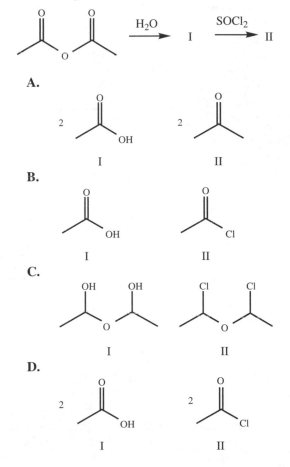

A.
   2 (acetic acid) — I
   2 (acetone) — II

B.
   (acetic acid) — I
   (acetyl chloride) — II

C.
   (structure with OH, OH, O) — I
   (structure with Cl, Cl, O) — II

D.
   2 (acetic acid) — I
   2 (acetyl chloride) — II

PASSAGE 4 (QUESTIONS 17–20)

Emmetropia is the state of human vision in which the crystalline lens performs its function as intended by focusing parallel rays of light on the retina at the back of the eye after being refracted by the cornea. An eye that is not emmetropic is said to be ametropic, a condition observed when the crystalline lens has an inherent spherical or cylindrical error.

Spherical errors in the lens can be categorized as either myopia or, as shown in Figure 1(A), hyperopia. Figure 1(B) shows how the refraction of parallel rays in a hyperopic eye is corrected with a convex lens. Glasses and contact lenses are the most common and inexpensive corrective measures for spherical ametropia. Laser vision correction (LASIK) and photorefractive keratectomy (PRK) are the most common surgical procedures used in its correction, although in patients with thin or otherwise fragile corneas, these procedures are not viable alternatives to corrective lenses. In patients with thin corneas, phakic intraocular lenses (PIOLs) can be inserted surgically to correct moderate to severe myopia.

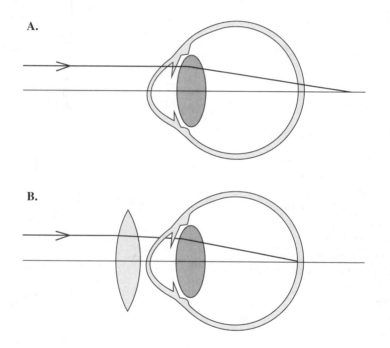

Figure 1. Refraction of parallel rays by the cornea and crystalline lens in a hyperopic eye (A) and with a convex lens (B).

In order to explore the causes of ametropia, a student made three postmortem measurements per patient in his sample. The first measurement was from the surface of the cornea to the surface of the retina. The second measurement was of the radius of curvature of the cornea. The third measurement was of the radius of curvature of the crystalline lens. He compared the average measurements of myopic, hyperopic, and emmetropic groups. The student discovered that myopic individuals have a greater distance from cornea to retina and hyperopic individuals have a lesser distance from cornea to retina than do emmetropic individuals. He found that, on average, myopic corneas had greater curvature and hyperopic corneas had lesser curvature. He did not, however, find any significant difference in the shape of crystalline lenses between the three groups.

17. A color-blind individual reports seeing close objects as blurry. The best option for restoring emmetropia in this individual is:

    A. concave contact lenses.
    B. PIOLs.
    C. diverging contact lenses.
    D. glasses with convex lenses.

18. Before passing through the cornea, which of the following wavelengths of light would have a frequency of $5.56 \times 10^{14} \text{ s}^{-1}$?

    A. Green light at 540 nm
    B. Green light at 180 nm
    C. Red light at 540 nm
    D. Red light at 180 nm

19. Vertex distance is the distance between the rear surface of a corrective lens and the cornea. What is the image length of the cornea for an individual wearing corrective lenses with a focal length of 5.5 mm focusing on an image 11 mm away, with a vertex distance of 14 mm if the crystalline lens makes no adjustments? (Note: The typical focal length of the human cornea is 17 mm.)

    A. 3.64 mm
    B. −3.64 mm
    C. 0.39 mm
    D. −0.39 mm

20. For a myopic individual, the crystalline lens and cornea project an image:

    A. in front of the retina and behind the crystalline lens.
    B. behind the retina and behind the crystalline lens.
    C. in front of the retina and in front of the crystalline lens.
    D. behind the retina and in front of the crystalline lens.

PASSAGE 5 (QUESTIONS 21–27)

Serous otitis media (SOM) is a condition characterized by a buildup of fluid in the middle ear. Typically, SOM follows a bacterial or viral infection and usually clears up without direct treatment. Sometimes, however, fluid accumulation persists or the fluid itself becomes infected. If left untreated, chronic otitis media (COM) can develop, potentially leading to hearing loss, deep ear pain, and continued ear drainage.

Hearing occurs as mechanical vibrations are transduced into electrical impulses that are transmitted to the brain. Sound waves are funneled into the pinna and travel through the ear canal to the tympanic membrane. The ossicles amplify the incoming signal and transmit it to the inner ear at the cochlea, a fluid-filled tube. The sound waves pass through the cochlear fluid to the basilar membrane, which is lined with hair cells. These hair cells are depolarized, indirectly stimulating the auditory nerve. Figure 1 shows the anatomy of the ear.

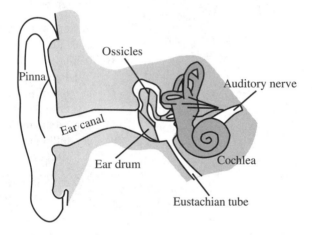

Figure 1. Anatomy of the ear.

The middle ear is lined with mucous membranes and is connected to the nasopharynx by the Eustachian tube. The Eustachian tube remains closed except during swallowing, when it temporarily opens, equalizing external pressure and the pressure in the middle ear. Congestion and swelling due to illness may cause the Eustachian tube to become completely blocked, preventing air pressure equalization. Over time, a negative pressure develops in the middle ear, which draws liquid from the mucosal cells. Eventually, the fluid thickens and the middle ear membranes become inflamed. Pressure builds on the tympanic membrane until it becomes distorted or perforated. At this stage, an individual is diagnosed with COM.

Preventative measures can limit the probability of developing COM. One such approach is a myringotomy (incision in the ear drum) to drain fluid followed by insertion of a grommet. By aerating the middle ear, fluid accumulation is remediated. The structure of a grommet is illustrated in Figure 2.

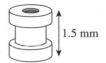

Figure 2. Structure of a grommet.

(Note: Unless otherwise indicated, assume that the effects of viscosity and turbulence are negligible.)

21. A patient with COM experiences significant hearing loss and is provided with a hearing aid. If the hearing aid amplifies sound intensity by 100 times, by how much is the decibel level increased?

    A. 10 dB
    B. 20 dB
    C. 40 dB
    D. 100 dB

22. How does the speed of sound waves moving through the ear canal compare to the speed of sound waves moving through cochlear fluid?

    A. Sound waves travel faster in the ear canal.
    B. Sound waves travel slower in the ear canal.
    C. Sound waves travel at the same speed in both the ear canal and the cochlear fluid.
    D. Sound waves do not travel in the ear canal at all.

23. Which of the following accurately describes the purpose of the third paragraph?

    A. To describe the significance of the Eustachian tube in proper ear function
    B. To explain the mechanism of air pressure equalization that occurs during swallowing
    C. To identify one potential cause of ear drum perforation
    D. To offer a mechanism for COM development.

24. A patient hears a beeping sound from ten meters away and decides to go closer to examine the source. If the patient is now one meter away, what is the ratio of the original intensity of the sound to the new intensity of the sound?

    A. 1:1
    B. 1:10
    C. 1:100
    D. 1:1,000

25. Which of the following best explains why a patient with a middle ear volume of 1.7 mL experiences a dramatic increase in pressure when 2 g of a fluid with a density of 1.08 g/mL accumulates in her middle ear?

    A. The Eustachian tube is typically closed, so fluid cannot escape the middle ear.
    B. The mucosal cells cannot take up more water.
    C. The ratio of fluid mass to volume is essentially constant.
    D. The tympanic membrane is inflexible.

26. Which of the following describes the main idea of the fourth paragraph?

    A. Aerating the middle ear will eliminate the possibility of COM.
    B. Failure to take preventative measures will likely cause COM.
    C. One treatment of COM is myringotomy followed by insertion of a grommet.
    D. The chance of acquiring COM is lessened with insertion of a grommet.

27. A man is on an airplane and notices that his ears keep "popping." What is the cause of this phenomenon?

    A. His Eustachian tube is blocked and pressure is building in his middle ear.
    B. His Eustachian tube is blocked and pressure is decreasing in his middle ear.
    C. External pressure is lower at a high altitude and air is rushing out of his middle ear.
    D. External pressure is greater at a high altitude and air is rushing into his middle ear.

PASSAGE 6 (QUESTIONS 28–34)

Styrene is used extensively in the manufacture of plastics, rubber, and resins. It is a colorless liquid with a sweet, aromatic odor at low concentrations, but with a sharp, penetrating, disagreeable odor at high concentrations.

In humans, the liver metabolizes styrene into styrene oxide via the cytochrome P450 system. Both enantiomers are toxic, although (R)-styrene oxide has more pronounced health effects in mice. Long-term human exposure to styrene via inhalation, ingestion, or skin contact can lead to lethargy, memory loss, and headaches. Because of the reactivity of its metabolite, styrene is further classified as a mutagen. Studies have not yet definitively proven that exposure leads to cancer, but a causal link is strongly suspected and the U.S. National Toxicology Program describes styrene as "reasonably accepted to be a human carcinogen."

Styrene can be synthesized in the lab by either reacting sulfuric acid with compound **A** ($C_8H_{10}O$) or using zinc metal with compound **B** ($C_8H_8Br_2$) in ethanol. Compound **B** can be made from compound **C** (C_8H_9Br) by generating Br_2 gas *in situ* from the reaction of potassium bromate and hydrobromic acid and irradiation with a lamp. Compound **A** is characterized by its mild hyacinth odor and the ester, compound **D** ($C_{10}H_{12}O_2$), formed by the reaction of compound **A** with acetic acid and sulfuric acid, has a fruity smell.

Compound **A** will undergo oxidation to compound **E** (C_8H_8O) in the presence of bleach and acetic acid. Compound **E**, which is characterized by its floral aroma, has a boiling point of 202°C and a refractive index of 1.5372. The semicarbazone derivative of compound **E** has a melting point of 198°C.

For styrene production on an industrial scale, the preferred method of synthesis involves taking compound **F** (C_8H_{10}) through a dehydrogenation reaction catalyzed by an amalgam of iron(III) oxide and potassium carbonate. Figure 1 shows selected syntheses and derivatives of styrene.

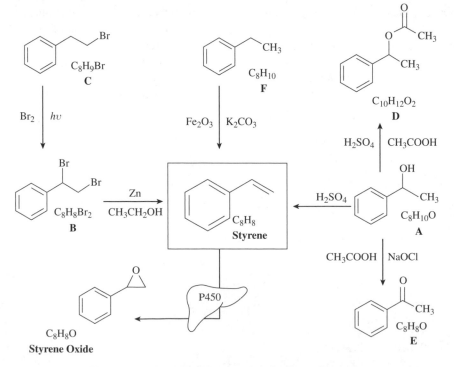

Figure 1. Selected syntheses and derivatives of styrene.

28. Which of the following compounds illustrated in the passage will have the lowest melting point?

    A. Compound A
    B. Compound D
    C. Compound E
    D. Compound F

29. What is the likely intermediate in the conversion of compound A to styrene?

    A. A carbene
    B. A carbocation
    C. A cyclic bromonium ion
    D. A radical

30. What is the likely first step in the conversion of compound A to compound D?

    A. Nucleophilic attack of acetic acid on the carbon bound to the –OH group
    B. Nucleophilic attack of compound A on the carbonyl carbon of acetic acid
    C. Protonation of the hydroxyl group of compound A
    D. Protonation of the carbonyl oxygen of acetic acid

31. Which of the following reagents would NOT convert compound A to compound E?

    A. CrO_3
    B. $K_2Cr_2O_7$
    C. PCC
    D. Tollen's reagent

32. CH_3CH_2OH, H_2SO_4, and CH_3COOH are all reagents illustrated in Figure 1. Which of the following is true?

    A. CH_3CH_2OH has a higher K_a than CH_3COOH.
    B. CH_3COOH has the lowest pK_a.
    C. CH_3COOH has a lower pK_a than CH_3CH_2OH.
    D. H_2SO_4 has the highest pK_a.

33. Which of the following correctly identifies the main idea of the second paragraph?

    A. (R)-Styrene oxide is more dangerous than (S)-styrene oxide.
    B. Further medical research is needed to effectively treat those poisoned by styrene.
    C. Styrene usage should be reduced to limit health risks.
    D. Styrene is likely a carcinogen with known health impacts.

34. Which of the following accurately reflects a statement made in the third paragraph?

    A. Compounds A and B can be used to synthesize styrene in the lab.
    B. Compounds A, B, C, and D are all effective means by which to synthesize styrene.
    C. Compounds A and B each have a unique associated smell.
    D. Synthesis of styrene requires either ethanol or a zinc catalyst.

PASSAGE 7 (QUESTIONS 35–41)

The cornea, at approximately 43 diopters, provides most of the focusing power of the eye, while the lens provides power for fine adjustments. The lens is a transparent, biconvex structure in the human eye that helps to refract light so it can be focused on the retina; it has a refractive index of approximately 1.42. The cornea has a slightly smaller refractive index, at 1.38. When the ciliary muscles are contracted, zonule fibers loosen, allowing the lens to relax to a more convex shape. In contrast, when the ciliary muscles are relaxed, zonule fibers tighten, causing the lens to become less convex. Through this process, the focal length of the lens can be changed to match the object's distance so that a clear, focused image forms on the retina. When the ciliary muscles are relaxed, the lens has a power of 15.8 diopters and is used for objects at infinite distances.

Myopia is an ocular pathology that includes good near vision and poorer vision for farther objects. Simple myopia results when the lens is too powerful for the eye's axial length, approximately 17 mm in most adults.

Corrective lenses for myopia diverge the light before it hits the lens, so the image still lies on the retina for faraway objects. Both contact lenses and eyeglass lenses can be used to correct for myopia; however, the distance between lenses needs to be taken into account for eyeglasses when deciding the appropriate corrective power. Eyeglass makers can change the power of lenses by adjusting their shape according to the equation below:

$$\frac{1}{f} = (n-1)\left(\frac{1}{r_1} - \frac{1}{r_2}\right)$$

In this equation, f is the focal length, n is the refractive index of the lens, r_1 is the external radius of curvature, and r_2 is the internal radius of curvature. The lensmaker equation can be used for approximating the power of thick, spherical lenses.

35. For a myopic person with a normal axial length, the image of a star appears 7 mm in front of the retina. When they put on corrective contact lenses, however, the image of the star appears focused. Assuming the distance between lenses is negligible, what is the approximate power of the contact lens?

    A. +58.8 diopters
    B. −41.2 diopters
    C. +29.4 diopters
    D. −29.4 diopters

36. If the external radius of curvature of an unaccommodated human lens is 10.2 cm and the internal radius of curvature is −6.0 cm, what is its total power?

    A. −0.556 diopters
    B. 0.111 diopters
    C. −5.56 diopters
    D. 11.1 diopters

37. What would be the effect of a muscle relaxant applied directly to the ciliary muscles of the eyes for people with normal vision?

    A. They'd have trouble focusing on faraway objects.
    B. They'd have trouble focusing on nearby objects.
    C. They'd have trouble seeing in the dark.
    D. They'd have trouble seeing in bright sunlight.

38. An object is situated in front of a glass lens with a power of +5 diopters. The object is moved from a distance of 100 cm to a distance of 5 cm. What would be the associated change in the image's appearance?

    A. It would get smaller, then disappear, then get bigger.
    B. It would get bigger, then disappear, then get smaller.
    C. It would get smaller.
    D. It would get bigger.

39. Hyperopia, or farsightedness, is when the lens is too weak and the image focuses behind the retina. Which of the following corrective lenses could be worn to improve hyperopic vision?

    A. Glasses that are thicker in the center and thinner along the edges, to help converge the rays
    B. Glasses that are thinner in the center and thicker along the edges, to help converge the rays
    C. Glasses that are thicker in the center and thinner along the edges, to help diverge the rays
    D. Glasses that are thinner in the center and thicker along the edges, to help diverge the rays

40. Which of the following properties will change as incident monochromatic rays refract from the air into the cornea?

    I. Frequency
    II. Wavelength
    III. Speed
    IV. Intensity

    A. I, II, and III only
    B. I, III, and IV only
    C. I, II, and IV only
    D. II, III, and IV only

41. Which of the following glass lenses could potentially be used to correct myopic vision?

    A. External radius of curvature of −15 cm, internal radius of curvature of 10 cm, refractive index of 1.4
    B. External radius of curvature of −10 cm, internal radius of curvature of −8 cm, refractive index of 2.4
    C. External radius of curvature of 8 cm, internal radius of curvature of −8 cm, refractive index of 1.5
    D. External radius of curvature of 10 cm, internal radius of curvature of 10 cm, refractive index of 1.8

DISCRETE PRACTICE QUESTIONS (QUESTIONS 42–44)

42. If a grandfather perceives sound as 100 times less intense than his grandchild, with what decibel level will the grandchild perceive a sound that his grandfather hears as 90 decibels?

   A. 70 dB
   B. 90 dB
   C. 100 dB
   D. 110 dB

43. A tone from a tuning fork travels down the ear canal of a listening musician. Given that the musician's ear canal can be thought of as a pipe with one closed end and with a length of 2.5 cm, what is the wavelength of this tone's third harmonic in the ear canal?

   A. 0.033 cm
   B. 0.67 cm
   C. 3.3 cm
   D. 6.7 cm

44. A sound wave of 100 decibels is incident upon an eardrum with a surface area of 5.5×10^{-2} m^2. Assuming no dissipation, what is the energy transmitted on the eardrum over 10,000 seconds? (Note: $I_0 = 10^{-12}$ W/m^2)

   A. 1.4 J
   B. 5.5 J
   C. 27 J
   D. 55 J

Extra practice for the next class session starts on the next page ▶ ▶ ▶

Bio/Biochem 3: Advanced Research & Experimental Design

PASSAGE 1 (QUESTIONS 1–6)

Hypercholesterolemia is a term used to describe abnormally high levels of cholesterol in the blood. Cholesterol is linked to proteins, termed lipoproteins, in the blood; hypercholesterolemia involves high levels of lipoproteins, including high-density lipoproteins (HDL) and very-low-density lipoproteins (VLDL). However, a high level of low-density lipoproteins (LDL) in the blood is the type most strongly associated with an increased risk of atherosclerosis and heart disease.

While hypercholesterolemia can be caused by environmental factors, familial hypercholesterolemia (FH) is caused by mutant alleles of genes associated with LDL uptake from the blood. The most common cause of FH is a mutation in the LDL receptor (LDLR) gene that follows autosomal dominant inheritance patterns. Normal LDL receptors are located on liver cells, where they bind LDL particles from the blood. After binding, both the receptor and LDL are taken into the cell; the LDL particle is released into the cell to be metabolized, and the receptor returns to the cell surface to bind more LDL. Several different LDLR gene mutations exist that can cause problems with either the synthesis or proper function of the LDLR protein.

A common cause of autosomal dominant FH is a mutation in the ApoB gene. ApoB is the main protein component of LDL particles that forms the connection with LDLR. Mutant ApoB proteins are unable to bind to LDLR; therefore, the LDL particles remain in circulation. Finally, the LDLR adaptor protein ARH interacts with the LDL receptor within the cell, helping it to be taken into the cell after it has attached to an LDL particle. A diagram of the interaction between LDLR, ApoB, and ARH is shown in Figure 1. Autosomal recessive mutations in ARH inhibit the uptake of LDLR into the cell, thereby keeping the receptor from removing the particles from circulation. Typical plasma LDL levels from these mutations are shown in Table 1.

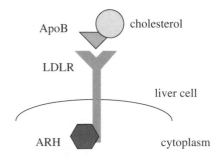

Figure 1. Interaction of ApoB, LDLR, and ARH.

Genotype	Blood LDL (mg/dL)
Wildtype	80
Heterozygous LDLR	170
Homozygous LDLR	450
Heterozygous ApoB	190
Homozygous ApoB	250
Heterozygous ARH	90
Homozygous ARH	200

Table 1. Average plasma LDL profiles of individuals who are either homozygous or heterozygous for alleles associated with familial hypercholesterolemia.

1. A child with FH exhibiting plasma LDL levels of 500 mg/dL is given a liver transplant from a wildtype individual and exhibits no improvement in plasma LDL after recovery. What is the most likely explanation for this occurrence?

   A. The child is heterozygous for an ARH mutation.
   B. Gene crossover occurs between the child's natural cells and the new liver cells, causing the liver to produce mutant LDLR protein.
   C. The child is homozygous for an ApoB mutation with high expressivity.
   D. The child eats fast food twice a week.

2. Individuals who are heterozygous for an LDLR gene mutation produce half the number of normal LDL receptors as a wildtype individual, while the other half are made by the mutant allele. This is an example of:

   A. codominance.
   B. penetrance.
   C. incomplete dominance.
   D. translocation.

3. There is a mutation in the main protein component of LDL particles that forms the connection with LDLR in a patient. How many copies of this mutation may this patient have?

   A. One copy
   B. Two copies
   C. One or two copies
   D. One, two, or three copies

4. A patient with parents who are both affected by familial hypercholesterolemia has fairly normal serum levels of LDL. What are possible genotypes that this patient could have?

   I. Heterozygous ARH
   II. Heterozygous ApoB
   III. Heterozygous LDLR

   A. I only
   B. I or II only
   C. II or III only
   D. I, II, or III

5. An unaffected woman's parents, two brothers, and one sister all suffer from FH. She marries a man who suffers from FH and one of their three children has FH. Which mutation from the passage could be the cause of the high cholesterol phenotype in the child?

   A. LDLR mutation
   B. ARH mutation
   C. ApoB mutation
   D. More than one cause is supported by the given information.

6. An unaffected woman whose sibling suffers from FH has parents and one sibling who do NOT suffer from the disease. What is probability that this woman is a carrier?

   A. 100%
   B. 75%
   C. 12.5%
   D. 67%

PASSAGE 2 (QUESTIONS 7–12)

The intestines have special structural features that allow them to function efficiently. These special features allow the intestines to maximize time for digestion and absorption.

Single-unit smooth muscle cells in the intestines have gap junctions. These gaps allow the muscles to work in syncytia. Gap junctions also play an important part in tissue homeostasis because they allow for the exchange of ions, signaling molecules, nucleotides, and other small molecules between adjacent cells. Other organs, including the stomach, are also known to have these features.

Ions are reabsorbed through channels in the small and large intestines. For instance, Na^+ enters into cells lining the colon via an epithelial sodium channel. Similarly, to adjust the fluidity of the luminal contents and to allow mixing and movement, Cl^- is secreted into the lumen. Depending on the relative osmotic pressures in the luminal and circulatory compartments, water can move in either direction across the epithelial lining via the paracellular pathway. Under normal physiological conditions, the osmotic pressure is slightly higher in the circulation than in the lumen.

Cancers of the small intestine are fairly rare. Factors that can protect against these types of cancers include having a lower bacterial count and a more alkaline pH in the small intestine. Another protective factor is the presence of benzopyrene hydroxylase, an enzyme that is thought to break down polycyclic aromatic hydrocarbons.

7. Gap junctions differ from desmosomes in that they:

   A. link cells to the basement membrane.
   B. are composed of multiple families of proteins.
   C. permit conduction of electricity from one cell to another.
   D. may link cells that serve similar functions.

8. Which of the following could be a direct response by the body to a low-sodium diet?

   A. Increased reabsorption of water
   B. Increased active secretion of sodium
   C. Increased expression of epithelial sodium channels
   D. Decreased expression of epithelial sodium channels

9. Cholera is an infection caused by the bacterium *Vibrio cholerae*. It is known to increase cAMP to activate Cl^- secretory channels in the small intestine. Based on the passage, what would be a consequence of this pathology?

   A. Increased fluid retention in the body
   B. Increased sodium reabsorption in the small intestine
   C. Increased potassium reabsorption in the small intestine
   D. Loss of fluids from the body

10. Which of the following is the most likely molecule to pass through a gap junction that connects two cells of the intestine?

    A. An antibody
    B. A hormone
    C. An amino acid
    D. An enzyme

11. Why would having the enzyme benzopyrene hydroxylase present in the small intestine potentially protect against cancer?

    A. Benzopyrene hydroxylase decreases the amount of carcinogenic polycyclic aromatic hydrocarbons in the lumen.
    B. Benzopyrene hydroxylase increases the amount of carcinogenic polycyclic aromatic hydrocarbons in the lumen.
    C. Benzopyrene hydroxylase increases the amount of carcinogenic Cl^- in the lumen.
    D. Benzopyrene hydroxylase decreases the amount of carcinogenic Cl^- in the lumen.

12. A bacterial infection causes the paracellular pathway in the small intestine to be fully blocked. Assuming physiological conditions are otherwise normal, what effect would this have on intestinal material by the time it reaches the colon?

    A. Increased Na^+ in the lumen
    B. Decreased water in the lumen
    C. Increased fluidity of the material in the lumen
    D. Decreased fluidity of the material in the lumen

PASSAGE 3 (QUESTIONS 13–17)

The major histocompatibility complex (MHC) is a protein complex found on the surface of most cells in the body. When proteins are degraded within a cell, small pieces of these proteins, called epitopes, are displayed on the cell surface via the MHC complex. Nonhost cells are digested by phagocytic cells of the immune system, such as macrophages and dendritic cells; these cells then present foreign antigens on MHC-II. MHC is critical in the development of adaptive immunity, as it is responsible for presenting foreign proteins to lymphocytes, which then retain knowledge of the epitopes.

MHC-II is expressed exclusively on the surface of antigen-presenting cells, including macrophages, B-cells, and dendritic cells. When these phagocytic cells take up and process an antigen, they display resulting epitopes on the surface via MHC-II. Epitopes on these complexes are recognized by naïve helper T-cells, which, during maturation in the thymus, are programmed to only recognize nonself epitopes. When they are exposed to these epitopes, the helper T-cells can then differentiate into memory T-cells (which retains knowledge of the epitope) or effector T-cells (which stimulate other immune cells to function, including cytotoxic T-cells).

MHC-I molecules are expressed on the surface of all nucleated cells in humans. These complexes present antigens on the cell surface, which are recognized by cytotoxic T-cells. If the antigen is nonself and is recognized by the T-cell receptor on the surface of the cytotoxic T-cell, the T-cell will cause the infected host cell to die.

Most of the multiple proteins subunits that make up MHC are encoded by genes located on chromosome 6. Diagrams of MHC-I and MHC-II are shown in Figure 1.

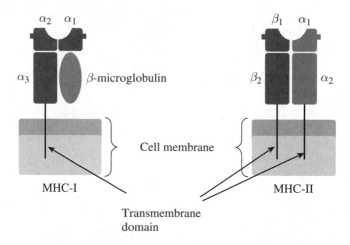

Figure 1. MHC structures.

13. Which of the following cell types is unable to initiate an immune response through the use of MHC?

    A. Adipocyte
    B. Erythrocyte
    C. Spermatogonium
    D. Myocyte

14. The two alleles for each subunit of MHC-II have equal expression levels. This is an example of:

    A. incomplete dominance.
    B. recessivity.
    C. codominance.
    D. pleiotropy.

15. Which of the following is a lymphocyte that primarily targets bacterial pathogens?

    A. Helper T-cell
    B. Natural killer cell
    C. B-cell
    D. Macrophage

16. An individual has mutations in both alleles for the α-3 subunit, rendering them nonfunctional. This mutation most directly impacts the individual's ability to:

    A. produce a humoral immune response.
    B. present epitopes to killer T-cells.
    C. produce lymphocytes.
    D. induce the production of memory T-cells.

17. Which of the following would most likely result in a decreased immune response?

    A. A mutation that causes increased expression of MHC-II on dendritic cells.
    B. A mutation rendering the transmembrane domain of MCH-II nonfunctional.
    C. A mutation that includes the MHC-I complexes on nonnucleated cell surfaces.
    D. A drug that increases the proliferation of macrophages within the body.

PASSAGE 4 (QUESTIONS 18–22)

Excessive accumulation of interstitial (extravascular) fluid in tissues is known as edema. Although edema can be caused by a wide variety of disorders, its character and location varies with the particular condition, which makes it a valuable diagnostic indicator. Abnormal capillary dynamics may result in edema via one of four general mechanisms, which are described below.

Mechanism I
The most frequent cause of edema is high capillary blood pressure, which results in excessive movement of fluid into tissue spaces. Continuous overexpansion of extracellular tissue space gradually compromises its elastic network and eventually forms large fluid reservoirs. Elevated capillary blood pressure can also cause fluid to leak into various natural body cavities, such as the peritoneal cavity.

Mechanism II
Another common cause of edema is a decrease in plasma protein concentration, especially that of albumin. Plasma proteins are produced by the liver and then released into the blood. A decrease in plasma protein concentration causes a decrease in plasma oncotic pressure, which leads to a loss of fluid retention in the capillaries.

Mechanism III
The most severe type of edema results from lymphatic obstruction, which can seriously impede the drainage of proteins from extracellular spaces. The two common causes of lymphatic obstruction are surgical removal of regional lymph nodes (which routinely accompanies excision of a malignant tumor) and infection of the lymph nodes with the larvae of certain tropical parasites (which produces inflammatory lesions and eventually results in permanent scarring).

Mechanism IV
Edema can also arise from abnormally high capillary porosity, which leads to leakage of proteins and excess fluid out of the capillary lumen. For instance, certain vasoactive substances, such as histamine, can make capillaries leaky by acting directly on specific endothelial receptors.

18. In addition to causing edema, which of the four mechanisms would most likely decrease the body's resistance to local infection?

    A. Mechanism I
    B. Mechanism II
    C. Mechanism III
    D. Mechanism IV

19. Based on information in the passage, which of the following conditions would NOT be expected to cause edema?

    A. Decreased fluid reabsorption by kidneys
    B. Decreased lymphatic fluid flow
    C. Increased protein excretion in urine
    D. Increased permeability of capillary endothelium

20. Based on the fact that Mechanism II and Mechanism IV both cause edema by way of decreased plasma protein concentration, it could be concluded that:

    A. capillaries are always fully permeable to albumin.
    B. interstitial fluid albumin concentration is normally greater than plasma albumin concentration.
    C. interstitial fluid albumin concentration is normally less than plasma albumin concentration.
    D. histamine decreases blood vessel permeability.

21. Cortisol, a steroid hormone, has been shown to enhance the activity of liver enzymes required for protein synthesis. Based on this information, would cortisol administration be an effective treatment for a patient suffering from edema?

    A. Yes, because cortisol would increase the concentration of plasma proteins and thus enhance fluid retention in the capillaries.
    B. Yes, because cortisol would decrease capillary blood pressure.
    C. No, because cortisol would decrease the concentration of plasma proteins by increasing metabolic rate.
    D. No, because cortisol would increase the risk of lymph node infection.

22. Which of the four classical characteristics of inflammation is histamine likely responsible for, based on information in the passage?

    A. Dolor (pain)
    B. Rubor (redness)
    C. Tumor (swelling)
    D. Calor (heat)

PASSAGE 5 (QUESTIONS 23–26)

Proper functioning of the respiratory system relies on the integrity of mechanical and chemical mechanisms that allow for the efficient exchange of oxygen and carbon dioxide. The lungs are individually enclosed in fluid-filled sacs that couple the lungs to the chest wall. Upon inhalation, the lungs, composed of alveoli, fill with oxygen-rich air, allowing oxygen to diffuse from the alveoli into the blood. However, the alveoli are prone to collapse due to surface tension from the air–liquid interface. This collapse, due to the hydrophilic pull of surface-lining water molecules toward each other, is prevented by the body's use of a special detergent called surfactant, composed of lipids and proteins. This surfactant, produced by type II pneumocytes, interrupts the attractive bonds between water molecules, reducing hydrophilic interactions and lowering surface tension. Normally, when an alveolus shrinks due to surface tension, the volume of the interstitial space between the alveolus and capillary increases, decreasing pressure in the interstitial space drawing fluid into it.

In respiratory distress syndrome of the newborn, premature babies are born without the ability to manufacture surfactant. These babies often exhibit collapsed alveoli. The collapse of alveoli increases the energy required to breathe and decreases the surface area through which gases can diffuse. Treatment of these babies often includes administering enough surfactant to prevent alveolar collapse. To determine how much supplemental surfactant these babies require, a scientist conducts an experiment to discover the dependence of alveolar surface area on surface tension within that alveolus. Three samples of lung tissue are placed into three separate dishes. In the first dish, pure water is injected into the lung tissue; the tissue is filled with oxygen gas, then deflated in order to calculate surface tension at different lung volumes. In the second dish, the same procedure is replicated, but Detergent A is added in addition to water. Finally, in the third dish, the same procedure is repeated, but surfactant, instead of Detergent A, is injected into the lung tissue in addition to the water. A force transducer is used to measure surface tension. The results are summarized in Figure 1.

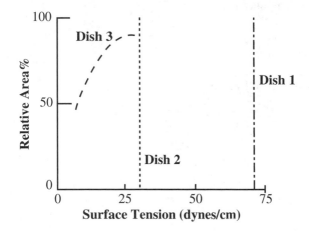

Figure 1. Surface tension results.

23. A premature baby is born without the ability to manufacture sufficient quantities of surfactant, which results in:

   A. increased pH in muscles of respiration.
   B. lactic acid buildup in muscles of respiration.
   C. increased pH in the blood leaving the lungs.
   D. increased oxygen pressure in the blood leaving the lungs.

24. Suppose a fourth dish of lung extract is prepared, but oxygen gas is not used to fill and expand the lung. If the scientist wishes to decrease the surface tension in the lung to a minimum value, oxygen should be replaced with:

   A. nitrogen gas.
   B. carbon dioxide gas.
   C. sodium chloride solution.
   D. water containing dissolved oxygen gas.

25. Which of the following explains the biologist's findings regarding the dependence of surface tension on surface area in the second and third dishes?

   A. Upon deflation of the lung, the number of Detergent A molecules on the surface of alveolar cells increases.
   B. As the surface area of an alveolar cell decreases, surfactant moves from the surface of the cell to the center.
   C. Detergent A is hydrophobic and loses its ability to interrupt water's attractive forces as the surface area decreases in the alveolar cell.
   D. The ratio of water to surfactant molecules on the surface of an alveolar cell decreases as the surface area of the cell decreases.

26. Fluid buildup in the lungs may impede blood flow, resulting in an immediate increase in blood pressure in the:

   A. pulmonary veins.
   B. pulmonary arteries.
   C. aorta.
   D. right atrium.

PASSAGE 6 (QUESTIONS 27–31)

Leigh syndrome (LS) is one of many mitochondrial encephalomyopathies—diseases that involve the nervous system and muscle tissue. It is an early-onset, fatal neurodegenerative disorder characterized by lesions in the brain stem, basal ganglia, thalamus, and spinal cord.

While most genetic causes of LS are nuclear DNA mutations, a sizable minority of mutations are found in the mitochondrial DNA. Mitochondrial DNA mutations are unique in that, if they are transmitted to the next generation, it is only through the mother. The severity of these disorders is affected by heteroplasmy, which refers to the variable copies of mitochondrial DNA within one cell due to the presence of many mitochondria.

Additionally, mutations in genes encoding for electron transport chain complexes I, II, and III have all been associated with LS. Specifically, missense mutations in the *SDHA* gene, which makes soluble proteins for complex II, have been found in families with autosomal recessive LS. These missense mutations do not appear to create new restriction sites that do not exist in wild-type individuals. The soluble proteins in complex II contain succinate dehydrogenase activity, while the membrane-associated subunits (*SDHC* and *SDHD* genes) contain cytochrome-binding sites for ubiquinone. The latter are responsible for transferring electrons into the ubiquinone pool from FAD-linked molecules. Thus, these mutations can cause less ATP per cytosolic NADH or $FADH_2$ to be made.

Case 1

A mother with a family history of LS goes to a genetic counselor concerned after she finds out that she is pregnant, according to an at-home pregnancy test. After identifying the type of mutation present in the mother's DNA, the counselor checks the status of the unborn child when it is feasible to do so. Additionally, he checks for the transcription rate of the mutated gene. Results are shown in Figure 1.

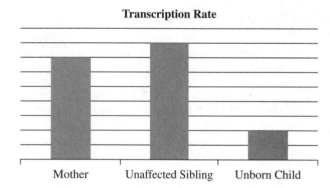

Figure 1. Transcription rate of the mutated gene.

Case 2

Another mother, with a family history of LS in her paternal grandfather, consults a doctor who decides to run a DNA gel electrophoresis to confirm an expected diagnosis of LS in the fetus. The doctor looks specifically for the presence of the *SDHA* mutation in the mother, father, unaffected sibling, and fetus. Figure 2 shows the results of the gel analysis.

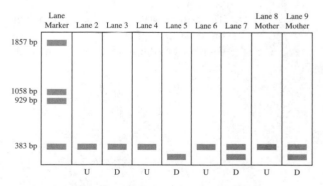

Figure 2. Results of gel analysis where U = undigested DNA and D = DNA digested with restriction enzyme specific to normal LS gene site.

27. A human geneticist working in the same laboratory as a microbiologist was working on elucidating the genetic sequence in the *SDHA* gene. After some abnormal results, he decided to test the nucleotide content to determine if contamination was present. His results were as follows:

> Adenine: 40%
> Guanine: 10%
> Cytosine: 10%
> Thymine: 40%

What can be concluded based on this finding?

A. The results show that bacterial DNA can be ruled out as a possibility for contamination.
B. The results are consistent with human DNA; thus, contamination can be ruled out.
C. The results show that all viral DNA can be ruled out as a possibility for contamination.
D. The results are consistent with DNA from multiple sources; therefore, another test should be performed.

28. According to the details found in Case 1 and Figure 1, what DNA site in this family is likely affected by a mutation that renders the genetic element nonfunctional?

A. Enhancer
B. Promoter
C. Silencer
D. Third codon leading to missense mutation

29. Which of the following correctly pairs an individual from Case 2 with one of his or her corresponding lanes in Figure 2?

A. Lane 3: unaffected sibling
B. Lane 5: unaffected sibling
C. Lane 5: father
D. Lane 7: fetus

30. Further testing reveals that the most common mutations causing Leigh syndrome decrease the activity of certain enzymes in Complex II with no notable effect on their substrate affinities. This mechanism of disease is most analogous to the action of:

A. a competitive inhibitor.
B. a mixed inhibitor.
C. a noncompetitive inhibitor.
D. an uncompetitive inhibitor.

31. The mutation in LS is a change from adenine to cytosine, which leads to an amino acid change from cysteine to tryptophan. A method of gene therapy was developed in which the original functional protein is made using a vector. In animal models, however, the subjects deteriorate more rapidly than is expected. Which of the following would most likely explain this finding?

A. The vector that was introduced was an infectious entity and induced an immune response that ultimately killed the host.
B. The stop codon UGG was created instead of the missense codon; the protein was truncated and completely nonfunctional.
C. The base change back to adenine was achieved, but the decrease in double-helix stability due to increased hydrogen bonding made the gene harder to access by RNA polymerase.
D. The change of one base was too difficult and precise to achieve and a nonsense codon was created unintentionally.

DISCRETE PRACTICE QUESTIONS (QUESTIONS 32–44)

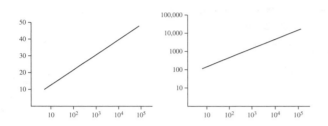

32. Which of the following best describes the graphs above?

    A. Both graphs represent a linear relationship.
    B. The first graph is a log–log plot; the second is a semilog plot.
    C. The first graph is a semilog plot; the second is a log–log plot.
    D. Both graphs represent an exponential relationship.

Questions 33–35 are based on the following data set:

Number of Nonsense Words Memorized

	Trial 1	Trial 2	Trial 3	Trial 4	Trial 5	Trial 6	Trial 7	Trial 8	Trial 9
Participant 1	4	5	4	8	6	8	9	8	9
Participant 2	6	7	7	6	7	9	10	9	9
Participant 3	4	3	5	4	8	6	6	13	9
Participant 4	5	6	5	5	6	7	7	8	7

33. Which of the participants has the lowest standard deviation?

    A. Participant 1
    B. Participant 2
    C. Participant 3
    D. Participant 4

34. Which of the following is an accurate comparison between the results for participants 1 and 2?

    A. Participant 1 has a lower median and a lower mean.
    B. Participant 1 has a lower median and a higher mean.
    C. Participant 1 has a higher median and a lower mean.
    D. Participant 1 has a higher median and a higher mean.

35. Should Trial 8 for Participant 3 be removed as an outlier?

    A. Yes, because it is more than two standard deviations from the mean.
    B. Yes, because it is more than 1.5 interquartile ranges from Q_3.
    C. No, because it is within 1.5 interquartile ranges from Q_3.
    D. No, because removing data decreases the validity of a study.

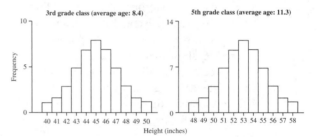

36. If the information in the above graphs were combined into one data set, which of the following would accurately describe the result?

    A. The standard deviation of the combined graph would be double that of the original graphs.
    B. The mean of the combined graph would remain the same as the mean in the original graphs.
    C. The value of n at each point would increase, but other statistical measures would remain largely unaffected.
    D. The combination would result in a different average and standard deviation, and the graph would be bimodal.

37. A hormone enters a cell and binds with an intracellular receptor. The receptor–hormone complex then enters the nucleus and causes a change in DNA expression. Which of the following is likely a characteristic of this hormone?

    A. It is synthesized from amino acids.
    B. It triggers a signaling cascade.
    C. It requires cholesterol as a precursor.
    D. It causes a rapid change in physiology.

38. A tumor located in the adrenal medulla results in high blood pressure that is resistant to treatment with multiple medications. Which hormone is likely to account for this effect?

   A. Aldosterone
   B. Cortisol
   C. Estrogen
   D. Epinephrine

39. Refeeding syndrome is a life-threatening complication that occurs when individuals with severe malnutrition are given large quantities of macronutrients very quickly, either in the form of oral intake or parenteral nutrition delivered by an intravenous line. Which element is likely to be depleted specifically by this condition?

   A. Iron
   B. Nitrogen
   C. Glucose
   D. Phosphorus

40. A university faculty member conducts a study in which he asks undergraduate students to use "ESP" to guess the shapes on randomly selected cards, which are hidden from the student's view but visible to the faculty member. If a student guesses incorrectly, an electric shock is administered, which the experimenter hypothesizes will motivate the student to guess more accurately in future trials. Which of the following is NOT a defensible objection to this study?

   A. The study, as described, lacks sufficient beneficence to justify harm done.
   B. Informed consent from participants, even if obtained, would be invalid given the nature of the study.
   C. The population being tested would not benefit from discovery of true "ESP."
   D. During the experiment, the faculty member might hint at the shapes on the cards in his speech or actions.

41. A study calls for random telephone calls to the home phone numbers of a sampling of individuals in a city between 1:00 p.m. and 3:00 p.m. One of the study's findings is that 72 percent of the city's residents are unemployed. Which of the following is a likely source of error in this study?

   A. The Hawthorne effect
   B. Lack of blinding
   C. Selection bias
   D. Detection bias

42. Two people throw darts at a dartboard. Person A always hits the dartboard, but the distance of the shots from the center varies. Person B misses the dartboard entirely, but his darts always land in the same spot below the bottom of the board. Which of the following describes the types of error demonstrated?

   A. Both Person A and Person B are imprecise.
   B. Both Person A and Person B are inaccurate.
   C. Person A is precise, while Person B is accurate.
   D. Person A is accurate, while Person B is precise.

43. In human subjects research, experimenters must honor requests from participants for:

   A. other participants' contact information.
   B. withdrawal from the study.
   C. placement in a particular experimental group.
   D. reimbursement for travel to the laboratory.

44. Assuming informed consent is given by all participants, which of the following is the LEAST acceptable risk in its respective study?

   A. Providing a drug with reversible side effects to volunteers who do not have the disease the drug treats
   B. Infecting healthy participants with the common cold
   C. Administering a potentially harmful treatment to a terminal cancer patient
   D. Requiring volunteers to take actions that have been consistently traumatic in previous experiments

Science Capstone: MCAT Skills in the Laboratory

PASSAGE 1 (QUESTIONS 1–6)

Carbon monoxide reacts with nitrogen dioxide according to the following equation:

$$CO\ (g) + NO_2\ (g) \rightleftharpoons CO_2\ (g) + NO\ (g) \qquad\qquad \Delta H = +33\ \text{kJ/mol}$$

While carbon monoxide, carbon dioxide, and nitric oxide are colorless, nitrogen dioxide is reddish-brown in color. By shining light rays of a specific wavelength and intensity at a colored compound, the concentration of that compound can be determined from its absorbance, the negative logarithm of the ratio of the transmitted intensity to the incident intensity. A spectrophotometer can be used to measure the rate of a reaction by determining a solution's absorbance at regular intervals.

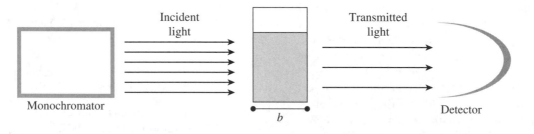

Figure 1. A spectrophotometer.

The Beer–Lambert law ($A = bc\varepsilon$) shows that A (absorbance of the solution) is equal to b (the length of the measurement cuvette) multiplied by c (the concentration of colored compound in solution) multiplied by ε (the molar extinction coefficient, a constant indicating the absorption strength of the colored compound).

A chemistry student decides to study the kinetics of the above reaction by completing the following experiment. A solution of known NO_2 concentration was measured at 390 nm to determine NO_2's molar extinction coefficient. The ε value was calculated as $5.04 \times 10^2\ \text{cm}^{-1}\ M^{-1}$, the intensity of incident light as 998 W/m^2, and the cuvette length as 1 cm. All subsequent measurements were also taken spectrophotometrically at 390 nm.

In Trial 1, the student adds 11 mmol CO to 5.5 mmol NO_2 in a rigid one-liter container and measures the initial rate of reaction. In Trial 2, the student repeats the experiment at the same temperature, but with twice the initial pressure. In Trial 3, the student adds 66 mmol CO to 5.5 mmol NO_2 at STP. Table 1 shows the results.

Trial Number	Initial Change in Absorption/Time
1	-7.64×10^{-2}
2	-3.10×10^{-1}
3	-7.59×10^{-2}

Table 1. Kinetics experiment results.

1. What would be the effect of increasing the temperature after the system reaches dynamic equilibrium?

   A. The system would become redder.
   B. The system would become less red.
   C. The forward rate of reaction would decrease.
   D. The reverse rate of reaction would decrease.

2. Which of the following is the best description for the reaction studied in the passage?

   A. Combustion
   B. Double-displacement
   C. Hydrolysis
   D. Oxidation–reduction

3. Based on the passage, which of the following is a reasonable rate law for the reaction?

   A. $d[NO]/dt = +5\,M^{-2}\,s^{-1}\,[NO_2]^2$
   B. $d[NO]/dt = +5\,M^{-2}\,s^{-1}\,[NO_2]^2[CO]$
   C. $d[CO_2]/dt = +5\,M^{-1}\,s^{-1}\,[NO_2]^2$
   D. $d[CO_2]/dt = +5\,M^{-3}\,[NO_2]^2[CO]^2$

4. If the initial concentrations of NO, NO_2, CO, and CO_2 are all 0.1 M, and the K_{eq} for this reaction were 0.5, what would the graph of absorbance *vs.* time look like if the system were allowed to reach equilibrium?

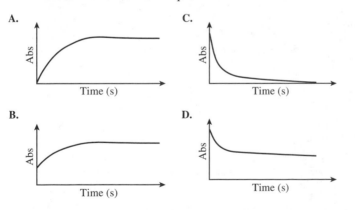

5. A final trial is conducted using unspecified concentrations of NO_2 and CO. If the intensity of light transmitted at $t = 0$ s is 11.0 W/m^2 and the intensity of light transmitted at $t = 20$ s is 63.4 W/m^2, what is the initial rate of the reaction? (Note: Assume the rate is constant over the first 20 seconds of this reaction.)

   A. rate $= 1.51 \times 10^{-5}\,M\,s^{-1}$
   B. rate $= 7.54 \times 10^{-5}\,M\,s^{-1}$
   C. rate $= 3.88 \times 10^{-3}\,M\,s^{-1}$
   D. rate $= 1.94 \times 10^{-2}\,M\,s^{-1}$

6. Which of the following conditions is/are always true for exothermic reactions?

   I. If ΔS is positive, $Q < K_{eq}$.
   II. If ΔS is negative, the reaction is spontaneous.
   III. If ΔG is positive, $Q < K_{eq}$.
   IV. The forward rate of reaction is equal to the reverse rate of reaction.

   A. I only
   B. II only
   C. II and III only
   D. I, II, and IV only

PASSAGE 2 (QUESTIONS 7–10)

Cyclohexanol is used in a variety of industrial cases. It can be used as a precursor for various chemical processes, including the formation of nylons. It can also be used as a plasticizer or, in miniscule amounts, as a solvent. Because of this, many chemical companies keep cyclohexanol around as chemical reaction "feedstock." Cyclohexanol undergoes the acid-catalyzed elimination of water to form cyclohexene, as shown in Figure 1.

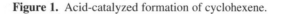

Cyclohexanol   Cyclohexene

Figure 1. Acid-catalyzed formation of cyclohexene.

The reaction takes place via the conjugate acid of cyclohexanol, which loses a molecule of water in the rate-limiting step to form the secondary carbocation, which then transfers a proton to the solvent to give the alkene.

In contrast to the dehydration of cyclohexanol, which can give only a single alkene upon dehydration, a mixture of as many as four alkenes results from the dehydration of 2-methylcyclohexanol, as shown in Figure 2.

A chemistry student wishing to investigate elimination reactions studied the dehydration of 2-methylcyclohexanol. In the reaction, the student heated 2-methylcyclohexanol with 85 percent phosphoric acid to produce a mixture of alkenes, which was subjected to gas chromatographic analysis. A summary of the starting materials used and the results obtained are shown in Table 1.

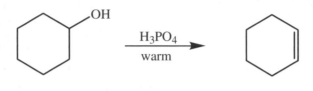

2-methylcyclohexanol

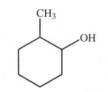

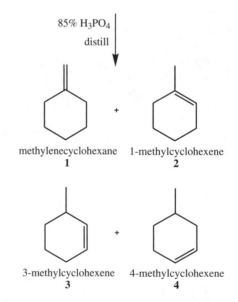

Figure 2. The dehydration of 2-methylcyclohexanol.

Compound	2-methylcyclohexanol	1	2	3	4
mmol used	50				
bp (°C)	161	103	110	103	102
% yield		5	73	20	3

Table 1. Results of the dehydration of 2-methylcyclohexanol.

7. Compound 2, 1-methylcyclohexene, is the major product of the dehydration of 2-methylcyclohexanol because:

   A. the secondary carbocation formed in the rate-determining step transfers a proton to the solvent.
   B. the primary carbocation formed in the rate-determining step transfers a proton to the solvent.
   C. the secondary carbocation formed in the rate-determining step rearranges to a more stable tertiary carbocation, which transfers a proton to the solvent.
   D. the tertiary carbocation formed in the rate-determining step rearranges to a more stable secondary carbocation, which transfers a proton to the solvent.

8. The 2-methylcyclohexanol used in this experiment is actually a mixture of two diastereomers, *cis*-2-methylcyclohexanol and *trans*-2-methylcyclohexanol. Does this fact make any difference in the product composition?

   A. Yes, because the *cis* isomer will react preferentially over the *trans*.
   B. Yes, because the *trans* isomer will react preferentially over the *cis*.
   C. No, because the reactive site within the intermediate exhibits sp^2 hybridization.
   D. No, because the intermediate carbocation will undergo rearrangement.

9. The dehydration of 2-methylcyclohexanol illustrates Zaitsev's rule, which states that in a β-elimination reaction, the most highly substituted alkene will be the major product. Assuming the following reaction follows an E2 mechanism, what is the predicted product distribution?

   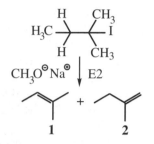

   A. Compound 1 will be the major product and Compound 2 will be the minor product.
   B. Compound 2 will be the major product and Compound 1 will be the minor product.
   C. Both products will be formed in equal amounts.
   D. The product distribution is impossible to predict without experimental evidence.

10. If Compound 2, 1-methylcyclohexene, were treated with Br_2, the product of the reaction would be:

    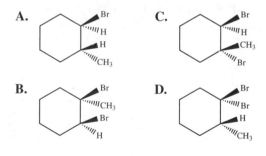

PASSAGE 3 (QUESTIONS 11–15)

A young boy had been playing with his neighboring family's several children and two dogs during a party. The next day, the young boy was found to be suffering from vomiting and severe diarrhea. The boy's parents took immediate action and rushed the boy to the local hospital. Given the occupation of the family whose children and dogs this young boy had been playing with, a family friend suspected ricin poisoning. Clinicians performed experiments to investigate this possibility, given that the identification of ricin poisoning could affect treatment options.

The ricin protein is derived from castor beans. It is composed of two subunits, one with a molar mass of approximately 32 kDa (267 amino acids) and the other with a molar mass of 34 kDa (262 amino acids). It functions by blocking ribosome function. Signs of ricin poisoning are consistent with the symptoms displayed by the patient.

Another toxin found in castor beans, ricinine, is also known to cause diarrhea. Its structure is depicted in Figure 1. Ricinine's presence in urine is an indicator of ricin poisoning.

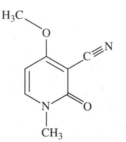

Figure 1. Ricinine.

There are no proven antidotes for either toxin. Treatment is limited to supportive care, including IVs and drugs to maintain blood pressure. Exposure is usually fatal.

11. Which of the following would be the easiest method to separate the two subunits of the ricin polypeptide?

A. Polyacrylamide gel electrophoresis

B. Distillation

C. Gas chromatography

D. Extraction in a 70% ethanol in water solution

12. Is this the IR spectrum for the alkaloid ricinine?

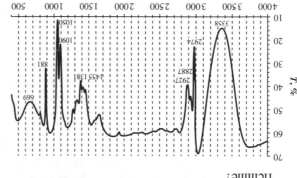

A. Yes, as confirmed by the presence of the peak at 3300 cm^{-1}

B. Yes, as confirmed by the absence of the peak at 1750 cm^{-1}

C. No, as confirmed by the absence of the peak at 1750 cm^{-1}

D. No, as confirmed by the presence of the peak at 1000 cm^{-1}

13. Which molecule could be used for the detection of the ricin protein in a sample?

A. Cholesterol

B. Theobromine

C. Acetyl-coenzyme A

D. An antibody

14. The effects of ricin are not immediate; it can take several hours for its effects to be seen. Which of the following statements best explains this discrepancy?

A. Ricin, like all proteins, is poorly soluble in water and is not transported by the blood very well.

B. Ricin is polar, so it takes time for it to cross the nuclear membrane and bind to DNA.

C. Ricin shuts down new protein production but does not affect already synthesized proteins.

D. Ricin is immediately filtered from the blood by the kidneys and excreted in urine.

15. Which of the following is the most effective method for isolating benzoic acid from a solution also containing an alcohol?

A. Extraction with a strong acid

B. Extraction with a weak acid

C. Extraction with a strong base

D. Extraction with a weak base

PASSAGE 4 (QUESTIONS 16–20)

1-Propanol exhibits low toxicity, but intoxication may occur when individuals with alcohol dependence ingest common household chemicals containing 1-propanol. Its effects include extreme alcoholic intoxication and possible high-anion gap metabolic acidosis.

Two students attempted to oxidize 1-propanol to propionaldehyde (propanal) using dichromate. Because dichromate is a strong oxidizing agent, both students decided to monitor the reaction by measuring the amount of dichromate in the reaction mixture using UV–Vis spectroscopy. By recording the UV–Vis spectrum of the reaction mixture at intervals, the students hoped to prevent the 1-propanol from being oxidized beyond the aldehyde, propanal, to the carboxylic acid, propanoic acid. The oxidation of 1-propanol to propanal in the presence of dichromate is shown in Equation 1.

$$CH_3-CH_2-CH_2-OH \ + \ Cr_2O_7^{2-} \ + \ H^+$$

b.p. = 97.2°C

$$\uparrow$$

$$CH_3-CH_2-\overset{\overset{\displaystyle O}{\|}}{C}-H \ + \ 2\,Cr^{3+} \ + \ 7\,H_2O$$

b.p. = 49.0°C

Equation 1. Oxidation of 1-propanol to propanal.

Student A used the following procedure. He combined 0.1 moles of potassium dichromate (0.5 M $K_2Cr_2O_7$) and 0.25 moles of 1-propanol in a round-bottom flask. He then measured the UV–Vis absorption spectrum of the reaction mixture at 350 nm over 30-second intervals. When the peak at 350 nm disappeared, he distilled the reaction mixture under reduced pressure. In order to determine if he obtained the intended product, he recorded an IR spectrum of the distillate in CCl_4.

Student B used a modification of Student A's procedure. She increased the amount of 1-propanol used to 0.40 moles and distilled the propionaldehyde off the reaction mixture as it was produced. Like Student A, she used the UV–Vis absorption spectrum of the reaction mixture at 350 nm to determine when the reaction was complete.

The IR data obtained from the distillates of both students is shown in Table 1.

Student	IR Data of Distillate, ν (cm^{-1})
A	3637 (sh), 3333 (br), 2963 (mult), 1466 (mult), 1383 (mult), 1250 (sh), 1090 (sh)
B	2900 (mult), 1730 (sh), 1450 (mult), 1370 (mult), 1270 (mult), 1106 (sh)

Note: sh = sharp, br = broad, mult = multiple peaks, w = weak

Table 1. IR data obtained from distillates of Student A and Student B.

16. The distillate obtained by Student A is likely to be:

    A. propanal.
    B. propanal and water.
    C. propionic acid.
    D. 1-propanol.

17. The distillate obtained by Student B is likely to be:

    A. propanal.
    B. propanal and water.
    C. propionic acid.
    D. 1-propanol.

18. Why is UV–Vis spectroscopy a useful tool for monitoring the oxidation of 1-propanol to propanal using chromic acid?

    I. The oxidation state of chromium changes during the reaction.
    II. All of the dichromate ion is consumed during the reaction.
    III. As 1-propanol is consumed, the absorption spectrum of the dichromate ion is shifted to another wavelength.
    IV. The other compounds in the reaction mixture do not interfere with the absorption spectrum of dichromate.

    A. I only
    B. I and II only
    C. III only
    D. I, II, and IV only

19. If the students had been using proton NMR to confirm the identity of their products, what unique peak would they be looking for to confirm the presence of an aldehyde?

    A. A peak at 1.2 ppm
    B. A peak at 9.8 ppm
    C. A peak at 39.3 ppm
    D. A peak at 200.2 ppm

20. In a second experiment, Student A follows the same procedure using 2-propanol instead of 1-propanol. He measures the IR spectrum of the distillate and records the following data:

    ν (cm^{-1}): 2970 (w, mult), 2950 (mult), 1750 (sh), 1430 (mult), 1230 (sh), 1080 (sh)

    What product does he obtain?

    A. 2-Propanol
    B. Propionic acid
    C. 2-Propanone
    D. Propanal

PASSAGE 5 (QUESTIONS 21–27)

In order for a titration to yield concentration data with an acceptable level of accuracy, standardized solutions with precisely known normalities must be prepared. This is no small accomplishment, as most commonly used titrants are difficult to handle in the pure state. Sodium hydroxide, for example, is a common basic standard; it is hygroscopic as a solid and thus absorbs water from the atmosphere. Hydrogen chloride, a common acidic standard, is a gas at ambient temperatures and pressures; saturated aqueous solutions can be prepared simply by bubbling the gas through deionized water, but temperature effects on solubility and volatility generally limit the significance of concentration calculations to the nearest $0.1\ M$.

To overcome the difficulties inherent in the preparation of standard solutions, one usually resorts to the use of a primary standard, such as sodium carbonate (Na_2CO_3) or potassium hydrogen phthalate (KHP). The primary standard is used to determine the concentration of a newly prepared solution, the concentration of which can then be adjusted via dilution. The fundamental criteria for the selection of a primary standard are listed below:

1. It must be stable in light, in air, and in the solution to be titrated.
2. It must be free of any significant quantity of impurities.
3. It must be sufficiently soluble in the solution to be titrated.
4. It must react with the substance to be titrated by a single known pathway.
5. Its reaction with the titrated substance must be rapid.
6. It should be nontoxic and present few disposal problems.
7. It should be readily available and relatively inexpensive.

A student preparing to perform a series of titrations on a group of vitamin samples produced a secondary standard of $0.01000\ N$ NaOH (aq) by first making a more concentrated solution. She dissolved approximately 2.5 mg of NaOH (s) in enough water to make 250.0 mL of solution. This solution was then standardized against KHP according to the reaction:

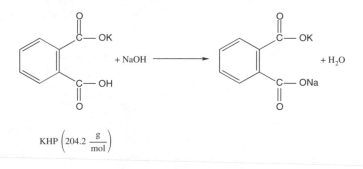

KHP $\left(204.2\ \dfrac{g}{mol}\right)$

Figure 1. Neutralization of KHP

The student placed 385.43 mg of KHP into a clean flask, added 50 mL of deionized water and two drops of phenolphthalein solution, and then titrated with the freshly prepared NaOH solution. The endpoint was reached upon addition of 25.10 mL of the basic solution. From this titration data, the student calculated the concentration of the NaOH solution as $0.07520\ N$; then, using a pipette and a volumetric flask, diluted the NaOH solution as needed to a final concentration of $0.01000\ N$.

21. The student decides to study venous [Cl^-], but must first prepare a $AgNO_3$ secondary standard. Which of the following compounds would be an acceptable primary standard for the titration of a $AgNO_3$ solution?

    A. NaCl
    B. HCl
    C. KOH
    D. Hg_2Cl_2

22. $Ca(OH)_2$ is commonly used to treat tooth infections. If a solution of $Ca(OH)_2$ were prepared, the addition of 0.5 mol/L of which of the following fully soluble hypothetical compounds would result in the LEAST change in [Ca^{2+}] in a 0.01 N $Ca(OH)_2$ solution? (Note: X represents an unidentified element besides calcium.)

    A. XOH
    B. $X(OH)_2$
    C. $X(OH)_3$
    D. $X(OH)_4$

23. In addition to being an indicator, phenolphthalein can be used to detect the presence of blood, as it turns pink upon binding to hemoglobin. When used in the titration of NaOH, phenolphthalein has a pK_a closest to which of the following?

    A. 3.8
    B. 5.5
    C. 7
    D. 9.3

24. A student is preparing a NaOH solution to titrate a folic acid (vitamin B_9) solution. She adds 5 g NaOH (s) to 1 L of water. Which of the following is likely to be the molarity of the resulting solution?

    A. 0.120 M
    B. 0.125 M
    C. 0.130 M
    D. 0.135 M

25. While analyzing samples for vitamin B content, a student found it necessary to titrate for niacin. If a 5.00 mL sample containing no other acidic compounds required the addition of 3.75 mL of 0.01000 N NaOH solution to reach the equivalence point, how many moles of niacin would be found in one liter of the sample solution?

    A. 18.75
    B. 0.75
    C. 1.3×10^{-2}
    D. 7.5×10^{-3}

26. Commercially available KHP must be prepared in a "dry box," usually under an argon atmosphere. One likely reason for this necessity is that:

    A. freshly prepared KHP is hygroscopic, and thus must be kept in an inert atmosphere.
    B. the phthalic acid from which it is made is extremely volatile, and thus must be used in the absence of oxygen.
    C. the KOH used in the preparation is hygroscopic, and thus must be weighed in an anhydrous environment.
    D. very pure KHP is extremely toxic, and thus requires careful handling.

27. According to the information contained in the passage, which of the following reactions would be the best choice for the standardization of an aqueous nitric acid solution?

    A. Al_2O_3 (s) + 6 HNO_3 (aq) → 2 $Al(NO_3)_3$ (aq) + 3 H_2O (l)
    B. $ZnCl_2$ (aq) + 2 HNO_3 (aq) → $Zn(NO_3)_2$ (aq) + 2 HCl (aq)
    C. 2 Cu (s) + 6 HNO_3 (aq) → 2 $Cu(NO_3)_2$ (aq) + NO (g) + NO_2 (g) + 3 H_2O (l)
    D. NaOH (s) + HNO_3 (aq) → $NaNO_3$ (aq) + H_2O (l)

DISCRETE PRACTICE QUESTIONS (QUESTIONS 28–31)

28. A mutated protein contains all of the correct amino acids until the middle of the protein; the rest of the protein is prematurely truncated and substantially altered in terms of the amino acid sequence. Which of the following types of mutation best accounts for all of the changes observed in the protein?

   A. Insertion
   B. Substitution
   C. Nonsense
   D. Missense

29. Which of the following is NOT a mechanism by which genetic variability may be decreased?

   A. The founder effect
   B. Inbreeding
   C. Point mutations
   D. Bottlenecks

30. Which of the following compounds will produce the given ^1H–NMR spectrum?

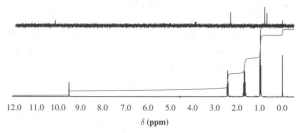

   A. 2-Chloropentane
   B. Butanal
   C. Benzoic acid
   D. Methanal

31. Which of the following compounds will produce the given ^1H–NMR spectrum?

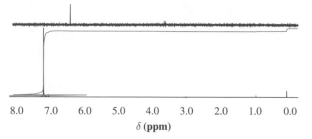

   A. Benzene
   B. Benzoic acid
   C. Acetone
   D. Methane

Extra practice for the next class session starts on the next page ▶ ▶ ▶

Countdown to Test Day

PASSAGE 1 (QUESTIONS 1–4)

The Ultimatum Game is a scenario in which two people are asked to split a certain amount of money. The first player determines how the money is to be divided, and the second decides whether or not to accept the proposed split. The first player can either split the money in half Fairly (F) or leave a less sizable portion of the money for his partner Unfairly (U). The second player can either Accept (A) or Reject (R) the offer. The "extensive form" of this game, using a total amount of $10 and an example unfair split of $8/$2, can be seen in Figure 1.

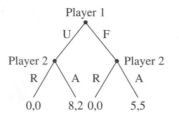

Figure 1. "Extensive form" of the game.

Experimental evidence demonstrates that Player 2 will rarely play optimally, routinely rejecting offers of 30 percent or less. This punishment behavior initially perplexed evolutionary theorists, but can be understood when it is considered that a "game" such as this one is rarely played just once between individuals. In subsequent iterations, Player 1 will tend toward more fair splits, and cooperation develops.

One such variation of the Ultimatum Game is the Big Monkey/Little Monkey game. In this scenario, two monkeys can cooperate to shake a fruit that contains 10 kCal of energy from a branch of a tall tree. Either monkey can choose to climb (C) the tree to help shake the fruit down or to wait (W) on the ground for the fruit to fall. The Big Monkey must expend 2 kCals of energy to climb the tree, while the Little Monkey can do so with negligible energy loss. The Big Monkey is also capable of hogging the fruit and eating more than the Little Monkey, such that if both climb and shake the fruit down together, they will reach the ground at the same time and split the fruit 7:3 in favor of the Big Monkey. If either monkey is waiting on the ground when the fruit falls, it will begin eating while the other monkey is climbing down. The extensive form of these two versions can be seen in Figure 2.

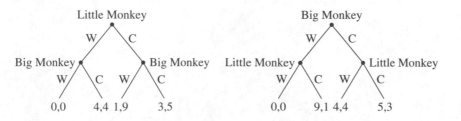

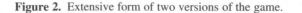

Figure 2. Extensive form of two versions of the game.

1. In the ultimatum game, Player 2's rejection of an $8/$2 split is an example of:

   A. spite.
   B. selfishness.
   C. reciprocal altruism.
   D. negative reinforcement.

2. Assuming both monkeys are rational and capable of computing kCal outcomes, which of the following describes the optimal strategy for the Little Monkey when going first and second, respectively?

   A. Climb; do the same thing Big Monkey does
   B. Climb; wait no matter what Big Monkey does
   C. Wait; climb no matter what Big Monkey does
   D. Wait; do the opposite of what Big Monkey does

3. In the Big Monkey/Little Monkey game, imagine that both monkeys decide their strategies by flipping a fair coin simultaneously. Which of the following is the expected payout for the Big Monkey?

   A. 2
   B. 4.5
   C. 6.5
   D. 9

4. Ecologists observing a population of rhesus monkeys find that members of the population are expected to signal others when they find food, and transgressors are so severely punished by the group that signaling has become an evolutionarily stable strategy. Which of the following is a consequence of this scenario?

   A. The population's genes encode instincts in such a way that natural selection will prevent individual cheaters from invading the group.
   B. An individual rhesus monkey could probably infiltrate the group and take advantage of the altruism displayed by the population.
   C. Selfishness in food gathering and consumption is the optimal strategy for each individual within the population.
   D. If disturbed by a change in environment or invasion by another large population of monkeys, the altruism strategy should return through natural selection.

PASSAGE 2 (QUESTIONS 5–9)

Chemical fixation is a process by which biological tissues are preserved from decay. One of the most popular chemical fixatives is formaldehyde.

Formaldehyde preserves tissue by driving cross-linking reactions in the tissue. These are reactions that result in the fusion of proteins. From a molecular perspective, cross-linking preserves protein structure and anchors proteins to the cytoskeleton. In addition, other biological molecules associated with proteins may remain trapped within a "web" of cross-linked proteins. Cross-linking results in an increase in the mechanical strength, rigidity, and stability of the tissue, improving a specimen's longevity.

Interestingly, when an aqueous formaldehyde solution is used as a chemical fixative, the molecule formaldehyde itself is not, strictly speaking, actually a reactant in cross-linking reactions. This is because formaldehyde spontaneously reacts with water to form methanediol ($K_{eq} = 2000$), which is the molecule that drives cross-linking reactions. Figures 1 and 2 show a cross-linking reaction between the amino acid lysine and the amino acid glutamine. Figure 1 shows the first half of this reaction: a hydroxyl group is eliminated from methanediol to form an oxocarbenium intermediate, which is then attacked by the amino group on lysine. The product of this reaction undergoes a second elimination step, forming an imine intermediate.

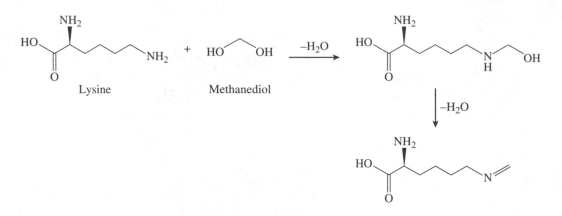

Figure 1. First step of the cross-linking reaction.

In the second half of the reaction, shown in Figure 2, this imine intermediate is attacked by the amide group on glutamine. This step completes the formation of the cross-link between lysine and glutamine. The mechanism for amino acid residues in gross proteins is similar.

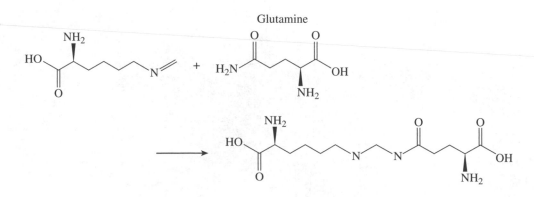

Figure 2. Last step of the cross-linking reaction.

5. Methanediol spontaneously polymerizes with formaldehdye, as shown below.

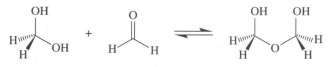

This reaction is an example of:

A. nucleophilic addition.
B. hydration.
C. bimolecular substitution (S_N2).
D. unimolecular substitution (S_N1).

6. Formaldehyde spontaneously forms methanediol in aqueous solution. This reaction is an example of:

A. hemiacetal formation.
B. hydration.
C. bimolecular substitution (S_N2).
D. unimolecular substitution (S_N1).

7. The first step in the cross-linking reaction is an example of what reaction type?

A. Nucleophilic acyl substitution
B. Hydration
C. Aldol condensation
D. Ammonia derivative condensation

8. If 0.1 mol formaldehyde is added to 100 mL of water and allowed to come to equilibrium, what will be the approximate methanediol concentration?

A. 0.01 M
B. 0.1 M
C. 1 M
D. 10 M

9. The rate of the first step in the cross-linking reaction will be increased by acidic conditions. This is because acidic conditions:

A. cause lysine's amino group to protonate, making it more nucleophilic.
B. hinder the conversion of formaldehyde to methanediol.
C. decrease the rate at which imine intermediate is formed.
D. make the formation of an oxocarbenium intermediate more likely.

PASSAGE 3 (QUESTIONS 10–15)

Oxidative phosphorylation, the final step in the aerobic utilization of glucose for energy, depends on sufficient concentrations of various substrates. Insufficient concentrations of any "essential substrates" can limit the rate of oxidative phosphorylation. Specifically, the concentration of ADP present influences the extent of mitochondrial activity within a cell: mitochondria increase their oxidative phosphorylation activity in the presence of high ADP concentrations. This increase in oxidative phosphorylation can be shown experimentally.

To study mitochondrial activity experimentally, a biochemist prepares a plate of mitochondria without the addition of external substrates. Initially, the biochemist records the basal rate of oxygen consumption by measuring the amount of oxygen present at different times. Next, the biochemist adds 1.0 μmol of glutamate, an amino acid, and records the change in oxygen consumption. The biochemist then adds 0.3 μmol of ADP. After this initial quantity of ADP is consumed, another 0.6 μmol of ADP is added. It is found that the amount of ADP present is directly proportional to the amount of oxygen taken up by the mitochondrion. Figure 1 summarizes the results.

In another experiment, the biochemist repeats the preparation of a mitochondria-rich plate. Initially, 1.0 μmol of glutamate is added, followed shortly thereafter by the addition of approximately 0.8 μmoles of ADP. Next, the biochemist adds oligomycin, which inhibits oxidative phosphorylation. Finally, the biochemist adds dinitrophenol (DNP), which acts to dissipate the proton gradient in the mitochondria. Figure 2 summarizes the results.

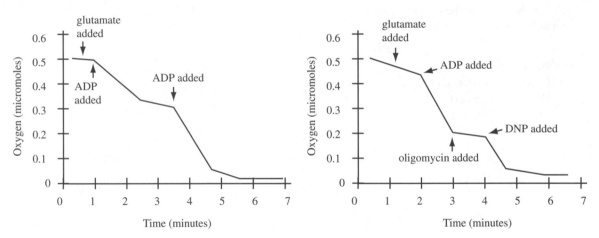

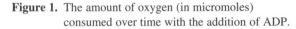

Figure 1. The amount of oxygen (in micromoles) consumed over time with the addition of ADP.

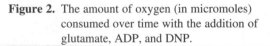

Figure 2. The amount of oxygen (in micromoles) consumed over time with the addition of glutamate, ADP, and DNP.

10. Based on the data in Figure 1, between which times would the rate of acetyl coenzyme A production be lowest?

    A. 0.5 to 1.1 minutes
    B. 2.8 to 3.3 minutes
    C. 4.6 to 5.1 minutes
    D. 5.8 to 6.3 minutes

11. Suppose a biochemist begins an experiment by measuring 1.5 μmoles of oxygen in a plate of mitochondria. After adding 1.2 μmoles of ADP, the amount of oxygen left in the plate is:

    A. 0.31 μmoles.
    B. 0.56 μmoles.
    C. 0.94 μmoles.
    D. 1.19 μmoles.

12. The absence of which of the following substrates would NOT be expected to limit the rate of oxidative phosphorylation?

    A. NAD^+
    B. O_2
    C. $FADH_2$
    D. Inorganic phosphate

13. According to Figure 2, oxygen consumption nearly ceased upon the addition of oligomycin. Why did the addition of DNP allow the resumption of oxygen consumption?

    A. ATP synthase was no longer blocked by DNP, so ATP production could resume.
    B. Protons provided a bypass pathway for DNP to enter the matrix.
    C. DNP provided a bypass pathway for protons to enter the matrix.
    D. DNP halted any protons from entering the matrix.

14. The chemical valinomycin inserts into membranes and causes the movement of K^+ into the mitochondria. According to Figure 1, if mitochondria are treated with valinomycin, the rate of ATP synthesis in the mitochondria will most likely:

    A. decrease, because the K^+ will compete with protons at the active site on ATP synthase.
    B. decrease, because movement of K^+ into the mitochondrial compartments will hinder proton movement into the mitochondrial matrix.
    C. increase, because the net positive charge in the mitochondria will increase the movement of protons into the mitochondrial matrix.
    D. increase, because the additional positive charge will further activate ATP synthase.

15. According to Figure 1, oxygen consumption was very poor in the absence of ADP. Why?

    A. In the absence of ADP, the flow of protons into the matrix via ATP synthase is blocked.
    B. In the absence of ADP, protons are too positive to pass through ATP synthase.
    C. In the absence of ADP, ATP synthase begins to work backwards.
    D. In the absence of ADP, the flow of electrons into the matrix via ATP synthase is blocked.

PASSAGE 4 (QUESTIONS 16–19)

Hemoglobin is the protein within erythrocytes that transports oxygen to body tissues. In adults, hemoglobin molecules are composed of two α-chains and two β-chains ($\alpha_2\beta_2$). Thalassemias are a class of inherited diseases caused by impaired synthesis of hemoglobin subunits. There are two types of thalassemia: thalassemia minor and thalassemia major. Thalassemia minor is found in heterozygotes, who are generally asymptomatic or have mild anemia, and also possess a resistance to malaria. Thalassemia major is found in homozygotes and causes serious symptoms.

α-Thalassemias are caused by deletions of one or more of the α-globin genes in an α-gene cluster. In the most severe form, where the patient is left without any α chains, fetal γ hemoglobin chains and adult β hemoglobin chains form homotetramers (γ_4 or β_4). These abnormal hemoglobin molecules cannot release oxygen under physiological conditions.

Heterozygotes with β-thalassemia are asymptomatic, while homozygotes have severe anemia. When levels of fetal hemoglobin drop, patients often require frequent blood transfusions. Anemia in these patients is due not only to the lack of β-chains, but also to the surplus of α-chains, which precipitate and damage erythrocyte membranes.

β-Thalassemias are generally caused by a diverse set of point mutations that alter β-chain levels. For example, mutations in the β-chain promoter region, nonsense mutations, frameshift mutations, mutations that alter sequences at the intron/exon boundary, and mutations that alter the AAUAAA cleavage signal at the mRNA 3' end all cause β-thalassemia.

16. A man with thalassemia major marries a woman with thalassemia minor. If they have three children, what is the probability that all three children will have thalassemia major?

    A. 12.5%
    B. 25%
    C. 50%
    D. 100%

17. A point mutation in the promoter region of a β-chain gene would have what effect?

    A. Translational repression would occur.
    B. Transcriptional repression would occur.
    C. Neither type of repression would occur.
    D. Both types of repression would occur.

18. In a certain nonevolving population, 16% of the individuals have thalassemia major. What percentage of this population is heterozygous for the thalassemia gene?

    A. 4%
    B. 24%
    C. 36%
    D. 48%

19. Transcriptional repression occurs in what region within the cell?

    A. Cytoplasm
    B. Ribosomes
    C. Rough endoplasmic reticulum
    D. Nucleus

PASSAGE 5 (QUESTIONS 20–24)

The biological cell membrane is a complex structure known for its function as a tightly managed gatekeeper for the cell. The cell membrane can be modeled as an electrical circuit consisting of a capacitor in parallel with four pathways, each consisting of a variable conductor in series with a battery. Figure 1 shows this equivalent circuit model for the cell membrane.

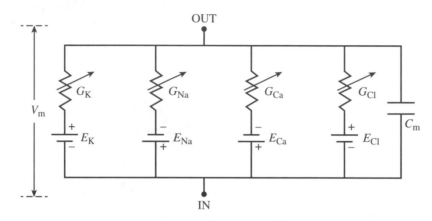

Figure 1. Equivalent circuit model for the cell membrane.

Cytoplasm and extracellular fluid are two electrically conducting regions separated by a thin dielectric, the lipid bilayer, which, at about 8 nm thickness, is thin enough so that the accumulation of charges on one side of the bilayer creates a coulombic force strong enough to attract opposite charges on the other side. The cell membrane thus acts as a capacitor, C_m, with a constant value estimated to be about 2 μF/cm^2.

A concentration gradient corresponding to each of the four principal biological ions—potassium, sodium, calcium, and chloride—exists across the plasma membrane. This creates an electromotive force that drives the ion through its ion-specific channel at a constant rate. The Nernst potential for that ion is the electrical potential difference across the channel, which can be represented in the equivalent circuit of the cell membrane as a battery.

The hydrophobic portion of the lipid bilayer impedes the movement of charges across it, which gives rise to the electrical resistance of the cell membrane. The conductance of a pure lipid bilayer is so low that the movement of ions across the membrane is almost entirely through alternative pathways provided by embedded molecules like leakage channels, ligand-gated channels, and voltage-gated ion channels. Thus, the conductances corresponding to each of the principal ions vary with the number and type of ion channels present in that patch of the cell membrane.

20. If $[K^+]_{cytoplasm} = 400$ mM and $[K^+]_{extracellular}$ $_{fluid} = 20$ mM for the neuron of a giant squid, what is the value of $|E_k|$ in the equivalent circuit for this neuron? (Note: Assume standard conditions. RT/F $= 0.025$ V/mol, ln $0.05 = -3$)

A. 0 mV
B. 25 mV
C. 50 mV
D. 75 mV

21. What is the value of G_{Cl} if the current flowing through the pathway corresponding to the chloride ion is 0.5 μA, $V_m = 10$ mV, and $E_{Cl} = 5$ mV?

A. 5×10^{-5} Ω^{-1}
B. 1×10^{-4} Ω^{-1}
C. 5×10^{-2} Ω^{-1}
D. 1×10^{-1} Ω^{-1}

22. Which of the following statements about the movement of ions across the plasma membrane is true?

A. Ions with high permeability move through a low-resistance pathway and ions with low permeability move through a high-resistance pathway.
B. Ions with high permeability move through a high-resistance pathway and ions with low permeability move through a low-resistance pathway.
C. Ions with high permeability move through a high-resistance pathway and ions with low permeability move through a high-resistance pathway.
D. Ions with high permeability move through a low-resistance pathway and ions with low permeability move through a low-resistance pathway.

23. Which of the following statements about the equivalent circuit model for the plasma membrane is true?

A. The capacitance of the membrane is relatively unaffected by the molecules that are embedded in it.
B. The capacitance of the membrane is directly proportional to the area of the membrane.
C. The resistance of the membrane is relatively unaffected by the molecules that are embedded in it.
D. The resistance of the membrane is directly proportional to the area of the membrane.

24. Which of the following statements about the electromotive force created by the concentration gradient of an ion across a membrane is true?

A. Its unit of measurement is newtons, or kg · m/s^2.
B. It is the potential difference associated with moving a unit charge around a complete circuit.
C. Its positive terminal is closer to the side with the higher ion concentration.
D. It is analogous to the voltage generated by a concentration cell, which is a special type of electrolytic cell.

DISCRETE PRACTICE QUESTIONS (QUESTIONS 25–26)

25. One of the major functions of the mitochondrial genome is to produce proteins necessary for the electron transport chain. Which complex is only fed electrons initially from NADH?

    A. Complex I
    B. Complex II
    C. Complex III
    D. Complex IV

26. Dinitrophenol (DNP) can allow protons to pass through holes in the inner mitochondrial membrane other than the one within ATP synthase. What effect would this have on ATP production?

    A. Production would decrease because H^+ movement is no longer coupled to ATP generation.
    B. Production would increase because H^+ movement is now coupled to ATP generation at a higher rate.
    C. Production would decrease because H^+ movement stops synthesis of ATP at these new holes.
    D. Production would increase because H^+ movement synthesizes ATP at these new holes.